NURSING THEORIES

The Base for Professional Nursing Practice

third edition

N̲URSING
T̲HEORIES

The Base for Professional
Nursing Practice

third edition

Editor:

Julia B. George, RN, PhD
Professor and Chair
Department of Nursing
California State University, Fullerton
Fullerton, California

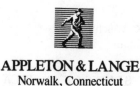

APPLETON & LANGE
Norwalk, Connecticut

0-8385-7051-8

Notice: Our knowledge in clinical sciences is constantly changing. As new information becomes available, changes in treatment and in the use of drugs become necessary. The authors and the publisher of this volume have taken care to make certain that the doses of drugs and schedules of treatment are correct and compatible with the standards generally accepted at the time of publication. The reader is advised to consult carefully the instruction and information material included in the package insert of each drug or therapeutic agent before administration. This advice is especially important when using new or infrequently used drugs.

90 91 92 93 94 / 10 9 8 7 6 5 4 3 2 1

Prentice Hall International (UK) Limited, *London*
Prentice Hall of Australia Pty. Limited, *Sydney*
Prentice Hall Canada, Inc., *Toronto*
Prentice Hall Hispanoamericana, S.A., *Mexico*
Prentice Hall of India Private Limited, *New Delhi*
Prentice Hall of Japan, Inc., *Tokyo*
Simon & Schuster Asia Pte. Ltd., *Singapore*
Editora Prentice Hall do Brasil Ltda., *Rio de Janeiro*
Prentice Hall, *Englewood Cliffs, New Jersey*

Library of Congress Cataloging-in-Publication Data

Nursing theories: the base for professional nursing practice /
    editor, Julia B. George.—3rd ed.
        p.   cm.
    Includes bibiographies and index.   ISBN 0-8385-
7051-8   1. Nursing—Philosophy. I. George, Julia B.
    [DNLM: 1. Philosophy, Nursing. WY 86 N9755]
    RT84.5.N89 1989
    610.73'01—dc20
    DNLM/DLC
    for Library of Congress   89-6825
                                                            CIP

Acquisitions Editor: Marion K. Welch
Production Editor: Susan Meiman
Designer: Janice Barsevich

PRINTED IN THE UNITED STATES OF AMERICA

CONTRIBUTORS

Janice Ryan Belcher, RN, MS
Doctoral Student
Medical College of Virginia/Virginia Commonwealth University
Richmond, Virginia

Agnes M. Bennett, RN, MS
Assistant Professor, Retired
Department of Nursing
Miami University
Oxford, Ohio

Mary Disbrow Crane, RNC, MS
Formerly Family and Community Health Clinical Specialist
Potomac, Maryland

Joanne R. Cross, RN, MSN, MS Counseling
Assistant Professor
Wright State University–Miami Valley School of Nursing
Wright State University
Dayton, Ohio

Suzanne M. Falco, RN, PhD
Associate Professor
School of Nursing
The University of Wisconsin, Milwaukee
Milwaukee, Wisconsin

Lois J. Brittain Fish, RN, MSN
Supportive Home Services Specialist
Riverside School and R.T. Industries, Inc.
Troy, Ohio

Peggy Coldwell Foster, RN, MSN
Coordinator, Childbirth Education for Adults and Children
Coordinator of Maternity Discharge Program
Bethesda Hospital
Cincinnati, Ohio

Chiyoko Yamamoto Furukawa, RN, PhD
Associate Professor
College of Nursing
University of New Mexico
Albuquerque, New Mexico

Julia Gallagher Galbreath, RN, CS, MS
Assistant Professor
Edison State Community College
Piqua, Ohio
Certified Clinical Nurse Specialist
Upper Valley Medical Center
Piqua, Ohio

Julia B. George, RN, PhD
Professor and Chair
Department of Nursing
California State University, Fullerton
Fullerton, California.

Janet S. Hickman, RN, EdD
Chairman and Associate Professor
Department of Nursing
Eastern College
St. Davids, Pennsylvania.

Joan K. Howe, RN, MS
Lecturer in Nursing
Lima Technical College
Lima, Ohio

Nancy P. Janssens, RN, MS,
Formerly Assistant Professor and Director of Continuing Education
Wright State University–Miami Valley School of Nursing
Dayton, Ohio

Mary Kathryn Leonard, RN, MS, PhD Candidate
Assistant Administrator
Southeast Volusia Hospital
New Smyrna Beach, Florida

Marie L. Lobo, RN, PhD
Assistant Professor
Department of Family & Community
College of Nursing
The Ohio State University
Columbus, Ohio

Charlotte Paul, RN, PhD
Professor and Chairperson
Director of Nursing Programs
Edinboro University of Pennsylvania

Susan G. Praeger, RN, EdD
Associate Professor
Wright State University–Miami Valley School of Nursing
Dayton, Ohio

Joan S. Reeves, RN, DrPH
Assistant Clinical Professor
Department of Public Heath Nursing
College of Nursing
University of Illinois at Chicago
Chicago, Illinois

Marjorie Stanton, RN, EdD
Consultant in Nursing Education
Mountaintop, Pennsylvania

Barbara Talento, RN, EdD
Associate Professor
Department of Nursing
California State University, Fullerton
Fullerton, California

Gertrude Torres, RN, EdD
Chair, Nursing Division
College Misericordia
Dallas, Pennsylvania

REVIEWERS

Rinda Alexander, PhD, RN, CS
Associate Professor of Nursing
Department of Nursing
Purdue University Calumet
Hammond, Indiana

Mary L. Lovering, RNC, EdD
Professor
Department of Nursing
Worcester State College
Worcester, Massachusetts

CONTENTS

PREFACE

As an emerging profession, nursing continues to be deeply involved in identifying its own unique knowledge base. In identifying this base of knowledge, various concepts, models, and theories specific to nursing are being recognized, defined, and developed. Although these concepts, models, and theories have been published in a variety of journals and books, there is a need for them to be gathered in one volume and applied to nursing practice through the nursing process.

This book is designed to consider the ideas of eighteen nursing theorists and relate the work of each to the nursing process of assessing, diagnosing, planning, implementing, and evaluating. It must be recognized that the book serves as a secondary source in relation to the statements and purposes of the individuals whose writings are discussed. It is intended for use as a tool for the thoughtful and considered application of nursing concepts and theories to nursing practice.

There are essentially three areas of focus. First, Chapters 1 and 2 present the place of concepts and theories in nursing and discuss the nursing process. These chapters provide a common base for the next twenty chapters and should be read first.

Next, Chapters 3 through 20 present the major components of the work of Florence Nightingale, Hildegard E. Peplau, Virginia Henderson, Lydia E. Hall, Dorothea E. Orem, Dorothy E. Johnson, Faye Glenn Abdellah, Ida Jean Orlando, Ernestine Wiedenbach, Myra Estrin Levine, Imogene M. King, Martha E. Rogers, Sister Callista Roy, Josephine E. Paterson and Loretta T. Zderad, Jean Watson, Rosemarie Rizzo Parse, and Madeleine Leininger. Each chapter presents one theorist (or pair of theorists). Although an effort has been made to present the information chronologically, these chapters may be read in any order. Each chapter gives the historical setting of the nurse theorist and the specific components that she identified as meaningful to nursing. This material is drawn from the work of each theorist. The components are then interpreted and discussed by the chapter author(s) in relation to the four basic concepts: (1)The human or individual, (2)health, (3)society/environment, and (4) nursing and to the use of these concepts in the nursing process. In addition, the work of each theorist is discussed in relation to the characteristics of a theory. This discussion is not to be considered a comprehensive critique of the work but rather an effort to give one view of the strengths and weaknesses of the work and to stimulate the reader's thought processes about the characteristics of a theory and those of the particular work. The terms *theory, model, conceptual framework,* and *conceptual model* are not used consistently in the nursing literature. Thus the work being presented may meet the characteristics of a theory as described in this book and still not be generally accepted as a theory.

Chapter 21 is an aid to the reader for using several or all of these theories in the nursing process in a given situation. This chapter gives some examples of application of the components as a guide and stimulus to the reader's utilization of theory and the nursing process for professional nursing practice. Chapter 21 will be most meaningful if it is read after becoming familiar with the contents of chapters 1 through 20. Finally, chapter 22 presents an overview of theories that have built on, or been influenced by, the theories or theorists presented in more detail in this book. These theorists are Evelyn Adam, Betty Jo Hadley, Joyce Fitzpatrick, and Margaret Newman. A glossary is also provided for quick reference to some common terms and to terms specific to the work of particular theorists.

Some of the theorists, as appropriate to their times, used *she* to refer to the nurse, and *he* to refer to the recipient of care. In some chapters, it would have been awkward to change the theorist's use of such words. In these situations, we have indicated that the use is that of the original author. In like manner, we have tried to reflect the original author's use of the terms *patient* and *client.*

A special "thank you" is due the staff at Appleton & Lange for their help and encouragement during the process of developing the third edition of this book. They have been patient, understanding, and supportive.

Suggestions and comments from users of this text are requested and welcomed.

Julia B. George

CHAPTER 1

The Place of Concepts and Theories Within Nursing

Gertrude Torres

Basic to any professional discipline is the development of a body of knowledge that can be applied to its practice. Such knowledge is often expressed in terms of concepts and theories, especially in the area of the behavioral or social sciences. Thus, nursing as a young, evolving profession is developing a body of knowledge in terms of the concepts and theories that support its practice.

DEFINITION OF TERMS

The use and meanings of the terms *concept* and *theory* within nursing and other disciplines are often conflicting. This confusion can be caused by differences of opinion. However, such confusion is more likely to be caused by the frequent use of the terms in a broad nondefined sense, leaving the listeners or readers uncertain as to the purpose of the presentation and encouraging them to focus on details or specifics rather than on concepts.

In 1920, Lavinia Dock and I. M. Stewart, in discussing the education of nursing for the future, stated that the *concept* of public health and the normal healthy individual should be taught before the care of the sick individual. Although they did not define what was meant by *concept*, one can conjecture that the term was used because they apparently viewed public health as a concept.[1]

In 1933, the New York League of Nursing Education prepared a *concept* of nursing that defined nursing as "using skillfully scientific methods in adapting prescribed therapy and preventive treatment to the specific physical and psychic needs of the individual."[2] A year later in the *American Journal of Nursing*, Effie Taylor spoke of the prevailing concept of nursing as practical, having real depths through love, sympathy, knowledge, and culture.[3] In 1969, Faye Abdellah proposed that nursing theories are the basis for nursing sciences. Among those she identified as being pioneers in the development of nursing theories were Ida Jean Orlando, Ernestine Wiedenbach, and Hildegard Peplau.[4]

The use of the word *concept* is not a new phenomenon; it is one that has been part of nursing's historical background. This is also true in other disciplines within and outside the health care fields. Nursing has used the word *concept* for over fifty years without its having a specific meaning and probably will continue to do so for several more decades.

The main purpose of this chapter is to present some understanding of the words *concepts* and *theories*. This is important in order to grasp what is being said in the chapters that follow. Again, be aware of the differences of opinions and meaning of the terms.

Concepts are basically vehicles of thought that involve images.[5] They are abstract notions and are similar in definition to ideas.[6] Impressions received by sensing our environment evolve into concepts.[7] Chinn and Jacobs define a concept as "a complex mental formulation of an object, property or event that is derived from individual perception and experience."[8] Individuals vary in the specific images or notions they perceive in relation to a given concept.

For the purposes of this text, *concepts are words that describe objects, properties, or events and are the basic components of theory.* Concepts are said to be empirical, inferential, or abstract depending on their ability to be observed in the real world. Empirical concepts are those that can be easily observed in the real world, such as a boat or a drinking glass; inferential concepts are those that are indirectly observable, such as pain or blood pressure; and abstract concepts are those that are nonobservable, such as health or stress. For example, the concept man, when used to represent all humans, is basically abstract since we cannot directly observe all humans. The concept in relation to a male or a particular man is empirical since one can observe a male person. At times, there is disagreement as to whether a particular concept is inferential or abstract. What is important to understand is that the more abstract the concept, the more difficult it is to clearly understand its meaning.

Within this text, in the discussion of nursing theories, many concepts will be identified such as stress, adaptation, stimuli, needs, empathy, and environment. Basically, these are abstract concepts that require much clarification if they are to be used for practice or research. For the most part such clarity is missing. Questions to ask in relation to the use of such concepts are:

- What is the theorist's definition of the concept?
- What are the characteristics of the concepts?
- What terms are closely related in meaning to the concept and what are their differences?
- Is there adequate clarity of abstract concepts so that they can be useful for practice?

In nursing, the most significant concepts that influence and determine its practice include: (1) the human or individual, (2) society/environment, (3) health, and (4) nursing (see Fig. 1–1). Among these four concepts, the core of the practice of nursing is the individual. It is from the patient that the other nursing concepts arise. Without any of these concepts, nursing cannot evolve either as a science or as a professional practice field. For example, the concepts of nursing and the individual may have little relationship unless one recognizes some aspect of health, such as its promotion or restoration, as part of a mutual concern. Also, to attempt to envision the individual without a society is impossible.

Since concepts create images abstract in nature, these concepts tend to have different meanings and can lead to different interpretations. Concepts are strongly influenced by previous learning experiences. Thus, the concept of the individual creates an almost endless supply of notions and ideas. For example, it creates images related to woman, soldier, client/patient, daughter, father, son, and so forth. This kind of word association also leads to identifying related concepts so that increased clarification can occur. In communicating, nurses often use concepts followed by some explanation or description in order to increase the clarity of the message. Misinterpretation, which can lead to misunderstanding, is caused by lack of clarification in the meaning of words representing concepts. It is not essential to agree on the meaning of a particular term, but it is important to describe it sufficiently so that the image one attempts to project becomes

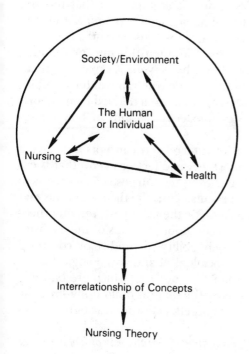

Figure 1–1. Concepts essential to practice.

more explicit. Undefined concepts tend to be too generalized in nature to assist in understanding specifics of our unique experience, and defined concepts do not necessarily indicate a plan for implementation. For this reason, the use of concepts alone without theories is of little assistance in influencing nursing practice.

If nursing accepts the idea that concepts are the elements used to develop theories—theories that form the basis for nursing practice—the profession must then have a thorough understanding of the meaning of the word *theory.*

Within nursing and many disciplines, the meaning of the word *theory* varies. This variety of interpretations is a method of searching and exploring for truths and clarity. Although the lack of precise definition may lead some to a state of confusion and frustration, it allows the option of developing a definition of *theory* that is functional for nursing practice. As the nursing profession matures, sophistication in the understanding and utilizing of nursing theories will probably increase.[8]

In order to give some clarity to the word *theory* so that it can be functional throughout this book, a review of some of the literature is necessary. The word evolves from the Greek word *theoria* signifying a "vision." Based on this sensory nature, the development of theories should be viewed as rational and intellectual and leading to the disclosure of truth. Involved in this intellectual process is comparing, experimenting, and uncovering relationships.[9] This approach to the meaning of theory makes most individuals in nursing potential theory builders. Thus, it is important that nursing recognize that anyone who is capable of speaking is a potential theorist. Nursing practitioners frequently claim to have visions or truths about beliefs that strongly influence their actions. Although this interpretation is helpful in allowing the profession to believe that anyone is capable of theorizing as an intellectual human being, it is of little true value in the development of a sound body of knowledge based on research derived from theory. Theories need to do more than foster intellectual visions of how nurses might practice.

Kerlinger views theories as a set of interrelated concepts that give a systematic view of a phenomenon (an observable fact or event) that is explanatory and predictive in nature.[10] Basically, the purpose of theories is to describe, explain, predict, and control events. Thus the theories in this text will serve one or more of these purposes. For the most part, nursing theories do describe and explain the human condition in terms of the environment and illness but are limited in their ability to predict or control a nursing situation. This is also true of sociological and psychological theories. Keep in mind that theories are not laws or facts, which are basically verifiable and exist as truths. Nor is theory the same as philosophy since the latter deals with more logical reasoning and ethical issues through analysis rather than research.

For the purposes of this text. *theories are a systematic way of looking at the world in order to describe, explain, predict, or control it.* Theories are composed of concepts, definitions, models, and propositions and are based on assumptions. The concepts and their definitions are basic to the understanding of a theory. *Models are representations of the interaction among and between the concepts showing patterns.* You will note within the text a variety of diagrams, representing models, used to show the relationship between the various concepts within the theory. Some models have been developed by the theorist and some are the writers' interpretation of what the theorist's model might be. *Propositions are statements that explain the relationship between the concepts.* Thus, in a way, a model is a pictorial representation of a proposition. Review Figure 1–1, which is a model of the concepts essential to nursing practice, and see if you agree with the following propositions:

* Humans relate to the society/environment, nursing, and health.
* Nursing relates to society and health as well as to humans.
* Health relates to nursing, society, and humans.

Although the model does not offer any differences in the relationships between the concepts, through research such differences could be discovered. For example, review the following research questions which stem from the model and the propositions:

* Does increased nursing care affect the level of health of the individual?
* Do changes within the environment affect the health of the individual?
* Are individuals more affected by the environment or by nursing?

RELATIONSHIP BETWEEN THEORY, RESEARCH, AND PRACTICE

It is important to understand how theory, research, and practice relate to and are supportive of each other. As noted, theories do lead to propositions that need to be tested. In nursing, practice is the basic purpose of the discipline. As a profession, nursing has the responsibility to assist individuals, groups, families, and communities to retain, obtain, and maintain a state of health. In order to assume such a responsibility, nursing must have a foundation of theoretical knowledge which is based on research findings. It is not good enough to practice based on intuition, habit, or traditions as a basis for making nursing decisions.

Research is the *formal, systematic process of gathering data from the real world to gain solutions, discover answers, and interpret new ideas, facts, or assumptions and relationships.* The more research that has been done in relation to a particular theory, the more useful that theory is to practice. Recently, in nursing, there is a greater emphasis on doing research in relation to nursing theories rather than attempting to validate psychological theories such as Maslow's Need theory. In summary, *practice is based on the theories of a discipline which are validated through research.* This is true in relation to all the health disciplines. The extent of predictability depends on the amount of research available and on the theorist's skill in studying existing knowledge and in linking concepts and theories to form new knowledge.

For example, in caring for a person with a particular need or problem, using a particular nursing theory should give strong clues as to the outcomes of nursing care. If we relate this to the use of a particular drug, given the correct data about the person and the drug, we can expect certain results to occur from the administration of the drug. Thus, the outcome has the element of prediction. In nursing, we should view a theory as a way of relating concepts through the use of definitions that assist in developing significant interrelationships to describe or classify approaches to practice (see Fig. 1–1). Classification is used to relate facts and to generalize about them. This will assist in explaining events.[11] From this approach we can develop the important predictive ingredients of a theory and can view nursing theories as a way of assisting and explaining approaches to practice.

In other fields, especially the biological sciences, there are laws as well as theories. Laws are truly *predictable* and can be utilized with assurance because they provide a sound body of knowledge in which to function. For example, in chemistry, if one correctly places a salt and an acid in the same vehicle, one can predict the results. Laws compose the basis of the most mature sciences. On the other hand, since nursing is a behavioral *and* a new science, its knowledge is based primarily on theories that have not yet been validated and are not predictable. In the future, the predictability of nursing theories will become more reliable as concepts are better defined and as the research from which theories develop grows.

In reviewing theories, it is important to understand their basic characteristics. These are reviewed below.

BASIC CHARACTERISTICS OF A THEORY

1. Theories can interrelate concepts in such a way as to create a different way of looking at a particular phenomenon. Theories are constructed from concepts, which are abstract ideas or mental images that represent reality. A theory is only a theory if more than one major concept is identified and defined, and if explicit or clearly stated relationships are projected between these concepts. The definitions of the concepts should provide a clear mental picture of the events or experiences that the theory is designed to explain, and should clarify how these experiences fit together to describe, explain, and predict reality. Theory provides a way of viewing our everyday experiences in a way that is not always evident based on our limited experience, and it also provides a way of looking at possible goals that might not otherwise occur to us.

For example, a theory might identify the two concepts "need" and "nursing." The concept of need may be described in terms of actual experiences that a person might encounter that interfere with an optimal health state. The concept of nursing may be defined in terms of actions that can be taken to reach an optimal health state such as touch, listening, or teaching. The theory, in turn, may connect the two concepts of need and nursing in such a way that nursing actions can be deliberately viewed as meeting needs, and in so doing reach a goal of optimal health. Without the theory, we may not perceive the relationship between a need and a nursing action, but the theory should provide a unique way of viewing nursing actions as meeting a particular goal: a specific relationship.

With the theory, we begin to look more closely at a need and relate our nursing actions more directly to that need, rather than simply doing what we think we should be doing in a situation because someone says that is what we should do. For example, we can approach a typical care giving situation by providing information because we have been taught that a young mother must be given information about how to feed her infant. If we have a theory on which to base our nursing practice that relates the abstract ideas of "need" and "nursing action," and these concepts are defined in the theory so that our experiences with this young mother are consistent with the theory, then we can begin to look for evidence that she *needs* this information, and can provide the type of information that is viewed as consistent with her need. If the theory includes a concept of family or society, then we would also integrate our notions about families or societies into our view of this situation.

2. Theories must be logical in nature. Logic involves orderly reasoning. Interrelationships must be sequential and must follow principles of reasoning. Theories must have clearly defined concepts, and the concepts and their relationships must be consistent; that is, there must not be any apparent contradictions between the definitions of the concepts, the relationships within the theory, and the goals of the theory. Theories all have basic underlying assumptions that must be consistent with the goals and the relationships of the theory. For example, a theory might be based on the underlying assumption that humans are basically good in nature. Then all the concepts and the relationships must be consistent with this basic assumption. Therefore, if the theory defines human beings as basically good, but then goes on to describe relationships that focus on sick or unhealthy goals or outcomes, the theory lacks logical consistency. Such a theory would be logical only if it describes, explains, and predicts the natural and healthy outcomes as well as the hazards that threaten these naturally healthy or good outcomes or goals.

3. Theories should be relatively simple yet generalizable. A theory that is thought of as a "good" theory is stated in the most simple terms possible, but at the same time it includes a wide range of possible experiences in nursing practice. The concept of motion is a relatively simple term in that it can be applied to a wide range of experiences, such as or including blood flow, muscles, objects (air, automobiles, etc.), and even ideas. Likewise, the concept of time can be simply defined in relation to the moon or sun cycles, but it can also be generalized to include how people perceive its passage as slow or fast. If a theory relates the relatively simple concepts of time and motion, then it is said to be simple yet generalizable to a wide range of specific events and experiences in the real world. Such theories that are both simple and generalizable may be referred to as *parsimonious*.

4. **Theories can be the bases for hypotheses that can be tested.** If a particular theory cannot be tested, it offers little as a base of knowledge. The definitions of the concepts in the theory should suggest precise experiences that can be observed or measured in some way. A broad concept such as need might have many possible real-world experiences that can be measured either directly or indirectly. For example, an imbalance of electrolytes might imply a direct observation of need for electrolyte substances that would restore balance in the physiological system. An indirect measurement might be indicated for something more abstract such as attachment or adaptation. If the concepts of the theory cannot be measured, observed, or demonstrated in some way, then the theory cannot be tested empirically. On the other hand, if the theory suggests some means of measuring or observing the abstract concepts that form the relationships, then research can be designed that tests the precision of the theory in predicting relationships, and the theory grows in meaning and significance.

5. **Theories contribute to and assist in increasing the general body of knowledge within the discipline through the research implemented to validate them.** Theories that are not tested empirically (through measurement or observation of real-world events) contribute little to the body of knowledge of a discipline. If the theory stimulates research, then this research and the theory on which it is based will contribute to the present body of knowledge of the discipline. Since all research raises additional questions for investigation, the research and the theory on which it is based lead to the development of other scientific theories from which new hypotheses can be drawn. Thus theories, if sound, assist in developing nursing hypotheses that can be used to develop new theories.

6. **Theories can be utilized by the practitioners to guide and improve their practice.** One of the most significant characteristics of a theory is its usefulness to the practitioner. A theory should provide an indication of the goal that is to be attained if the relationships of the theory are accurate in reality. If the goal of the theory is high-level wellness, and the relationships of the theory are accurate in reality, then if the practitioner provides for the conditions and realities implied in the theory, the goal of high-level wellness should be attained. Although theories are not principles or rules for practice but rather serve to stimulate further testing of reality, they can provide guidelines that can be used in the ongoing process of improvement of nursing practice. As the theories of nursing are tested with research and

shown to be reliable, the profession will continue to grow and develop new and evolving approaches to its practice.[12]

7. Theories must be consistent with other validated theories, laws, and principles but will leave open unanswered questions that need to be investigated. Unless nursing theories build upon scientific findings that have been validated, much confusion will occur. The logic of theory is based on the underlying laws, previously validated knowledge, and humanitarian values that are generally accepted as "good" and "right." Theory within nursing must be consistent with previously established knowledge; however, the tentative nature of theory continues to raise questions that challenge aspects of that knowledge that have not yet been challenged. For example, most previous research has demonstrated that adaptation is a response that leads to an improved state of health. However, the question still persists as to whether this is always the case or under what conditions adaptation best exists. Nursing theory will build on and support previously developed knowledge about adaptation but will leave open the possibility of new knowledge that has not yet been explored about adaptation.

THEORETICAL APPROACH TO NURSING PRACTICE

By examining the following situation, one can identify how a theoretical approach can be used in nursing practice.

Situation. Mrs. Mary Dolphin is nine months pregnant and is expecting her first child within a week. She is visiting her obstetrician for an examination. The office nurse has been requested to do health teaching either during the office visits or in Mrs. Dolphin's home. Mrs. Dolphin is an executive career woman of Irish descent who has been married for one year. Mr. Dolphin is in governmental service and travels a great deal, frequently leaving Mrs. Dolphin alone. During the entire pregnancy, Mrs. Dolphin has been cooperative and enthusiastic. No complications or unusual problems (other than morning sickness, which lasted for six weeks during her first trimester) have occurred during the pregnancy.

In reviewing the above situation, many theories, especially those related to the sciences, can be identified that would show the need of special knowledge in order to practice professional nursing. The following kinds of theories reflect only a sample.

KINDS OF THEORIES

Stress Theories
The nurse needs to assess Mrs. Dolphin's previous ability to deal with stress. Theories that give clues as to how individuals deal physiologically and

psychologically with stress will assist the nurse in understanding how people can be expected to react. Stress theories will also enable the nurse to differentiate between typical and atypical reactions to stress, thus leading to more appropriate nursing diagnoses.

Developmental Theories
Theories relating to the development of each member of the family will give the nurse an appropriate knowledge base on which to assess specific developmental levels and tasks for each member of the family. For example, during Mrs. Dolphin's pregnancy, it is important for the nurse to teach her what is the "normal" physical, intellectual, and emotional development of the newborn and the infant, as well as the "normal" development of the pregnant family.

Family Theories
The structure and function of the family unit and the interrelationships of a family group are reflected in theories relating to the family. Although the office nurse may not have seen Mr. Dolphin, the nurse is able to assess Mrs. Dolphin's relationship with her husband as perceived by Mrs. Dolphin and the impact that a new child may have on the family relationships. Theories concerning family structure and needs will assist the professional nurse in health teaching and nursing diagnoses.

Interactive Theories
The professional nurse must have a sound base of theoretical knowledge about interactions since the base of health teaching relates to the nurse's ability to interact with Mrs. Dolphin and Mrs. Dolphin's ability to interact with others.

Adaptation Theories
Mrs. Dolphin needs to be assessed in terms of her ability to adapt to both her pregnancy and the birth of a child. The nurse needs to be able to explain and hypothesize physical and emotional changes in Mrs. Dolphin.

Other Theories
Other theories can also be identified that will offer the nurse insight into both assessing and planning care. For example, *role* theories will assist in explaining both the role of the nurse and Mrs. Dolphin's role as a mother. *Change* theories will offer insight into the expected behaviors that evolve when significant change occurs within an environment. *Nursing* theories that explain phenomena and guide the nurse in giving care would be instrumental as guidelines to care. Also, involved in the care of Mrs. Dolphin is a variety of scientific knowledge related to physiology, such as fetal nourishment, labor, and delivery.

In caring for Mrs. Dolphin, the nurse needs a breadth of knowledge.

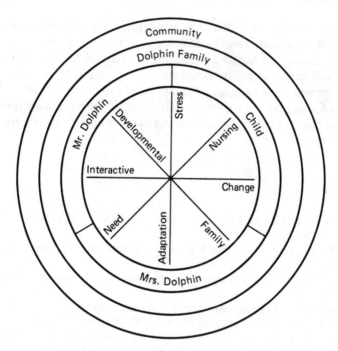

Figure 1-2. Theories—Base of knowledge.

The greater the nurse's sophistication and expertise in theories, the greater the potential for the use of appropriate approaches to care. A strong theoretical knowledge base assists the nurse in providing quality nursing care.

Figure 1-2 gives us a visual reference point by which to identify how various theories assist the nurse in the care of Mrs. Dolphin. Other theories can be identified that would enhance the knowledge base upon which to provide care for Mrs. Dolphin. A beginning student in nursing should review theories that are foundational to nursing.

SUMMARY

Concepts represent abstract notions and ideas that, when interrelated, provide the foundation of a theory. Theories may be viewed as visions giving intellectual insight into phenomena, but for maximum significance and impact they should be explanatory and predictive in nature so as to guide professional practice. Nursing theories need to be viewed in the context of how they describe or classify approaches to practice by interrelating the four concepts of (1) the human or individual, (2) society/environment, (3) health, and (4) nursing. Nursing research, through testing hypotheses derived from theories and through assisting in the development of more predictive theories, will thus build a body of nursing science.

Within any given nursing situation, a variety of theories can be identified that will give the professional nurse a strong base of knowledge on which to practice and explain the approach to nursing care. The main function of this text is to demonstrate how nursing theories provide this knowledge base for professional nursing practice and ultimately for improving health care.

REFERENCES

1. Dock, L.L., & Stewart, I.M. *A Short History of Nursing* (4th ed.), New York: G. P. Putnam's Sons, 1920, p. 249.
2. New York League of Nursing Education, A concept of nursing. *The American Journal of Nursing*, 1933, *33*, 565.
3. Taylor, E.J. Of what is the nature of nursing? *The American Journal of Nursing*, 1934, *34*, 476.
4. Abdellah, F.G. The nature of nursing science. *Nursing Research*, 1969, *18*, 390.
5. Harre, R. The formal analysis of concepts. *Analysis of Concept Learning*, (eds. Klausmerer, H., Harris, C.), New York: Academic Press, Inc., 1966, pp. 3–4.
6. *Webster's New Collegiate Dictionary*, Springfield, Mass.: Merriam, 1974, p. 233.
7. Toffler, A. The psychology of the future. *Learning for Tomorrow—The Role of the Future in Education*, New York: Vintage Books, 1974, p. 12.
8. Chinn, P.L., & Jacobs, M.K. *Theory and Nursing: A Systematic Approach*, St. Louis: C. V. Mosby, 1983, p. 200.
9. Phenix, P.H. Educational theory and inspiration. *Educational Theory*, 1963, *13*, 1–2.
10. Kerlinger, F.N. *Foundations of Behavioral Research*, New York: Holt, Rinehart & Winston, 1965, p. 11.
11. Beauchamp, G. *Curriculum Theory* (2nd ed.), Wilmette, Ill.: Kagg Press, 1968, pp. 23–24.
12. Chinn & Jacobs, *Theory and Nursing*.

CHAPTER 2

An Overview of the Nursing Process

Marjorie Stanton
Charlotte Paul
Joan S. Reeves

This chapter is based on the assumption that professional nursing practice is interpersonal in nature. Recognizing the importance and effect of the nurse's relationship with the client/patient, professional nurses use this knowledge in proceeding through each phase of the nursing process.

It is also assumed that professional nurses view human beings as holistic, thereby acknowledging that mind and body are not separate but function as a whole. People respond as whole beings. What happens in one part of the mind or body affects the person as a whole entity.

Given these two assumptions, it would be impossible for a nurse to view a client/patient as "the hysterectomy in room 201" or "the paranoid in bed 2." The woman who has experienced a hysterectomy may have physiological, spiritual, and psychological health problems, i.e., physiological and psychological adjustments due to induced menopause, and spiritual adjustments if her life style includes a religious orientation related to a life of childbearing. Or the person with symptoms of paranoia may refuse to eat, causing physiological changes related to malnutrition. These two assumptions, that nursing is interpersonal in nature and that professional nurses view human beings as holistic, give guidance and direction to the use of the nursing process.

The nursing process is the underlying scheme that provides order and direction to nursing care. It is the essence of professional nursing practice. It is the "tool" and methodology of the nursing profession and, as such, helps nurses in arriving at decisions and in predicting and evaluating consequences. The nursing process can be defined as a deliberate intellectual activity whereby the practice of nursing is approached in an orderly, systematic manner. Each of these terms for defining the process can be further delineated as follows:*

---

* This list is based on definitions found in the *American Heritage Dictionary*, 1975.

- *Deliberate:* Careful, thoughtful, intentional
- *Intellectual:* Rational, knowledgeable, reasonable, conceptual
- *Activity:* The state or condition of functioning, initiating, changing, behaving
- *Orderly:* A methodical, efficient, logical arrangement
- *Systematic:* Purposeful, pertaining to classification

The nursing process was developed as a specific method for applying a scientific approach or a problem solving approach to nursing practice.[1a,1b] Problem solving approaches are not unique to nursing. For example, health planners use a health planning process which is a problem solving approach aimed at planned social change.[2] The nursing process deals with problems specific to nurses and their clients/patients. In nursing, the client/patient may be an individual, family, or community and the nursing process has been adapted for use with each type of client/patient.[3]

Students of nursing using the nursing process are learning to behave as professional nurses in practice behave. Since the nursing process is the essence and tool (methodology) of professional nursing practice, students must become familiar with and adept at using the nursing process as their basis for practice. The nursing process also provides a means for evaluating the quality of nursing care given by nurses and assures their accountability and responsibility to the client/patient. In order to use the nursing process effectively, nurses need to understand and apply appropriate concept and theories from nursing, from the biological, physical, and behavioral sciences, and from the humanities, in order to provide a rationale for decision making, judgments, interpersonal relationships, and actions. These concepts and theories provide the framework for nursing care.

FIVE PHASES

Many authors agree that four phases, or components, are considered necessary to the nursing process: assessment, nursing diagnosis or identification of problem, intervention or implementation, and evaluation.[4] However, some authors do not mention the nursing diagnosis as such, and some consider the nursing care plan separately. In this book, because nursing diagnosis is considered an essential component of the nursing process and planning is included as an integral part of it, we will consider five different phases or components, as listed below:

1. Assessment
2. Nursing diagnosis
3. Planning
4. Implementation
5. Evaluation

Although this listing suggests a forward movement of the process through each discrete phase, this does not always occur in the actual process. Assessment must always begin the process, and it always leads to a nursing diagnosis. The assessment phase includes collection and analysis of data. The nursing diagnosis is derived from assessment. However, during the diagnosis, planning, implementation, and evaluation phases, *reassessment* can lead to immediate changes in each of these four stages. Reassessment, the further collection and analysis of data, is a continuous, ongoing process; and it is not to be confused with evaluation, which measures outcomes. Reassessment may also lead to a change in diagnosis, which could lead to a change in planning, implementation, and evaluation as the process continues (see Fig. 2–1).

Assessment

Assessment is the first phase in the nursing process and has two subphases, data collection and analysis or synthesis. Assessment consists of the systematic and orderly collection and analysis of data pertaining to and about the health status of the client/patient for the purpose of making the nursing diagnosis. It always leads to a nursing diagnosis. Thus insufficient or incorrect assessment could lead to an incorrect nursing diagnosis, which could mean inappropriate planning, implementation, and evaluation. Therefore, the importance of accurate assessment cannot be overemphasized. It is vital to the process and is the basis for all other stages in the process. Although assessment is the first phase, it may also occur as reassessment during any other phase of the process when new data are obtained.[5]

The systematic and orderly collection of data is essential in order for the nurse to know if sufficient data have been collected, and it also serves to provide a method of quick retrieval of information relative to the client/patient for auditing professional practice and for doing nursing research. Several authors have provided guidelines for the systematic collection of data.[6a–6d] The American Nurses' Association's (ANA) *Standards of Nursing Practice* also provides information.[7] A holistic view during the assessment

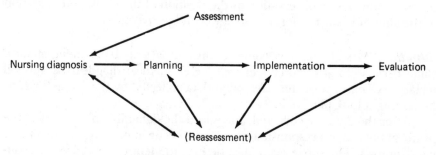

Figure 2–1. The nursing process.

phase ensures that the biological, psychological, social, and spiritual spheres of the individual are considered. Any assessment guidelines should include the following:

- Biographical data
- A health history including family and social history
- Subjective and objective data about the current health status, including reasons for contact with health care professional, medical diagnosis if the client/patient has a medical problem, and results of diagnostic studies

By using these guidelines, the data collected are classified into discrete areas that can be compared, contrasted for relationships, and clustered during the analysis of the data.

The biographical data are generally provided during an interview with the client or the person responsible for the client.[8] Such data are necessary to appropriately identify the client as an individual and may provide clues to the client's health status. For example, the age of clients gives an indication of their growth and developmental status.

A health history is "the client's story of past and present events which may affect current and future health status."[9] The history is obtained through interviewing the client, the individual responsible for the client, i.e., parent, or both, and by reviewing previous health records of the client if available. Clients may, if able, fill out part of the biographical data and health history forms. Interviewing the client is essential for discerning clues and cues and for beginning the establishment of a therapeutic relationship.

The current health status of the client is also ascertained through interviewing the client or person responsible for the client (subjective data) and through examination and observation of the client to obtain data that can be seen or measured objectively (objective data). For example, a client's description of pain is considered to be subjective data, whereas vital signs are an example of an objective measurement of physiological data.[10] When possible, objective data should be obtained to verify subjective data. For example, the client complains of abdominal pain (subjective data), which the nurse verifies by observation of the position of the client and palpation of the abdomen for tenderness or rigidity (objective data).

Situation. Mrs. James has come to the outpatient department medical clinic because "I just don't feel well." Her medical diagnosis is general malaise. An excerpt of the assessment data collected by the nurse for Mrs. James might look like Table 2–1.

After the data are collected, analysis of the data takes place. This is the professional nurse's responsibility and *must* occur in order to make a nursing diagnosis. The nurse examines the data to identify, compare, and contrast the relationship of one piece of data to another. The data collected are

TABLE 2–1. ASSESSMENT OF MRS. JAMES

Biographical Data	Health History	Subjective Data	Objective Data
Client—Mrs. James Age 45 Housewife Husband Philip, age 46 electrical helper Daughters Ann, age 18 Jean, age 15	Italian/Spanish heritage. Mother of Mrs. James had diabetes in older years. "All family are overweight." Shops at local fast-food market. Usually shops daily. Mrs. James responsible for cooking. Family does not have regular mealtimes.	"Fingernails break easily." Favorite foods are pizza, pasta with butter, french fries, biscuits with gravy. Drinks are coffee and Tab. Dislikes milk, meats, and vegetables.	Height—5'2" Weight—180 lb Skin pale, dry to touch. Hair lifeless and dry to touch. Nails are ragged and broken.

also compared to societal norms to identify an actual or potential health problem. For example, a four-year-old who is unable to walk does not meet the developmental standards for four-year-olds, and this is an example of an actual health problem.

It is during the analysis stage of assessment that the nurse uses her or his knowledge of various theories and concepts to cluster the collected data. Clustering the data is the grouping of data pieces that fit together and show relationships. Nursing diagnoses are derived from clusters of data that show relationships, make sense, and lead to a logical conclusion. The clustering of data in Table 2–2 indicates that the client may have a potential health problem in relation to diabetes based on age, family history of diabetes, and obesity problem.

When analyzing the data related to age, the nurse needs to know what is expected of people during each stage of development. Abraham Maslow's hierarchy of needs,[11] E. H. Erikson's eight stages of man,[12] and other sources in the literature are useful references to consider in looking at the data.

Identification of gaps in the data should occur during the analysis stage in order to ensure that all important information has been supplied and that the nursing diagnosis is based on actual data and not on inaccurate assumptions. For example, assessing a young child without talking to the mother or to the person responsible for the child will immediately tell the nurse that there are gaps in the data. An analysis of the data should also give clues as to the kinds of patterns developing. In the case of Mrs. James, there is a pattern of poor eating habits, poor selection of foods, and little understanding of diet for good health. These patterns may be handed down from generation to generation.

TABLE 2–2. COMPARISON AND RELATIONSHIP OF DATA FOR MRS. JAMES

Biographical Data	Health History	Current Health Status
45 years old	Mother had adult onset diabetes	Height—5'2" Weight—180 lb

Nursing Diagnosis

Nursing diagnosis, the second phase of the nursing process, is recognized in the ANA definition of nursing as "the diagnosis and treatment of human responses to actual or potential health problems."[13] Nursing diagnosis may be defined here as the identification of the human responses and resource limitations of the client for the general purpose of identifying and directing nursing care. The diagnostic statement identifies the client's actual or potential health problem, deficit, or concern, which can be affected by nursing actions. Models for these diagnostic statements have been provided in the reports of the National Nursing Diagnosis Conferences and by Campbell and Gordon.[14a–14f] For most clients, there will be more than one nursing diagnosis.

These diagnostic statements are derived from the nurse's inferences, based on the assessed and validated data coupled with nursing, scientific, and humanistic concepts and theories. As one proceeds through the analysis of data, certain patterns develop, and the use of relevant concepts and theories is appropriate. Nursing diagnoses are formulated after conclusions or decisions have been reached based on analysis of the data. Each nursing diagnosis can be considered a client-related behavioral statement that identifies the area for the focus of nursing action. A diagnosis may deal with an actual (present-oriented) or a potential (future-oriented) health problem.

After the nursing diagnoses are identified, they should be ranked in order of priority. This ranking should take into consideration both the client's and the nurse's opinions. Those areas that have the greatest impact on the client, the family, or both, should receive particular attention. The nurse also determines priorities based on past nursing experience and on scientific knowledge of the needs and functions of human beings. Therefore, a continuum of priorities of nursing diagnoses is developed, based on the degree of threat to the level of wellness of the client.

The nursing diagnosis can be considered a decisive statement concerning the client's nursing needs. It is important to remember that diagnoses are based on the client's concerns as well as on actual or potential problems that may be symptoms of physiological disorders or of behavioral, psychosocial, or spiritual problems.

Situation. Mrs. James's medical diagnosis has been altered to: adult onset diabetes mellitus. She asks the nurse if this means she will need to make any changes in how she lives. She says she remembers her mother "took some kind of shots."

For Mrs. James, an actual health problem can be identified as a lack of information regarding diabetes management. This is based on data about her height, weight, and family nutrition patterns, and the status of her integumentary system. In this case, the nursing diagnosis could be: "Inadequate information relating to diabetes management: lack of information regarding cause, effect, and therapeutic action associated with diabetes management (more specific nutritional needs)."[15] This statement indicates the client has inadequate information, as determined from assessed validated data.

The nursing diagnosis also states the categories where lack of information is pertinent. This assists the nurse in developing a plan of action. Another way to state the diagnosis would be: "Alterations in nutrition (eating and drinking)." This statement identifies the need to investigate the client's eating habits, her motivation to change, and her knowledge of nutritional needs.

Other nursing diagnoses for Mrs. James may deal with potential problems that can be identified through assessment or reassessment. These problems are related to significant risk factors that can be modified to reduce the impact of the illness. In this case, a nursing diagnosis could be: "Inadequate knowledge relating to diabetic skin care: lack of information regarding special skin care, peripheral circulation and the healing process."[16] This nursing diagnosis establishes the potential problem and identifies the categories where lack of knowledge can create problems to assist the nurse in developing the plan for care. Another way to state this diagnosis could be: "Potential for alterations in skin integrity." This diagnosis implies the need to evaluate the knowledge base of the client about special skin care and the healing process in persons with diabetes. These diagnoses, the needs, and the problem categories they represent are presented in Table 2–3.

Planning

Planning is the third phase of the nursing process. The plan for providing nursing care can be described as the determination of what can be done to assist the client, and involves the mutual setting of goals and objectives, judging priorities, and designing methods to resolve actual or potential problems.[17]

The first stage in the planning is setting goals and objectives. These goals and objectives are derived from the nursing diagnoses and are established for each nursing diagnosis listed.

In preparing to write the plan, the client and his or her family should be consulted before formulating the goals and objectives. The goals and objectives should be realistic and attainable, supportive of the client's needs, and mutually acceptable. It is important to consider the need for objectives

TABLE 2–3. CLASSIFICATION OF NURSING DIAGNOSES

Nursing Diagnosis Statement	Type of Need	Problem Category	
		Actual (present)	Potential (future)
I.			
Inadequate information relating to diabetes management; lack of information regarding cause, effect, and therapeutic action associated with diabetes management (more specific nutritional needs)	Biopsycho-social	Lack of information regarding diabetes management	
or			
Alterations in nutrition (eating and drinking)	Biological	Lack of knowledge pertaining to nutrition, eating habits; lack of motivation to change	
II.			
Inadequate knowledge relating to diabetic skin care: lack of information regarding special skin care, peripheral circulation, and the healing process	Biopsycho-social		Lack of knowledge regarding the need for special skin care
or			
Potential for alterations in skin integrity	Biological		Implies the need to evaluate knowledge base of client regarding special skin care and healing process in diabetics

that can be defined and stated concisely in an "act-of-being" phrase. This phrase should contain a performer (the client), a performance (action), and a change in behavior to be accomplished (objectives). The expected end behavior needs to be identified and be placed in the proper time frame, and can be used as a means for evaluation.

Goals are stated in broad terms in order to identify effective criteria for evaluating nursing action. These goals can pertain to rehabilitation, prevention of complications associated with stressors, the ability of the client to adapt to these stressors, or all three. Other goals may deal with the achievement of the highest potential for wholeness of the system. A sample of a goal statement would be, "Mrs. James will have an adequate understanding of the basic food groups and their relationship to recommended daily allowance (RDA) requirements within one month."

From the goals, objectives are determined that need to be stated in observable behavioral terms. Objectives should define the conditions under which the expected end behaviors are to occur and should specify the performance level and specific behaviors that will be accepted as being evidence of meeting the desired outcomes. The behaviors in question refer to psychological, physiological, social, and intellectual activities and other observable responses. Objectives related to the above goal for Mrs. James could be:

1. Identify the basic four food groups from a chart by the end of Week I.
2. Prepare a shopping list to include at least two necessary foods from each group by the end of Week I.
3. Prepare family menus for three days using the basic four food groups as a guide by Week II.
4. Make substitutions in family menus for three days using the basic four food groups chart as guide by Week III.
5. Evaluate eating patterns of family for one week using the basic four food groups chart as guide and identify at least two problem areas to discuss with nurse by Week IV.

Desired behavioral outcomes (objectives) should be stated in a manner that everyone is able to understand without having to seek clarification. Robert Mager in his book on preparing objectives indicates that a meaningfully stated outcome would be one that communicates to the staff the intent of the individual who stated it.[18] "The statement which communicates best will be one which describes the terminal behavior of the learner well enough to prevent misinterpretation."[19]

Time is another consideration when specifying desired outcomes. The time limits should be precise for evaluation purposes but should not be so rigid that changes cannot readily be made based on reassessment of the priorities and necessary outcomes. It is important to remember to state the desired outcomes in terms of client behaviors rather than nurse behaviors, in keeping with the ANA *Standards of Nursing Practice*.[20]

The second stage in nursing care planning is the identification of nursing actions for each nursing diagnosis, based on carefully thought out scientific rationale. The nursing action specifies what kind of nursing care is to be done to effectively meet the client's problem. Nursing actions should be precisely spelled out. These actions are part of the scheme for providing good nursing care.

Nursing actions can be said to be hypotheses established for testing if they contribute to the solution of the problem. It is up to the nurse in conjunction with the client, the family, or both to select appropriate actions to produce the desired results. In selecting these nursing actions, it is important to analyze the options available and to determine the probability of success in reaching the objective. Sometimes compromises must be made in order to provide the best care for the client, and the nurse needs to be aware of this when specifying nursing actions.

The nursing care plan deals with actual as well as potential problems. Nursing actions are based on scientific principles and theories of nursing and need to be specific. The plan serves as a means for resolving the problems and for meeting established goals in an orderly fashion. Also, it provides a means for organization, giving direction and meaning to the nursing action used in helping the client, the family, or both to resolve the health problems. A plan of action is essential in that it aids in the efficient use of time, thus saving time and energy by providing essential data for those individuals responsible for giving care.

Since the client's condition is continuously changing, the written nursing care plan needs to reflect these changes. Therefore, planning becomes a continuous process based on evaluation and reassessment and is the most efficient way of keeping all individuals involved in the client's care informed of modifications in the plan of nursing care.

Implementation

After planning, implementation is the next or fourth phase of the nursing process. Implementation refers to the action or actions initiated to accomplish the defined goals and objectives. Implementation is often considered as the actual giving of nursing care. It is putting the plan into action. Other terms used to describe this part of the process are *action* or *intervention*. According to *The Random House Dictionary*, the words *implementation* and *intervention* are not synonymous.[21] The definition of implementation is "to put into effect according to or by means of a definite plan or procedures." Intervention is defined as "interposition or interference of one state in the affairs of another, a coming between." Therefore the term *implementation* seems more appropriate to describe this phase of the process if nursing actions are to follow from stated goals and objectives.

Since the nursing process is interpersonal in nature, it must take place between the nurse and the client. The client may be a person, a group, a family, or even a community. The beliefs that the nurse and the client have about human beings, nurses, and clients, and about interactions between nurses and clients will affect the types of actions that both consider appropriate. If human beings are considered unique, then nursing actions should reflect this uniqueness. Therefore, the philosophy of nursing that a nurse develops will affect the nursing actions that he or she uses in meeting the needs of clients. Helen Yura and Mary Walsh in their book *The Nursing Process* indicate that the implementation phase of the nursing process draws heavily on the intellectual, interpersonal, and technical skills of the nurse.[22]

Even though the focus is on action, the action is intellectual, interpersonal, and technical in nature.

The implementation phase begins when the nurse considers various alternative actions and selects those most suitable to achieve the planned goals and objectives. Just as goals and objectives have priorities in the plan, actions may also have priorities. Nursing actions may be carried out by the nurse who developed the nursing care plan or by other nurses or nursing assistants. Nursing actions may also be carried out by the client or family. To carry out a nursing action, the nurse refers to the written plan for specific information. Many nursing actions fall into the broad categories of counseling, teaching, providing physical care, carrying out delegated medical therapy, coordination of resources, referral to other sources of help, and therapeutic communication (verbal and nonverbal).

Based on the goals and objectives for Mrs. James, as discussed on page 21, there are several nursing actions that could be implemented. For example, under objective 1 (identify the basic four food groups from a chart), the following actions could be considered:

1. Establish an agreed upon time when Mrs. James and her family could meet with the nurse in their home during the next week.
2. Establish base-line knowledge about Mrs. James's and the family members' understanding of basic food groups.
3. Bring chart and booklets containing information about the four basic food groups to Mrs. James's home.
4. Teach family about using the four basic food groups for good nutrition (base teaching on information gained from base-line knowledge).
5. Focus on the value of the food groups for each family member based on age, height, weight, and activity.
6. Request a return demonstration in which Mrs. James and other family members will identify foods by placing the food in a food group and will state why each food group is important.

In Campbell's study of nursing diagnoses and nursing actions, seven categories of nursing actions were developed. These are: assertive, hygienic, rehabilitative, supportive, preventive, observational, and educative.[23] Campbell also points out that almost all nursing actions are initiated by nurses without medical direction. Nurses can initiate and carry out all activities that fall within the nursing domain. In the hospital setting, nurses are also asked to assist physicians in carrying out medical prescriptions. Therefore, nurses need to be clear about their dependent and independent functions.

For every nursing action, the client responds as a total person or as a whole. The concept of *holism,* which states that a person is more than the sum of that person's parts, means that the nurse may be treating a person's leg, but the person will respond as a whole person.[24] The concept is useful in thinking about the consequences of any nursing actions. For example, the simple action of turning the patient every two hours will have a variety of consequences. Some of these consequences should or could be: (1) increased circulation, (2) improved muscle tone, (3) improved breathing, (4) less flatus (gas) in the intestinal tract, (5) prevention of pressure sores, (6) increased or decreased pain, (7) opportunity for communication with care giver, (8) increased ability to socialize with patient in next bed, and (9) increased or decreased ability to reach articles at bedside. There may be other consequences that could not have been predicted, such as an opportunity to express values or beliefs. Therefore, in planning nursing actions, it is important to consider the cluster of consequences of both positive and negative value that can be expected to occur with and following each action.[25] Using this knowledge will help the nurse in selecting the most appropriate actions. Even though not all consequences are predictable for a specific client, it is possible to develop a general knowledge of expected consequences. Knowledge of consequences is an important aspect of the implementation phase of the nursing process. The implementation phase is completed when the nursing actions are finished and results are recorded.

Evaluation

Evaluation is the fifth and final phase of the nursing process. It may be defined as the appraisal of the client's behavioral changes due to the action of the nurse.[26] Although evaluation is considered to be the final phase, it frequently does not end the process. As mentioned earlier in this chapter, evaluation may lead to reassessment, which in turn may result in the nursing process beginning all over again. The main questions to ask in evaluation are: Were the goals and objectives met? Were there identifiable changes in the client's behavior? If so, why? If not, why not? Were the consequences of nursing actions predicted? These questions help the nurse to determine which problems have been solved and which problems need to be reassessed and replanned. Unsolved problems cannot be assumed to reflect faulty data collection or inadequate data collection; rather each part of the nursing process may need to be evaluated to determine the cause of ineffective actions.

The key to appropriately evaluating nurse–client actions lies in the planning phase of the process. When objectives are described in behavioral terms with clearly stated expected outcomes, it is easy to determine whether or not the nurse–client actions were successful. These objectives become the criteria for evaluating nurse–client actions. Just as goals should be mutually set with a client whenever possible, it is also important for the nurse and client to mutually establish the objectives (criteria for evaluation).

According to Dolores Little and Doris Carnevali, evaluation consists of three sequential steps.[27]

1. Selecting criteria (objectives) that will guide the nurse's observation to specified areas of the client's anticipated behavioral changes related to the diagnosis and goals
2. Collecting specific evidence (data) after goals have been set and client–nurse activities have taken place
3. Comparing the evidence collected to the criteria and base-line data (if available); then making judgments about the nature of the behavioral change (such as direction, stability, achievement)

Step 1 has been briefly discussed in relation to the planning phase of the process. In addition to stating the desired behavior change, it is also important for the nurse to decide how the change will be measured and when it will be measured.

Step 2 involves the collection of evidence (data). Although data are collected in both assessment and evaluation, the data collection during evaluation is used differently from data collected during assessment. In assessment, data are collected for the purpose of making a nursing diagnosis. In evaluation, data are collected as evidence to determine whether the goals and objectives were met. This is an important difference to note in using the nursing process.

Step 3 in evaluation is the one that often is the most difficult because it is easy to use different measurements in making judgments. For example, if a nurse observed that a client "ate well," would this mean the same thing to the client or to another nurse? "Ate well" could be interpreted that the client was able to chew, swallow, and digest the food with no difficulty, or it could refer to the amount and kind of food consumed. Therefore, in evaluation it is not only important to determine the criteria (objectives) but also to determine the exact way(s) in which evidence will be gathered and interpreted to ascertain whether the criteria were met.

In the third step, base-line data refer to information that should be collected in the assessment of the client. To observe a change and to measure a change, the nurse must know the current status of the client or the base from which the change will take place. An example of base-line data could be the weight of the client on initial contact.

In the situation regarding Mrs. James, objectives can be mutually set in measurable terms. Using Little and Carnevali's Step 1, it would be possible to select criteria for measuring the first objective (identify the basic four food groups from a chart). The criteria set could include eighteen out of twenty foods correctly identified. If at the end of Week 1, Mrs. James could identify nineteen foods correctly by food groups, then objective 1 would be evaluated as "accomplished." Specific evidence could then be collected (Step 2) and compared to the criteria (Step 3). Base-line data could be obtained so that change in knowledge about food groups could be measured.

Under objective 2 (prepare a shopping list to include at least two foods from each group by the end of Week 1), the criteria established could be:

1. The shopping list will include all foods essential for preparing three meals per day for seven days.
2. Two foods from each food group would be included on the shopping list.

In looking at the shopping list, the nurse may discover that no red meats were included, therefore creating a limited use of one food group. (Mrs. James revealed that her husband did not believe in eating red meat.) This information would then be included as reassessment data, and the nurse would collect information about foods containing protein that the family could eat. By evaluating the family eating patterns (objective 5), the nurse would have information to enable him or her to help Mrs. James in choosing high protein foods, thereby meeting objective 2.

When objectives have not been met, reassessment should occur, and the process will begin again. If the evaluation shows that the nurse–client objectives have been met, the nursing process is complete at that particular point in time.

Evaluation that is based on behavioral changes is called *outcome evaluation*. There are two other types of evaluation that may also be considered: (1) structure and (2) process. *Structure evaluation* relates to such things as appropriate equipment to assess the client or carry out the plan. For example, if the scales were inaccurate, then correct base-line data could not be obtained. Structure evaluation may also relate to the organization within which the nurse works. If the nurse is unable to carry out the nursing process appropriately due to agency time limitation, this must be considered as part of the evaluation.

Process evaluation, which focuses on the activities of the nurse, can be done during each phase of the nursing process, or it may be carried out at the end of the process. The following are examples of process evaluation questions that could be used in evaluating each phase of the process:

Assessment:

1. Were historical data that might be related to health problems collected?
2. Was a physical examination carried out and the results recorded?
3. Was the analysis logical? Did it make use of data collected? Were significant findings mentioned in the analysis?

Diagnosis:

1. Was the diagnosis based on the analysis?
2. Is the diagnosis a logical conclusion from the data collected?

Planning:

1. Are goals and objectives stated?
2. Does the plan rationally follow from the diagnosis?
3. Were goals and objectives mutually established with the client?

Implementation:

1. What activities did the nurse carry out?
2. What activities did the client carry out?
3. Were the activities consistent with the objectives?

Evaluation:

1. Were the goals and objectives accomplished?
2. What evaluation methods were used?

The nurse and the client are responsible for carrying out outcome evaluation. Structure and process evaluations are typically carried out by the nurse, others in nursing administration, or both within an agency.

SUMMARY

In summary, the nursing process is the "tool" or methodology of professional nursing that helps nurses arrive at decisions and helps them predict and evaluate consequences. To use the nursing process successfully, a nurse needs to apply concepts and theories from nursing: from biological, physical, and behavioral sciences; and from the humanities, in order to provide a rationale for decision making, judgments, interpersonal relationships, and actions. The five components considered necessary to the nursing process are: assessment, nursing diagnosis, planning, implementation, and evaluation.

It is expected that students learning about the use of the nursing process will need to use many references and resources to augment their knowledge and skills as they proceed through their nursing program.

REFERENCES

1.(a) Yura, H. & Walsh, M.B. *The Nursing Process: Assessing, Planning, Implementing, Evaluating* (2nd ed.), New York: Appleton-Century-Crofts, 1973, p. 69.
1.(b) Griffith, J.W. & Christensen, P.J. *Nursing Process—Application of Theories, Frameworks, and Models,* St. Louis, Mo: C. V. Mosby, 1982, p. 4.
2.   Blum, H.L. *Planning for Health* (2nd ed.), New York: Human Sciences, 1981, pp. 54–55.

28 NURSING THEORIES: THE BASE FOR PROFESSIONAL NURSING PRACTICE

3.   Griffith & Christensen, *Nursing Process*, p. 3.

4.(a) Yura, H. & Walsh, M.B. *The Nursing Process: Assessing, Planning, Implementing, Evaluating* (2nd ed.), New York: Appleton-Century-Crofts, 1973, p. 69.

4.(b) Bower, F.L. *The Process of Planning Nursing Care—A Model for Practice*, St. Louis, Mo.: C. V. Mosby, 1977, p. 11.

4.(c) Mitchell, P.H. *Concepts Basic to Nursing*, New York: McGraw-Hill, 1973, p. 71.

4.(d) Marriner, A. *The Nursing Process: A Scientific Approach to Nursing Care*, St. Louis, Mo.: C. V. Mosby, 1975, p. 1.

5.   Bower, *The Process of Planning*, pp. 10–11.

6.(a) Walter, J.B., Pardee, G.P., & Malbo, D.M. *Dynamics of Problem-Oriented Approaches: Patient Care and Documentation*, Philadelphia: Lippincott, 1976, pp. 32–39.

6.(b) Bower, *The Process of Planning*, pp. 11–13, 48–70.

6.(c) Zimmerman, D.S. & Gohrke, C. The Goal-Directed Nursing Approach: It Does Work. *The Nursing Process: A Scientific Approach*, Ann Marriner, compiler, St. Louis, Mo.: C. V. Mosby, 1975, p. 150.

6.(d) Lewis, L. *Planning Patient Care*, Dubuque, Iowa: Brown Publishers, 1976, Chapter 3.

7.   Congress for Nursing Practice, *Standards for Nursing Practice*, Kansas City, Mo.: American Nurses' Association, 1973.

8.   Mahoney, E.A., Verdisco, L., & Shortridge, L. *How to Collect and Record a Health History*, Philadelphia: Lippincott, 1976, pp. 9–52.

9.   Ibid, 5.

10. Little, D. & Carnevali, D. *Nursing Care Planning* (2nd ed.), Philadelphia: Lippicott, 1976, p. 12.

11. Maslow, A. *Motivation and Personality*, New York: Harper & Row, Publishers, Inc., 1954.

12. Erikson, E.H. *Childhood and Society*, New York: W. W. Norton & Co., Inc., 1963, pp. 247–74.

13. American Nurses' Association. *Nursing: A Social Policy Statement*, Kansas City, Mo.: American Nurses' Association, 1980, p. 3.

14.(a) Gebbie, K.M., ed. *Summary of the Second National Conference: Classification of Nursing Diagnoses*, St. Louis, Mo.: Clearinghouse, 1976.

14.(b) Gebbie, K.M. & Lavin, M.A. *Classification of Nursing Diagnoses*, St. Louis, Mo.: C. V. Mosby, 1975.

14.(c) Gordon, M. *Manual of Nursing Diagnosis*, New York: McGraw-Hill, 1982.

14.(d) Gordon, M. *Nursing Diagnosis: Process and Application*, New York: McGraw-Hill, 1982;

14.(e) Kim, M.J. & Moritz, D.A., eds. *Classification of Nursing Diagnoses*, New York: McGraw-Hill, 1982.

14.(f) Campbell, C. *Nursing Diagnosis and Intervention in Nursing Practice*, New York: Wiley, 1980.

15. Campbell, *Nursing Diagnosis*, p. 849.

16. Ibid, 829.

17. Torres, G., & Stanton, M. *Curriculum Process in Nursing: A Guide to Curriculum Development*, Englewood Cliffs, N.J.: Prentice-Hall, 1982, pp. 128–29.

18. Mager, R. *Preparing Instructional Objectives*, Palo Alto, Calif.: Fearon Publishers, Inc., 1962, p. 12.

19. Ibid, 11.
20. Congress for Nursing Practice, *Standards of Nursing Practice*, Kansas City, Mo., 1973.
21. *The Random House Dictionary of the English Language*, New York; Random House, 1966.
22. Yura & Walsh, *The Nursing Process*, p. 108.
23. Campbell, *Nursing Diagnosis*, pp. 21–22.
24. Smuts, J.C. *Toward a Better World*, New York: World Book Company, distributed by Duell, Sloan and Pearce, 1944, pp. 123–33.
25. Byrne, M.L. & Thompson, L.F. *Key Concepts for the Study and Practice of Nursing*, St. Louis, Mo.: C. V. Mosby, 1972, pp. 67–75.
26. Ibid, Chapter 6.
27. Little & Carnevali, *Nursing Care Planning*, p. 230.

CHAPTER 3

Florence Nightingale

Gertrude Torres

Florence Nightingale (1820–1910) was born to English parents while they were on a trip to Florence, Italy. Her greatest achievement was the establishment of the concept of formal preparation for the practice of nursing; thus, the profession of nursing started with her commitment to the care of the sick.

Miss Nightingale's fame spread rapidly after she and a group of devoted women cared for the sick during the Crimean War. She was a proficient bedside nurse with a great concern for the soldiers. An account of her nightly rounds with her lamp ("The Lady with the Lamp") was given special attention by Henry Wadsworth Longfellow.

Organized nursing began in the mid-1800s with the leadership of Florence Nightingale. Before her era, nursing care was done by paupers and drunkards, persons unfit for any other type of work. Hospitals were placed where the poor frequently suffered more from the environment than from the disease that brought them there. Surgery without anesthesia, little or no sanitation, and filth within hospitals were prevalent everywhere.

Nightingale's beliefs about nursing form the basic foundation on which nursing care is practiced today. Her religious convictions and military nursing experience during the Crimean War had a strong influence on her approach and beliefs about the care of the sick. Her writing ability, which is well demonstrated in her *Notes on Nursing*,[1] can be attributed to her education, which was achieved mainly through her father's tutoring. She traveled extensively and had the ability to deal in government and politics. Many have called her a genius. Thus, in understanding her theoretical approach to professional nursing, the reader needs to keep in mind her unique characteristics in relation to the place of a woman of the mid-nineteenth century.

Nightingale did not specifically approach her writings in the context of today's terminology, that of concepts and theories. Yet these writings about nursing care can be interpreted to reflect the present emphasis on a theoretical approach to the nursing process. There may be the temptation to see her ideas as "old-fashioned" or "out-of-date." This must be avoided since many of her sound ideas about nursing are still not being universally carried out in contemporary practice.

NIGHTINGALE'S ENVIRONMENTAL THEORY OF NURSING

The core concept that is most reflective of Nightingale's writings is that of environment. Although she tends to emphasize the physical more than the psychological or social environment, this needs to be viewed in the context of her time and her activities as a nurse leader in a war-torn environment. It is understandable that she, having witnessed in the early 1850s the filth, vermin, and death within an enormous barracks hospital, would focus so heavily on improving the environment to assist soldiers to merely survive. Through such an emphasis, the death rate went from a staggering 42 per 100 to a low of 22 per 1000. This success gave her a strong data base on which to view nursing in her own unique way.

The environment is viewed as all the external conditions and influences affecting the life and development of an organism and capable of preventing, suppressing, or contributing to disease or death.[2] Nightingale's writing speaks of providing such things as ventilation, clean air and water, cleanliness, and warmth, so the reparative process that nature has instituted will not be hindered. Assisting patients toward the retention of their vital powers by meeting their needs is viewed as a goal of nursing. The flavor of her beliefs is expressed when she speaks of the environmental elements that disturb health, such as dirt, dampness, chills, drafts, smells, and darkness.[3]

Medical practice is not viewed as a curative process but as having the function of assisting nature. Thus, nursing is also a noncurative practice in which the patient is put in the best condition for nature to act. This condition was seen by her as enhanced by providing an environment conducive to health promotion.

At this point, it is helpful to think of a patient who has had surgery, such as an appendectomy, and relate what Nightingale proposes. Medicine is seen as functioning to remove the diseased part, whereas nursing places the patient in an environment in which nature can assist postoperative patients to reach their optimum health condition. This approach to nursing is as valid today as it was over one hundred years ago, in spite of the fact that both in homes and in hospitals the environment today is more sophisticated in structure. This should be kept in mind as the theory is viewed in more detail. Much of Nightingale's theory is noted in her writing, *Notes on Nursing*.[3]

Table 3–1 demonstrates her major areas of environmental control: ventilation, warmth, effluvia, noise, and light. Keep in mind that it is the interrelationship of this concept of a healthy environment with the practice of nursing, as seen by Florence Nightingale, that offers us a basic theory of nursing practice.

Ventilation, especially with increased fresh air, provided without drafts, is of primary importance. *Light* refers to sunlight for the most part, and is secondary. *Warmth, noise,* and *effluvia* (smells) are seen as areas in which attention must be given in order to provide a positive environment.

TABLE 3-1. NIGHTINGALE'S ENVIRONMENTAL CONCEPTS

Major Areas of Concentration	Examples
Ventilation	Fresh air, which is of primary importance, can be achieved through open windows. Corrupt, stagnant, and musty air breeds disease. An outlet is needed for impure air. Drafts caused by open windows and doors are to be avoided. Dirty carpets and furniture are a source of impurity in the air.
Warmth	Guarding against the loss of vital heat is essential to the patient's recovery. Chilling is to be avoided. Hot bottles, bricks, and drinks should be used to restore lost heat.
Effluvia (smells)	Sewer air is to be avoided, and care is needed to get rid of noxious body odor caused by disease. Chamber utensils should be odor-free and out of sight. Fumigations and disinfectants should not be used but the offensive substance removed.
Noise	Intermittent sudden noise causes greater excitement than continuous noise, especially during the patient's first sleep. The more the patient sleeps peacefully, the greater his or her ability to sleep will be. Walking lightly, whispering, or discussing a patient's condition just ouside his or her room is cruel.
Light	Second only to the need for fresh air is the value of light. Beds should be placed in such a position as to allow the patient to see out the window—the sky and sunlight.

In using this basic concept—the environment—within the nursing process, it becomes evident that the practitioner must view the patient in a particular context. For example, review the following situation:

Situation 1. Mrs. Anderson, a public health nurse, has just visited Mrs. Rose, an eighty-year-old arthritic patient who lives alone in a rural community. Since Mrs. Rose has difficulty ambulating, her neighbors visit her often to assist her in any way they can. One of these neighbors requested that Mrs. Anderson visit to assess the situation.

On entering Mrs. Rose's home, Mrs. Anderson was made aware of the lack of fresh air, the darkness of the environment caused by old dusty drapes covering the windows, and a draft in the bedroom. Mrs. Rose was found sitting in an old chair that provided little or no view of the world around her.

After her visit, Mrs. Anderson contacted Mrs. Rose's neighbors to set up a plan to improve her environment. The drapes were to be removed and replaced with simple curtains that would let the morning sun enter the room. The windows were to be opened in keeping with the weather during specific periods of the day, with care given to reduce drafts. Mrs. Rose's favorite chair was to be placed in such a way that she could look out the window to watch the neighbors coming and going.

This example is not to be viewed as offering a complete assessment of Mrs. Rose, but to point out how Nightingale's basic environmental concept, interrelated with the nursing process, can give us specific directions.

To Nightingale the environment of the patient was quite encompassing. Although she did not specifically distinguish among the physical, social, or psychological environments as such, she speaks of all three in the practice of nursing.

Admittedly, emphasis is placed on the physical environment of the patient. In the context of her time, this was essential if lives were to be saved and nursing was to take its proper place as a profession. When an optimum physical environment exists, greater attention can be given to the emotional needs of the patient as well as to the prevention of disease.

Figure 3–1 offers a view of the theory created by Nightingale. The key point is diagrammed in the center of the triangle—patient condition and nature. Here the thrust of environment is on the patient and nature func-

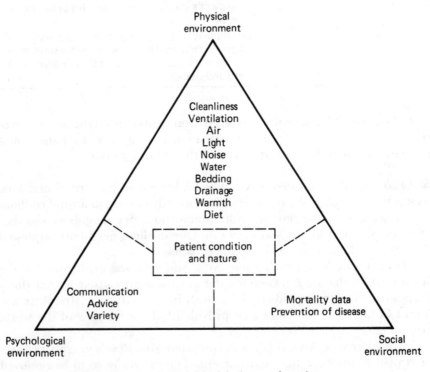

Figure 3–1. Nightingale's theory of nursing.

tioning together to allow the reparative process to occur. The three components—physical, social, and psychological—need to be viewed as interrelating rather than as separate distinct parts. The cleanliness of the physical environment has a direct bearing on the prevention of disease and mortality rates within the social environment of the community. (Also, all patients' psychological environments are strongly affected by physical surroundings.)

Physical Environment

As noted in Table 3–1, the basic environmental components are physical in nature and relate to such things as ventilation and warmth. These basic factors affect one's approach to all other aspects of the environment. Cleanliness is an encompassing notion related to all aspects of the physical environment in which the patient is found. The walls and entire room should not be dusty, smoky, or have a close odor.

A patient's bed must be clean, aired, warm, dry, and free from odor. One should provide an environment in which the patient can be easily cared for by others or self. The width, height, and placement of the bed should facilitate the activities of the patient. The bed should be placed in the best lighted spot, away from sudden noises and the odor of drainage. The position of the patient on the bed should be viewed in the context of supporting ventilation.

Psychological Environment

The effect of the mind on the body was fairly well accepted in Nightingale's time. However, there was a lack of understanding of exactly how the condition of the body as affected by the environment could affect the mind. Nightingale did recognize that a negative environment could cause physical stress, thereby affecting the patient's emotional climate. Therefore emphasis is placed on offering the patient a variety of activities to keep his or her mind stimulated. The view of the sunlight, the attractiveness of the food, and the offering of manual activities that stimulate the need to labor are all factors that assist the patient to survive emotionally. Boredom is viewed as painful.

Communication with the patient is viewed in the context of the total environment. Communication should not be hurried or allow for interruptions. When speaking with patients, it is important to sit down in front of them, unless other activities such as eating are occurring. The place one communicates with the physician and family about the patient is in the context of the environment of the patient. Outside the patients' rooms or within their hearing distance is viewed as inappropriate.

One should not encourage the sick by false hopes and advice about their illness. Rather the emphasis here is on communicating about the world around them that they miss, or about good news that visitors can share. Again, patients are viewed in the context of their total environment.

Social Environment

Observation of the social environment, especially as related to specific data collections relating to illness, is essential to preventing disease. Thus, each nurse must use observational powers in dealing with specific cases rather than be comfortable with data addressing the "average" patient.

Closely related to the community–social environment are those notions already discussed in relation to the individual patient—that is, physical environment such as clean air and water and proper drainage or sewage. The patient's *total* environment not only includes the patient's home or hospital room but the total community influencing that specific environment.

NIGHTINGALE'S THEORY AND THE FOUR MAJOR CONCEPTS

In reviewing how Nightingale relates her theory to the four major concepts, it becomes evident once again that the environment is the main focus of her theory. Figure 3–2 identifies the four major concepts as they are related in Nightingale's Theory. The *environment* affects the *human* condition, with *nursing* having the role of affecting that environment, so that *health/disease* becomes a reparative process.

Each of the major concepts impacts on the others. *Nursing* functions to influence the human environment to affect health. The *individual* is affected by the environment and by the nurse who influences his or her health. *Society/environment* has an impact on the nurse and on the health of the individual. *Health* is a process affected by nursing and by environmental and human conditions. These relationships give meaning to the theory by providing a view of the world in which we nurse.

The following list reflects Nightingale's view of the major concepts:

- *Human or Individual*—Has vital reparative powers to deal with disease.
- *Nursing*—The goal is to place the individual in the best condition for nature to act by basically affecting the environment.
- *Health/Disease*—The focus is on the reparative process of getting well.
- *Society/Environment*—Involves those external conditions that affect life and the development of the individual. The focus is on ventilation, warmth, odors, noises, and light.

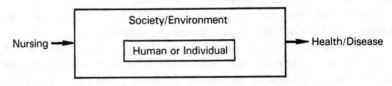

Figure 3–2. Nightingale's theory and the four major concepts.

Basically, these concepts are implicit rather than explicit, and thus they may be misunderstood and misinterpreted by those attempting to use the theory. The concept that is most clearly defined is the *society/environment*. Yet it is unclear how extensively or globally Nightingale viewed the environment. Other theories that will be discussed later within this book view the environment from a broad universal standpoint. Nightingale probably focused on the immediate environment in which humans find themselves. Today's view of clean air and water with our concern over environmental pollution is quite different than that held during the nineteenth century. Thus, although Nightingale's main focus is on the environment, she defines that concept in the context of her time only.

It is difficult to understand what the concept of *human/individual* really means to Nightingale. She is descriptive of humans only in terms of their healing process. However, one can draw certain assumptions that are basic to her theory such as humans need clean air, clean water, and proper nutrition. Thus, it is safe to describe individuals as responsive to the environment and having a healing power within themselves.

The concept of *health* is probably the most poorly defined. A view of health as the lack of disease offers us little understanding of what health really encompasses for Nightingale. One might assume that a healthy person is merely an individual who lacks a disease.

Nursing is described in relation to the other three concepts. Nightingale was the first to give clarity to the purpose of nursing. Thus, any description or explanation of this concept needs to be reviewed as an initial attempt to explain a professional role. By today's standards she gives a limited but rather clear picture of the meaning of nursing as a noncurative practice in which the patient is put in the best position for nature to act.

NIGHTINGALE'S THEORY AND THE NURSING PROCESS

In general, although Nightingale's theory has only rather vaguely defined concepts, it offers a lot in terms of guiding practice and research in its generalizability and simplicity. An example of application to practice follows.

Situation II. Mrs. Kerr is a seventy-year-old resident who lives in an old local nursing home. She is rarely visited by her only living relative, a brother who is several years older. Several years ago, she became partially immobile on her right side and continues to have difficulty walking around the home. When reminded, she is able to go to the dining room for meals but eats very little. Her environment consists of a two-bed room, which she shares with an eighty-year-old woman who is unaware of her surroundings. On admission, Mrs. Kerr was not able to bring any of her own belongings except for a few clothes. When communicating with her, she remembers the "old" days when she taught at the local elementary school. She seldom initiates a conversation and spends most of her time sitting in a chair in the lounge, apparently watching television.

The above situation is quite typical of a resident within today's nursing homes. In using the nursing process with a focus on Nightingale's theory, it is essential to focus on Mrs. Kerr's environment and her reactions to it, rather than specifically on her as a resident. Table 3–2 reflects the use of the Nightingale theory.

The major emphasis in this situation is to restructure the immediate environment around Mrs. Kerr so that nature can act to maintain her optimum condition. With additional reassessment and evaluation, much can be done to prolong a healthy life and promote total comfort. It is possible, after such assessment, that the environment of the nursing home may be destructive to Mrs. Kerr's health. Alternatives may need to be sought. By the application of adaptation, need, and stress theories to this

TABLE 3–2. NIGHTINGALE'S THEORY APPLIED TO THE NURSING PROCESS

Nursing Process Phases	Case Example of Mrs. Kerr
Assessment— Data collection	Seventy-year-old woman who has partial paralysis of her right side. Can move about the environment. The home offers some alternatives to the resident's surroundings—a dining room, bedroom, and television lounge. Visitors from the outside are allowed. Residents are not encouraged to bring meaningful things with them to the home. The only sensory stimulation is one television set. During periods of eating, food intake is poor.
Analysis of data	Basically, there is a lack of specific data, especially relating to the total environment of the nursing home. Thus, an analysis at this time must be viewed as tentative in nature until a reassessment can be done.
Data gaps	Inadequate information on the following: adequacy of ventilation, presence of drafts, sudden noises, cleanliness of surroundings, variety of dietary offerings, opportunities to communicate with others, variety of stimulus provided, specific physical limitations, previous nursing observation, odors present throughout the home, method of disposal of human wastes, amount of sunlight and artificial light.
Nursing diagnosis	Nonstimulating environment.
Implementation	Increase communication. Provide for an optimum environment that will facilitate health. Increase stimulus through a greater exposure to sunlight and fresh air. Place Mrs. Kerr in a room that will increase the amount of interaction she has with others.
Evaluation	Observe effect of a changing environment on her health state.

situation, in terms of the environment, the base for the practice of nursing becomes more theoretically sound.

Some of the questions that might be used to guide the practitioner in implementing Nightingale's theory in situations like Mrs. Kerr's are:

1. Is the environment the most crucial factor in the effective care of Mrs. Kerr?
2. What adaptations can be made within such environments that will facilitate optimum nursing care?
3. Do adjustments within the environment lead patients to a more optimum state of health and prolong their life?
4. Does the amount of stress within such environments affect both the residents and the nurse?
5. What hierarchy of needs is met in such an environment?

As an approach to the practice of nursing, Nightingale's theory is as valid today as it was over one hundred years ago. Within the hospital environment, much can be done to reduce stress, improve adaptation, and meet patient needs through minor adjustments that can be made by the professional nurse. Some examples are the following: the placement of a patient's bed within the room to provide a view of the outside world or sunlight; the encouraging and educating of visitors to provide a greater amount of variety or stimulation within the environment; the less frequent, sudden awakening of patients; and the provision for a quiet, unhurried atmosphere. Although today's hospitals have clean air through the air conditioning, and clean water through more sophisticated plumbing systems, they still have drafty, odorous environments created by the lack of attention to such details.

Much of Nightingale's theory might be viewed as involving basic common sense, such as giving attention to the cleanliness of a patient's surroundings, keeping chills away, and providing adequate lighting to read. Yet such things are frequently taken for granted and are often forgotten.

NIGHTINGALE'S WORK AND THE CHARACTERISTICS OF A THEORY

Nightingale's theory of nursing has its strengths and weaknesses in relation to the characteristics of a sound theory presented in Chapter 1, as noted below.

1. Theories can interrelate concepts in such a way as to create a different way of looking at a particular phenomenon. As mentioned earlier, the four major concepts are not explicit in Nightingale's theory, and yet they do offer nursing a specific way of looking at a particular phenomenon. This is evident in the two examples described in this chapter. Viewed very simply, the theory does offer a prediction in relation to the outcomes of nursing care. Creating a positive environment will allow humans to become healthy. Yet we know today that, although the human environment is critical in relation to health, other variables such as genetics are also very significant.

2. Theories must be logical in nature. The relationship between each of the concepts is logical and consistent with similar assumptions. The assumption that the environment affects humans is consistent with Nightingale's explanation of the purpose and goal of nursing and the meaning of health.

3. Theories should be relatively simple yet generalizable. Nightingale's theory, although limited, has a lot of generalizability. It can be used in any environment such as hospitals, nursing homes, schools, the individual's home, or wherever human beings may be found. The ideas are also basically simple to apply and easy to measure in terms of outcomes.

4. Theories can be the bases for hypotheses that can be tested.

5. Theories contribute to and assist in increasing the general body of knowledge within the discipline through the research implemented to validate them.

6. Theories can be used by the practitioners to guide and improve their practice.

7. Theories must be consistent with other validated theories, laws, and principles but will leave open unanswered questions that need to be investigated.

Due to their similarity, these last four characteristics will be discussed together as they relate to Nightingale's theory. In spite of the simplicity and generalizability of her theory, nursing has not yet adequately incorporated much of it into practice or research. For example, in a way, her theory has been researched by scientists such as environmentalists. That is, we are increasingly becoming aware of how environmental pollution affects our health in a negative way. From a broad perspective, this should give Nightingale's theory validity. However, we have not yet adequately validated the theory within the context of the health care and nursing enviroment. Research questions that can lead to hypotheses need to be tested within clinical nursing. For instance, What effect does the hospital environment have on the pace of the healing process? Does the nurse have the authority to impact on the patient's environment adequately? Do sudden, frequent environmental changes affect patients' perceptions of their reparative process? These are only a few of the many possible questions that can be used to guide research. The answers to these questions could well be used to develop guidelines for nursing education and practice.

NIGHTINGALE'S THEORY OF NURSING AS RELATED TO SCIENTIFIC THEORIES

Nightingale's theory of nursing is closely related to scientific theories frequently used in nursing practice today. Most significant are the theories of adaptation, need, and stress.

Adaptation Theory

Adaptation reflects man's adjustments to forces that confront him. Such forces are viewed in the context of the total environment in which man finds himself. The success or nonsuccess of the adpatative responses of man can be seen by reviewing the environmental forces described by Nightingale. Man's ability to allow nature to act on his behalf as influenced by his environment may lead to either adaptive or maladaptive response. For example, a patient who finds himself or herself in a cold, dusty, poorly ventilated environment will have to use much of his or her available energy for adapting to his or her environment rather than for recovering from his or her illness.

To put this in the context of the present, one should note that during the Vietnam War, injured soldiers were quickly airlifted to casualty stations in which they were treated before being sent to nearby hospitals for more complete care. In comparison to previous treatment of the injured, this led to a much lower death rate. Admittedly, this closely relates to improved medical care, but it should also be noted that removing the injured from a poor environment as soon as possible allowed nature to act on the patient's behalf—the Nightingale theory.

Need Theory

Need theories, especially Maslow's,[4] basically recognize theories given emphasis by Nightingale: for example, the need for oxygenation viewed in the context of fresh air, ventilation, and the need for a safe environment as related to proper drainage and clean water. Need theories stress the ability of humans to survive in the context of how well these needs are met. An environment that strongly supports basic human physiological needs is essential. Maslow's emphasis on a hierarchical order of needs places physiological needs as primary, whereas emotional and social needs have less significance for survival.[4] Again, Nightingale's emphasis on the physical environment that affects the physiological functioning of humans supports Maslow's theory.

Need theories frequently emphasize providing novelty and activities and encouraging exploration of the environment. Nightingale advised against having the patient suffer boredom from staring at four blank walls all day long. Today the literature speaks of sensory deprivation—demonstrated by boredom, daydreaming, and a lack of concentration.

Stress Theory

Stress involves a threat or a change in the environment in which an individual must cope. Stress can be positive or negative depending on its end result. Stress can encourage a person to take positive action toward a desired goal or need, or it can cause exhaustion if the stress is so intense that the individual is unable to cope. Nightingale emphasized placing the patient in an optimum environment so that there would be a minimum of outside stressors. For example, slow quiet movements, whispering, or sudden noises were viewed as causing stress, whereas purposeful quick actions were seen as more appropriate. However, suddenly waking the patient causes great excitement and can be viewed as a negative stressor.

The number and duration of stressors also have a strong influence on the individual's ability to cope. In reviewing the major components of Nightingale's theory, the greater the degree of poor air, poor water, poor light, and other negative environmental factors, and the longer the duration, the lesser the potential for the patient to cope with his or her illness. As a matter of fact, given a healthy individual within a poor environment with multiple stressors of long duration, illness would soon occur.

SUMMARY

Nightingale's major focus was on the environment of the patient. Nursing was viewed as distinct from medicine and focused on providing an environment that allowed nature to act on behalf of the patient. Environmental factors involved clean air and water, control of noise, proper drainage, reduction of chills, and a variety of activities. Nightingale emphasized fresh air as primary and good lighting as secondary to the effective care of the patient. Other theories most closely related to her writings are adaptation, need, and stress. In utilizing her theory within the nursing process, the focus is on how the environment affects the patient. Implementation involves adjustments to inadequate environments. Nightingale's theory is as appropriate today as a theoretical base for practice as it was during her time of practice in the mid-1800s. It is the foundation on which all other theories in nursing should be viewed.

REFERENCES

1. Nightingale, F. *Notes on Nursing*, New York: Dover Publications, Inc., 1969.
2. Murray, R. & Zentner, J. *Nursing Concepts for Health Promotion*, Englewood Cliffs, N.J.: Prentice-Hall, 1975, p. 149.
3. Nightingale, *Notes on Nursing*.
4. Maslow, A. *Motivation and Personality*, New York: Harper & Row, Pub., 1954.

BIBLIOGRAPHY

Auld, M.E., and Birum, L.H. *The Challenge of Nursing: A Book of Readings*, St. Louis, Mo.: C. V. Mosby, 1973.
Byrne, M.L., and Thompson, L.F. *Key Concepts for the Study and Practice of Nursing*, St. Louis, Mo.: C. V. Mosby, 1972.

CHAPTER 4

Hildegard E. Peplau

Janice Ryan Belcher
Lois J. Brittain Fish

Hildegard Peplau (b. 1909) was born in Reading, Pennsylvania. Dr. Peplau graduated from a diploma program in nursing in Pottstown, Pennsylvania, in 1931. She graduated from Bennington College with a BA in Interpersonal Psychology in 1943, and from Columbia University in New York with a MA in Psychiatric Nursing in 1947, and an EdD in Curriculum Development in 1953. Dr. Peplau's nursing experience includes private and general duty hospital nursing, two years in the U.S. Army, nursing research, and part-time private practice in psychiatric nursing. She has taught graduate psychiatric nursing for many years and is a Professor Emeritus from Rutgers University. The first postbaccalaureate nursing program in central Europe was facilitated by Dr. Peplau in Belgium.

Hildegard Peplau published the book Interpersonal Relations in Nursing *in 1952.[1] She has also published numerous articles in professional magazines on topics ranging from interpersonal concepts to current issues in nursing. Her pamphlet "Basic Principles of Patient Counseling" was derived from her research and workshops.[2a,2b]*

Dr. Peplau has served with many organizations, including the World Health Organization, the National Institute of Mental Health, and the Nurse Corps. She is past Executive Director and past President of the American Nurses' Association and a Fellow of the American Academy of Nursing. She has served as a nursing consultant to various foreign countries and to the Surgeon General of the Air Force. Dr Peplau "retired" in 1974 and remains active in nursing. Her 1952 book was reissued in 1988 (personal communication, November 4, 1987). Her many contributions to nursing are the result of her pioneer qualities in communicating her perceptions concerning nursing.

Hildegard Peplau published *Interpersonal Relations in Nursing,* referring to her book as a "partial theory for the practice of nursing."[3] In this source, Peplau discussed the phases of the interpersonal process, roles in nursing situations, and methods for studying nursing as an interpersonal process. This chapter defines the crux of her nursing theory to be the phases of the interpersonal process and relates the other ideas to this central core.

According to Peplau, nursing is therapeutic in that it is a healing art, assisting an individual who is sick or in need of health care. Nursing can be viewed as an interpersonal process because it involves interaction between two or more individuals with a common goal. In nursing, this common goal provides the incentive for the therapeutic process in which the nurse and patient* respect each other as individuals, both of them learning and growing as a result of the interaction. Learning takes place when an individual selects stimuli in an environment and develops more fully as a result of reactions to these stimuli.[4]

The attainment of this goal, or any goal, is achieved through the use of a series of steps following a certain pattern. As the relationship of the nurse to patient develops in this therapeutic pattern, there is flexibility in the way in which the nurse functions in practice—by making judgments, by using skills founded in scientific knowledge, by using technical abilities, and by assuming roles.

When the nurse and patient first identify a problem and begin to focus on a course of action, they approach this path from diverse backgrounds and individual uniqueness. Each individual may be viewed as a unique biological–psychological–spiritual–sociological structure, one that will not react the same as any other. Each individual has learned differently from the distinct environment, mores, customs, and beliefs of that individual's given culture. Each person comes with preconceived ideas that influence perceptions, and it is these differences in perception that are so important in the interpersonal process. In addition, the nurse, from an educational background, contributes an understanding of developmental theories, of concepts of life's adaptations, and of conflict responses, as well as a greater insight of nursing's professional role in the interpersonal process. As nurse and patient continue the relationship, an understanding of one another's roles and the factors surrounding the problem increases until both nurse and patient are mutually sharing in a collaborative manner toward resolution of the problem.

The nurse and the patient work together, and as a result both become more knowledgeable and mature in the process. Peplau views nursing as a "maturing force and an educative instrument."[5] She believes nursing is a learning experience of oneself as well as of the other individual involved in the interpersonal action. This concept is supported by Genevieve Burton, another nursing author from the 1950s, who states, "Behavior of others must be understood in light of self understanding."[6] Thus persons who are more in touch with themselves will be more aware of the various types of reactions induced in another individual.

As the nurse guides the patient toward the solutions of the everyday encounters, the methods and principles used in the professional practice become increasingly more effective. Each encounter influences the nurse's personal and professional development. Thus, the kind of person the

---

* *Patient* will be used throughout this chapter since it is Peplau's definition of the individual who is in need of health care.

nurse becomes has a direct influence on the therapeutic, interpersonal relationship.

Peplau identifies four sequential phases in interpersonal relationships: (1) *orientation,* (2) *identification,* (3) *exploitation,* and (4) *resolution.* Each of these phases overlaps and interrelates as the process evolves toward a solution. Different nursing roles are assumed during the various phases.

These roles can be broadly described in the following manner:

Teacher	One who imparts knowledge in reference to a need or interest
Resource	One who provides specific, needed information that aids in the understanding of a problem or new situation
Counselor	One who, through the use of certain skills and attitudes, aids another in recognizing, facing, accepting, and resolving problems that are interfering with the other person's ability to live happily and effectively
Leader	One who carries out the process of initiation and maintenance of group goals through interaction
Technical expert	One who provides physical care by displaying clinical skills and has the ability to operate equipment in this care
Surrogate	One who takes the place of another

PEPLAU'S PHASES IN NURSING

Orientation

In the initial phase of *orientation,* the nurse and patient meet as two strangers. The patient and/or the family has a "felt need";[7] therefore professional assistance is sought. However, this need may not be readily identified or understood by the individuals who are involved. For example, a sixteen-year-old girl may call the community mental health center just because she feels "very down." It is in this phase that the nurse needs to assist the patient and family in realizing what is happening to the patient.

It is of the utmost importance that the nurse work collaboratively with the patient and family in analyzing the situation, so that they together can recognize, clarify, and define the existing problem. Take the previous example: The nurse, in the counselor role, helps the teen-age girl who feels "very down" to realize that these feelings are the result of an argument with her mother over last evening's date. As the nurse continues to listen, there is a pattern established of the girl arguing with her mother and feeling depressed. As these feelings are discussed, the girl recognizes the arguing as the precipitating factor that causes the depression. Thus the nurse and the patient have defined the problem. The daughter and the parents then agree to discuss the concern with the nurse. Thus by mutually clarifying and defining the problem in the orientation phase, the patient can direct the accumulated energy from the anxiety of unmet needs to more constructively dealing with the presenting problem. Rapport is established and continues to be strengthened while concerns are being identified.

While the patient and family are talking to the nurse, a mutual decision needs to be made regarding what type of professional assistance should be pursued. The nurse, as a resource person, may work with the patient and family. As an alternative the nurse might, upon mutual agreement of all parties involved, refer the family to another source such as a psychologist, psychiatrist, or social worker. In the orientation phase, the nurse, patient, and family plan what type of services are needed.

The orientation phase is directly affected by the patient's and nurse's attitudes about giving or receiving aid from a reciprocal person. Therefore, in this beginning phase, the nurse needs to be aware of her personal reactions to the patient. For example, the nurse may react differently to the forty-year-old man with abdominal pain who enters the emergency room quietly than to the forty-year-old man with a history of regular alcohol abuse who enters the emergency room boisterously after a few drinks. The nurse's, as well as the patient's, culture, religion, race, educational background, past experiences, and preconceived ideas and expectations all play a part in the nurse's reaction to the patient. The same influencing factors play a part in the patient's reaction to the nurse (see Fig. 4–1). For example, the patient may have stereotyped the nurse as performing only technical skills such as giving medications or taking blood pressures and therefore may not perceive the nurse as a resource person who can help define the

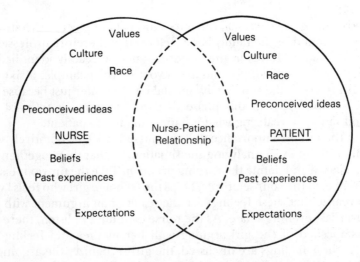

Figure 4–1. Factors influencing the blending of the nurse–patient relationship.

problem. Nursing is an interpersonal process, and both the patient and nurse have an equally important part in the therapeutic interaction.

The nurse, the patient, and the family work together to recognize, clarify, and define the existing problem. This in turn decreases the tension and anxiety associated with the felt need[8] and the fear of the unknown. Decreasing tension and anxiety prevents future problems that might arise as a result of repressing an event. Stressful situations are identified through therapeutic interaction. It is imperative that the patient recognize and begin to work through feelings connected with the events leading up to an illness.

Thus, in the beginning of the orientation phase, the nurse and the patient meet as strangers. At the end of the orientation phase, they are concurrently striving to identify the problem and are becoming more comfortable with one another. The patient is settling into the helping environment. The nurse and the patient are now ready to logically progress to the next phase.

Identification

The next phase, referred to as *identification*, is one in which the patient responds selectively to people who can meet his needs. Each patient responds differently in this phase. The patient might actively seek the nurse out or stoically wait until the nurse seeks him out. The response to the nurse is threefold: (1) participate with and be interdependent with the nurse, (2) be autonomous and independent from the nurse; or (3) be passive and dependent on the nurse.[9] An example would be that of a seventy-year-old man who wants to plan his new 1600 calorie diabetic diet. If the relationship is interdependent, the nurse and patient collaborate on the meal planning. Should the relationship be independent, the patient would plan the diet himself with minimal input from the nurse. In a dependent relationship, the nurse does the meal planning for the patient.

Throughout the identification phase, both the patient and nurse must clarify each other's perceptions and expectations.[10] Past experiences of both the patient and the nurse will have a bearing on what their expectations will be during this interpersonal process. As mentioned in the orientation phase, the initial attitudes of the patient and the nurse are important in building a working relationship for identifying the problem and deciding on appropriate assistance.

The perception and expectations of the patient and nurse in the identification phase are even more complex than in the preceding phase. The patient is now responding to the helper selectively. This requires a more intense therapeutic relationship.

To illustrate, a patient who has had a mastectomy may mention to the nurse her inability to understand the arm exercises that have been previously explained to her as an important regimen following surgery. The nurse observes the affected arm to be edematous (swollen). While the nurse is exploring possible reasons for the edema, the patient admits to not doing her arm exercises. The patient's reasoning is the result of being told by a friend that exercising after surgery delays healing. In order to facilitate the patient's understanding and subsequent resumption of the exercises, the nurse can identify professional people, such as the physical therapist, the nurse, and the physician, who will clarify the patient's misconceptions. Generally it is best if the nurse objectively discusses each person's role and the advantages and disadvantages of consulting with each of them. However, in this case, the patient may state that she does not care to discuss the exercises with the nurse or physical therapist because she perceives only the physician as having the necessary information. Thus previous perceptions of nursing and physical therapy can influence the patient's current decision on the selection of a professional person. In this situation, the nurse needs to be supportive of the patient's decision.

While working through this identification phase, the patient begins to have a feeling of belonging and a capability of dealing with the problem, which decreases her feelings of helplessness and hopelessness. This in turn creates an optimistic attitude from which inner strength ensues.

Exploitation

Following identification, the patient moves into the *exploitation* phase, in which advantage of all available services is taken. The degree to which these services are used is based on the interests and needs of the patient. The individual begins to feel an integral part of the helping environment. She or he feels as though some control over the situation is gained by extracting help from the services offered. Take the example of the woman with the edematous arm. During this phase the patient begins to absorb the information given to her for the arm exercises. She reads pamphlets and watches a film describing the exercises; she discusses questions with the nurse; and she may inquire about joining an exercise group through the physical therapy department.

During this phase some patients may make more demands than they did when they were seriously ill. They may make many minor requests or may apply other "attention-getting" techniques depending on their individual needs. These actions may often be difficult, if not impossible, for the health care provider to completely understand. The nurse must deal with the unconscious forces causing the patient's actions. The principles of interviewing techniques must be used in order to explore, understand, and adequately deal with the underlying problems. It is important that the nurse explore the possible causes for the patient's behavior. A therapeutic relationship must be maintained by conveying an attitude of acceptance, concern, and trust. The nurse must encourage the patient to recognize and explore feelings, thoughts, emotions, and behaviors by providing a nonjudgmental atmosphere and a therapeutic emotional climate.

Some patients may take an active interest in, and become involved in, self-care. Such a patient will become more self-sufficient and will demonstrate initiative by establishing appropriate behavior for goal attainment. Through self-determination, the patient progressively develops responsibility for self, belief in potentialities, and adjustment toward self-reliance and independence. These patients realistically begin to establish their own goals toward improved health status. They strive to achieve a pattern or direction to their lives and a feeling of wellness. This is accomplished by becoming productive, by trusting and depending on their own capabilities, and by becoming responsible for their own actions, thus becoming more fully themselves. As a result, as their unique personality continues to form, they develop sources of inner strength with which to face new problems or challenges.

Most patients fluctuate between dependence on others, as in the impaired health role, and the independence of functioning at an optimal health level. Using the previous example, this individual may want to actively exercise on schedule one day but will state she is too tired the next day. The nurse then needs to take the initiative to remind the patient of her scheduled exercises.

This type of intermittent behavior can be compared to the adjustment reaction of the adolescent in a dependency–independency conflict. The patient may temporarily be in a dependent role while the simultaneous need for independence exists. Various causes may trigger the onset of this psychological disequilibrium. The patient will vacillate unpredictably between the two states and will appear confused and anxious, protesting dependence while fearing independence. In caring for patients who fluctuate between dependence and independence, the nurse must deal with the particular behavior presented rather than trying to handle the composite problem of inconsistency. The nurse should provide an atmosphere that carries no threat, one in which a person can face himself or herself, recognize his or her weaknesses, use his or her strengths without imposing them on others, and accept help from others.

The nurse must also be fully aware of the various facets of communication including clarifying, listening, accepting, and interpreting. Correct use of all these factors will assist the patient to meet his or her challenges and will pave the way toward maximum wholesome adjustment. Thus the nurse aids the patient in exploiting all avenues of help, and progress is made toward the final step—the resolution phase.

Resolution

The last phase of Peplau's interpersonal process is *resolution*. The patient's needs have already been met by the collaborative efforts of the nurse and patient. The patient and nurse now need to terminate their therapeutic relationship and dissolve the links between them.

Sometimes dissolving these links is very difficult for both the patient and the nurse. Dependency needs in a therapeutic relationship often continue on psychologically after the physiological needs are met. The patient may feel that it "is just not time yet" to end the relationship. For example, the new mother has a desire to learn to take her baby's temperature. During the first home visit, the community health nurse and the new mother set their goal of having the mother take the baby's temperature correctly. After instruction and demonstration by the community health nurse on the first visit, the mother takes the temperature correctly on the second visit. Their goal is met. The relationship is ended because the mother's problem was solved. However, one week after the resolution, the mother telephones the community health nurse three times concerning minor questions on infant care. The mother at this point has not dissolved the dependency link with the community health nurse.

The final resolution may also be difficult for the nurse. In the above example, the mother may be willing to terminate the relationship, but the community health nurse may continue to visit the home to see how the baby is progressing. The nurse may be unable to become free of this bond in their relationship. In resolution, as in the other phases, anxiety and tension will increase in the patient and in the nurse if there is unsuccessful completion of the phase.

During successful resolution, the patient drifts away from identifying with the helping person, the nurse. This phase is a direct outgrowth of the successful completion of the other phases. The patient then breaks the bond with the nurse. A healthier emotional balance is demonstrated. The nurse also must establish independence from the patient. When the dissolving of the therapeutic interpersonal relationship is sequential to the previous phases, the patient and the nurse both become stronger maturing individuals. The patient's needs are met, and movement can be made toward new goals. Table 4–1 indicates the focus of each phase.

PEPLAU'S THEORY AND THE FOUR MAJOR CONCEPTS

Theories of nursing usually evolve around the four concepts of individual, health, society, and nursing. Peplau defines *man** as an organism who "strives in its own way to reduce tension generated by needs."[11] *Health* is defined as "a word symbol that implies forward movement of personality and other ongoing human processes in the direction of creative, constructive, productive, personal, and community living."[12]

Although Peplau does not directly address *society/environment*, she does encourage the nurse to consider the patient's culture and mores when the patient adjusts to the hospital's routine.[13] Currently when a nurse considers the patient's environment, she or he considers many more factors, such as cultural background and home and work environments, rather than just

* Peplau uses *man* and *he* in the generic sense.

TABLE 4–1. PHASES OF THE NURSE–PATIENT RELATIONSHIP

Phase	Focus
Orientation	Problem-defining phase
Identification	Selection of appropriate professional assistance
Exploitation	Use of professional assistance for problem-solving alternatives
Resolution	Termination of the professional relationship

considering a patient's adjustment to the hospital. Peplau's narrow perception of society/environment is a major limitation of her theory. The theory does not examine the broad environmental influences on the person but focuses more on the psychological tasks "within the person."[14] This view was timely in 1949 when the book was written. In examining the historical trend within psychiatric nursing, this view is categorized as "within the person," as contrasted to later views of "within the relationship" and "within the social system" which consider broader environmental influences on the person.[14]

Hildegard Peplau considers *nursing* a "significant, therapeutic, interpersonal process."[15] She defines it as a "human relationship between an individual who is sick, or in need of health services, and a nurse especially educated to recognize and to respond to the need for help."[16] The nurse assists the patient with this interpersonal process. Major concepts within this process are nurse, patient, therapeutic relationship, goals, human needs, anxiety, tension, and frustration.

RELATIONSHIP BETWEEN PEPLAU'S PHASES AND THE NURSING PROCESS

Peplau's continuum of the four phases of *orientation, identification, exploitation,* and *resolution* can be compared to the nursing process as discussed in Chapter 2 (see Table 4–2). The nursing process in Chapter 2 is defined as "a deliberate, intellectual activity whereby the practice of nursing is approached in an orderly, systematic manner" (see pg. 13).

There are basic similarities between the nursing process and Peplau's interpersonal phases. Both Peplau's phases and the nursing process are sequential and focus on therapeutic interactions. Both use problem-solving techniques for the nurse and patient to collaborate on, with the end purpose of meeting the patient's needs. Both go from general to specific, for example, the patient's vague feelings to specific facts concerning the vague feelings. Both include observation, communication, and recording as basic tools utilized by nursing.

There are differences, too, between Peplau's phases and the nursing process. When considering differences, it must be taken into account that

TABLE 4–2. COMPARISON OF NURSING PROCESS AND PEPLAU'S PHASES

Nursing Process	Peplau's Phases
Assessment Data collection and analysis Need not necessarily a "felt need"; may be nurse-initiated.	*Orientation* Nurse and patient come together as strangers; meeting initiated by patient who expresses a "felt need"; work together to recognize, clarify, and define facts related to need. (*Note:* Data collection is continuous.)
Nursing Diagnosis Summary statement based on analysis.	Patient clarifies "felt need."
Planning Mutually set goals.	*Identification* Interdependent goal setting. Patient has feeling of belonging and selectively responds to those who can meet needs. Patient-initiated.
Implementation Plans initiated toward achievement of mutually set goals.	*Exploitation* Patient actively seeking and drawing on knowledge and expertise of those who can help.
May be accomplished by patient, health care professional, or patient's family.	Patient-initiated.
Evaluation Based on mutually established expected end behaviors.	*Resolution* Occurs after other phases are successfully completed and have been met.
May lead to termination or initiation of new plans.	Leads to termination.

Peplau's book *Interpersonal Relations in Nursing* was published in 1952. Professional nursing today is functioning with more defined goals. Movement is away from the nurse as the physician's helper and toward the nurse as a consumer advocate. For instance, today part of the nursing process is nursing diagnosis. The American Nurses' Association, in the *Standards of Nursing Practice*, states: "Nursing diagnoses are derived from health status data."[17] Peplau, however, stated (in 1952) that the physician's primary function was "recognizing the full import of the nuclear problem and the kind of professional assistance that is needed," which results, for the physician, in "the task of evaluating and diagnosing the emergent problem."[18] This is in opposition to the present recognition of the independent nursing function.

Nursing functions, according to Peplau, include clarification of the information the physician gives the patient as well as collection of data about the patient that may point out other problem areas.[18] Today, however, with nursing's expanded roles, we have independent nurse practitioners who may or may not refer the patient to the physician, depending on the patient's need. Through expanded roles such as this, nursing is becoming more accountable and responsible, giving professional nursing greater legal independence. The nursing process provides a mode for evaluating the quality of nursing care rendered, which is the core of legal accountability.

Peplau gives the variables in nursing situations as needs, frustration, conflict, and anxiety. She further relates that these variables must be dealt with for growth to occur, as the nurse facilitates healthy development of each personality. It is readily seen that Peplau was influenced by some of the theories of the time, especially Harry S. Sullivan's interpersonal theory and Sigmund Freud's theory of psychodynamics.[19a,19b]

In nursing today, variables such as intrafamily dynamics, socioeconomic forces (e.g., financial resources), personal space considerations, and community social service resources should be taken into account for each patient. These variables provide a broader perspective for viewing nursing situations than Peplau's personal factors of needs, frustration, conflict, and anxiety. Currently, even a family, a group, or a community may be collectively defined as the patient.

Nursing has also broadened its perspective in helping the patient reach a fuller health potential through a greater emphasis on health maintenance and promotion. Martha Rogers states, "Maintenance and promotion of health, prevention of disease, nursing diagnosis, intervention, and rehabilitation encompass the scope of nursing's goals."[20] Nurses are actively seeking to identify health problems in a variety of community and institutional settings today.

The specific components of the nursing process and Peplau's phases will now be discussed. Refer again to Table 4–2. Peplau's orientation phase parallels the beginning of the *assessment phase* in that both the nurse and patient come together as strangers. This meeting is initiated by the patient who expresses a need, although the need is not always understood. Conjointly, the nurse and patient begin to work through recognizing, clarifying, and defining facts related to this need. This step is presently referred to as the data collection in the assessment phase of the nursing process.

In the nursing process the need is not necessarily a felt need. For example, the nurse may be currently functioning in the community by doing health assessments of people who perceive themselves to be healthy. A school nurse may do hearing screening for school children. If a hearing deficit is discovered, a referral is initiated by the nurse. The children do not usually seek out the nurse for this deficit. In this situation, the need must be identified for the child and for his or her parents in order to persuade them to seek assistance regarding the hearing deficit. Supplying the data on a note sent home to the parents might precipitate the parents' and child's perception of the need. This is congruent with the first part of Edgar H. Schein's model of change, the unfreezing of the established equilibrium so change can take place. Schein states, "If change is to occur, therefore, it must be preceded by an alteration of the present stable equilibrium which supports the present behavior and attitudes."[21] Supplying the data would be one stimulus for change. The nurse may also have to follow up the child's note with a telephone call or a home visit and additional data such as poor grades in order to facilitate the family's entry into the unfreezing stage or into Peplau's felt need phase of orientation.

Orientation and assessment are not synonymous and must not be confused. Collecting data is continuous throughout Peplau's phases. In the nursing process, the initial collection of data is the nursing assessment, and further collection of data becomes an integral part of reassessment (see Chapter 2, Fig. 2–1).

The *nursing diagnosis* evolves once the health problems or deficits are identified. The nursing diagnosis is a summary statement of the data collected. It delineates the patient's problem or potential problem. Peplau states that "during the period of orientation the patient clarifies his first, whole impression of his problem"[22]; whereas in the nursing process, the nurse's judgment forms the diagnosis from the data collected.

Mutually set goals evolve from the nursing diagnosis. These goals give direction to the plan and indicate the appropriate helping resources. When helping resources are discussed, the patient then can selectively identify with the resource persons. According to Peplau, the patient is viewed as being in the identification phase.

When the nurse and patient collaborate on goals, there may be a clash based on the preconceptions and expectations of each person, as described earlier in Peplau's identification phase. These discrepancies must be resolved before mutually stated goals can be agreed on. Goal setting should be an interdependent action between nurse and patient.

In the *planning* phase of the nursing process, the nurse must specifically formulate how the patient is going to achieve the mutually set goals. Patient input is actively sought by the nurse so that the patient feels an integral part of the plan and compliance is more likely to take place. In this step, the nurse considers the patient's own skills for handling his or her personal problems. Peplau stresses that the nurse wants to develop a therapeutic relationship so that the patient's anxiety will be channeled constructively to seek resources, thus decreasing feelings of hopelessness. This step in planning can still be considered within Peplau's identification phase.

The patient also begins to have a feeling of belonging because of mutual respect, communication, and interest. The feeling of belonging must be analyzed and should be a thrust toward a healthier personality and not imitative behavior.[23] Peplau states, "Some patients identify too readily with nurses, expecting that all of their wants will be taken care of and nothing will be expected of them."[24] In Peplau's identification phase, the patient selectively responds to people who can meet his personal needs. Therefore, the identification phase is patient initiated.

The planning stage of the nursing process gives direction and meaning to the nursing action toward resolving the patients' problems. The nurse uses the knowledge from her or his educational background to scientifically base the plan of nursing action.

In the *implementation phase*, as in exploitation, the patient is finally reaping benefits from the therapeutic relationship by drawing on the nurse's knowledge and expertise. In both phases (implementation and exploitation), the individualized plans have already been formed, based on the patient's interest and needs. Therefore, in both phases the plans are initiated toward completion of desired goals. There is a difference, however, between exploitation, where the patient is the one who actively seeks varying types of services in obtaining the maximal benefits available, and implementation, where there is a prescribed plan or procedure, holistic in nature, to achieve mutually predetermined goals or objectives based on the nurse's intellectual knowledge and technical skills. Exploitation is patient oriented, whereas implementation can be accomplished by the patient or by other persons including health professionals and the patient's family.

In Peplau's resolution phase, the other phases have been successfully worked through, the needs have been met, and resolution and termination are the end result. Although Peplau does not discuss *evaluation* per se, evaluation is an inherent factor in determining the status of readiness for the patient to proceed through the resolution phase.

In the nursing process, the evaluation is a separate step, and mutually established expected end behaviors are used as tools for evaluation. Time limits on attainment of these behaviors are set for the purposes of evaluation, although these limits need not be strictly adhered to. Circumstances may arise that require an adjustment on the time constraints.

In evaluation, if the situation is clear-cut, the problem moves toward termination. If the problem is unresolved, however, goals and objectives are not met; and if care is ineffective, a reassessment must be done. New goals, planning, implementation, and evaluation are then established.

PEPLAU'S WORK AND THE CHARACTERISTICS OF A THEORY

Currently in the literature, there is disagreement over whether Peplau's book is a theory as proposed in the 1980 edition of this text, a conceptual model,[25] or a grand theory.[26] Peplau's work will be compared to the characteristics of a theory introduced in this book's first chapter. Generally, Peplau's work is a theory of nursing.

1. Theories can interrelate concepts in such a way as to create a different way of looking at a particular phenomenon. The phases of orientation, identification, exploitation, and resolution interrelate the different components of each phase. This interrelationship creates a different perspective of the nurse–patient interaction and the transaction of health care.

The nurse–patient interaction can apply to the concepts of human being, health, society/environment, and nursing. For example, in the phase of orientation there are components of nurse, patient, strangers, problem, and anxiety.

2. Theories must be logical in nature. Peplau's theory provides a logical, systematic way of viewing nursing situations. The four progressive phases in the nurse–patient relationship are logical, beginning with initial contact in the phase of orientation and ending with termination in the phase of resolution. Key concepts in the theory, such as anxiety, tension, goals, and frustration, are clearly defined with explicit relationships among them and the progressive phases.

3. Theories should be relatively simple yet generalizable. The phases provide simplicity in regard to the natural progression of the nurse–patient relationship. This simplicity leads to adaptability in any nurse–patient interaction, thus providing generalizability. The basic nature of nursing is still considered an interpersonal process.

4. Theories can be the bases for hypotheses that can be tested. Peplau's theory has generated testable hypotheses. Most research has centered around the concept of anxiety, not the nurse–patient relationship which is the core of her work. Generally, nursing research has been scant and mostly descriptive (see Table 4–3). Much of the research has very small sample sizes and was conducted before 1970. For example, one study examined teaching the concept of anxiety to six female patients in a group setting.[27] Another study used Peplau's work on anxiety to develop a frame-

TABLE 4–3. NURSING RESEARCH USING PEPLAU'S WORK AS A FRAMEWORK

Date and Author	Research	Findings
1961 Hays, D.	Provided a description of phases and steps of experiential teaching to patients of a concept of anxiety. Sample size was 6 female psychiatric patients.	The verbal analysis of the group revealed that, when taught by the experiential method, the patients were able to apply the concept of anxiety after the group was terminated.
1963 Burd, S.F.	Developed and tested a nursing intervention framework for working with anxious patients. Sample was 25 psychiatric nursing students consisting of 15 freshmen and 10 graduate students.	Freshman students can develop beginning competency in interpersonal relationships. The earlier the student gains theoretical knowledge, the more the student is aware of his or her own anxiety. As students work with patients, patients respond by going through sequential phases including denial, ambivalence, and awareness of anxiety.

work and to conduct a study of twenty-five nursing students who worked with anxious patients.[28]

In examining Peplau's theory, one limitation is that some areas are not specific enough to generate hypotheses. One reason for this limitation may be that her theory was written in 1949, prior to a more organized thrust in nursing research that began in the 1950s. In general, in analyzing Peplau's theory, more concept development and concrete descriptions need to be made before the theory can be empirically tested. For example, the nurse–patient relationship describes a certain progressive relationship, but otherwise, more explicit relationships among the phases should be defined.

5. Theories contribute to and assist in increasing the general body of knowledge within the discipline through the research implemented to validate them. Peplau's work has contributed greatly to nursing's body of knowledge not only in psychiatric–mental health nursing, but also in nursing in general. An example is her work on anxiety. With regard to her contribution to research in psychiatric–mental health nursing, in the 1950s two-thirds of the nursing research concentrated on the nurse–patient relationship.[29] At Teachers College, Columbia University, Peplau's (1952) work influenced the interpersonal nature and direction of clinical work and studies.[29] Presently, as in the past, researchers continue to test her theory.[30]

6. Theories can be utilized by the practitioners to guide and improve their practice. Nursing is still defined as an interpersonal process built upon the progressive nurse–patient phases. As Peplau proposed, communication and interviewing skills remain fundamental nursing tools. Peplau's anxiety continuum is still used for nursing interventions in working with anxious patients.[31]

In applying Peplau's theory in clinical practice, one limitation is in working with the unconscious patient or a withdrawn individual. A major assumption in the theory is that the nurse and patient can interact. For example, the phase of orientation begins when the patient has a felt need and initiates interaction between the nurse and the patient. Nurse–patient interaction is extremely limited in working with the unconscious patient and seriously hampered with the withdrawn individual who does not communicate effectively.

7. Theories must be consistent with other validated theories, laws, and principles but will leave open unanswered questions that need to be investigated. In general, this theory is consistent with current theories and research. Interpersonal theories, including Sullivan's and Fromme's, are foundations in the theory.[32a,32b] Peplau's concepts and phases are consistent with other theories, such as Maslow's need theory and Selye's stress theory.[33a,33b] General system theory can also be broadly applied to the four phases of the nurse–patient relationship.[34] For example, the nurse and patient could each be defined as a system. Both systems (nurse and patient) interact with each other, processing inputs, throughputs, and outputs so a specific goal can be met.

In summary, a theory has seven characteristics. In examining these characteristics, Peplau's 1952 work has the characteristics of a theory. Strengths include creating a unique way of viewing nursing and increasing nursing's body of knowledge. Limitations of this theory are that some areas need to be more developed to be able to generate testable hypotheses, and that the theory is weak in the application to patients with certain characteristics. Nursing research should focus on testing this theory's hypotheses for validation.

SUMMARY

Peplau's text *Interpersonal Relations in Nursing,* published in 1952, is still applicable in theory and practice. The core of Peplau's theory of nursing is the interpersonal process, which is an integral part of present-day nursing. This process consists of the sequential phases of orientation, identification, exploitation, and resolution. These phases overlap, interrelate, and vary in time duration. The nurse and patient first clarify the patient's problem, and mutual expectations and goals are explored while deciding on appropriate plans for improved health status. This process is influenced by both the nurse's and patient's perceptions and preconceived ideas emerging from their individual uniqueness.

Both Peplau's phases and the nursing process are sequential and focus on therapeutic interactions. Through mutual exploration of the patient's difficulty and the nurse–patient relationship, a broader understanding of the patient's problem and new alternative approaches toward reaching the solution are uncovered.

When two persons meet in a creative relationship, there is a continuing sense of mutuality and togetherness throughout the experience. Both individuals are involved in a process of self-fulfillment, which becomes a growth experience.

Peplau focuses on a specific nurse and patient relationship. Today's nursing process, however, may view the patient collectively as a group, family, or community. Thus, today's nursing process takes the total environment more into account.

Peplau's nursing theory, the interpersonal process, has as its foundation theories of interaction. It has contributed to nursing in the areas of clinical practice, theory, and research, adding to today's nursing knowledge base. Thus Peplau's theory creates a unique view for understanding the nurse–patient relationship.

REFERENCES

1.   Peplau, H.E. *Interpersonal Relations in Nursing,* New York: G. P. Putnam's Sons, 1952.

2.(a) Peplau, H.E. Basic Principles of Patient Counseling, n.d.
2.(b) Profile: Hildegard E. Peplau, R.N., Ed.D., *Nursing '74*, 1974, *4*, 13.
3.   Peplau, *Interpersonal Relations*, p. 261.
4.   Ibid, 35.
5.   Ibid, 8.
6.   Burton, G. *Personal, Impersonal, and Interpersonal: A Guide for Nurses*, New York: Springer New York, Inc., 1958, p. 7.
7.   Peplau, *Interpersonal Relations*, p. 18.
8.   Ibid, 26–27.
9.   Ibid, 33.
10. Ibid, 37.
11. Ibid, 82.
12. Ibid, 12.
13. Ibid, 28.
14. Sills, G.M. Research in the Field of Psychiatric Nursing, 1952–1977. *Nursing Research*, 1977, *26*, 202.
15. Peplau, *Interpersonal Relations*, p. 16.
16. Ibid, 5–6.
17. Congress for Nursing Practice, *Standards for Nursing Practice*, Kansas City, Mo.: American Nurses' Association, 1973, p. 2.
18. Peplau, *Interpersonal Relations*, p. 23.
19.(a) Sullivan, H.S. *Conceptions of Modern Psychiatry*, Washington, D.C.: William Alanson White Psychiatric Foundation, 1947
19.(b) Freud, S. *The Problem of Anxiety*, New York: W. W. Norton & Co., Inc., 1936.
20. Rogers, M.E. *An Introduction to the Theoretical Basis of Nursing*, Philadelphia: F. A. Davis Company, 1970, p. 86.
21. Schein, E.H. The Mechanisms of Change, in *The Planning of Change* (2nd ed.), Bennis, W.G. et al., eds., New York: Holt, Rinehart and Winston, 1969, p. 99.
22. Peplau, *Interpersonal Relations*, p. 30.
23. Ibid, 30–31.
24. Ibid, 32.
25. Riehl, J.P. & Roy, Sr.C. *Conceptual Models for Nursing Practice* (2nd ed.), New York: Appleton-Century-Crofts, 1980, pp. 53–59.
26. Walker, L. & Avant, K. *Strategies for Theory Construction in Nursing*, Norwalk, Conn.: Appleton-Century-Crofts, 1983, p. 6.
27. Hays, D. Teaching a Concept of Anxiety, *Nursing Research*, 1966, *10*, 108–113.
28. Burd, S. Effects of Nursing Intervention in Anxiety of Patients, in *Some Clinical Approaches to Psychiatric Nursing*, Burd, S.F. & Marshall, M.A., eds., London: Macmillan, 1963, pp. 307–320.
29. Sills, G.M. Research in the Field of Psychiatric Nursing, 1952–1977, *Nursing Research*, 1977, *26*, 203.
30. Telephone interview with H. Peplau by J. Belcher, November 4, 1987.
31. Jandsick, E.H. & Davies, J.L. *Psychiatric Mental Health Nursing*, Boston: Jones and Bartlett Publishers, 1986, p. 447.
32.(a) Sullivan, H.S. *Conceptions of Modern Psychiatry;*
32.(b) Fromme, E. *Man for Himself,* New York: Rinehart & Company, Inc., 1947.
33.(a) Maslow, A. *Motivation and Personality*, New York: Harper & Row, 1954;
33.(b) Selye, H. *The Stress of Life*, New York: McGraw-Hill, 1956.

34.   von Bertalanffy, L. *General System Theory*, New York: George Braziller, Inc., 1968.

BIBLIOGRAPHY

Peplau, H.E., Is Nursing's Self-Regulatory Power Being Eroded? *American Journal of Nursing*, 1985, *85*, 140–143.

Peplau, H.E., Psychiatric Nursing: Role of Nurses and Psychiatric Nurses, *International Nursing Review*, 1978, *25*, 41–47.

Peplau, H.E., Psychiatric Skills. Tomorrow's World, *Nursing Times*, 1987, *83*, 29–33.

Peplau, H.E., Some Reflections on Earlier Days in Psychiatric Nursing, *Journal of Psychosocial Nursing and Mental Health Services*, 1982, *20*, 17–24.

Peplau, H.E., The Nurse as Counselor, *Journal of American College of Health*, 1986, *35*, 11–14.

Peplau, H.E., Theory: The Professional Dimension, Proceedings from the First Nursing Theory Conference, University of Kansas Medical Center, Department of Nursing Education, March 20–21, 1969. Reprinted in *Perspectives on Nursing Theory*, Nicholl, L.H. ed., Boston: Little, Brown and Company, 1986.

Thompson, L. Peplau's Theory: An Application to Short-Term Individual Therapy, *Journal of Psychosocial Nursing*, 1980, *24*, 26–31.

CHAPTER 5

Virginia Henderson

Chiyoko Yamamoto Furukawa
Joan K. Howe

Virginia Henderson was born in Kansas City, Missouri, in 1897, the fifth child of a family of eight children. Most of her formative years were spent in Virginia, where the family resided during the period her father practiced law in Washington, D.C.

Henderson's interest in nursing evolved during World War I from her desire to help the sick and wounded military personnel. She enrolled in the Army School of Nursing in Washington, D.C., and graduated in 1921. In 1926, Henderson began the continuation of her education at Columbia University Teachers College and completed her BS and MA degrees in nursing education. She taught clinical nursing courses with a strong emphasis on the use of the analytical process at Teachers College from 1930 to 1948. Since 1953, she has been a research associate at Yale University School of Nursing.

Henderson is the recipient of numerous recognitions for her outstanding contributions to nursing. She has received honorary doctoral degrees from the Catholic University of America, Pace University, University of Rochester, University of Western Ontario, and Yale University.

Her writings are far-reaching and have made an impact on nursing throughout the world. The publications The Nature of Nursing *and* Basic Principles of Nursing Care *are widely known, and the latter has been translated into many languages for the benefit of non-English-speaking nurses.[1a,1b] Although Henderson is in her eighth decade of life, she continues to contribute to the nursing literature. She has clarified her belief about nursing and nursing practice in view of recent technological and societal advances in publications, interviews, and personal appearances.[2a-2f]*

Questions about the exclusive functions of nurses provided the impetus for Virginia Henderson to devote her career to defining nursing practice. Some of these questions were: What is the practice of nursing? What specific functions do nurses perform? What are nursing's unique activities? The development of her definition of nursing communicated her thoughts on these questions. She believed an occupation that affects human life must outline its functions, particularly if it is to be regarded as a profession.[3] Her ideas about the definition of nursing were influenced by her nursing education and practice, by her students and colleagues at

Columbia University School of Nursing, and by distinguished nursing leaders of her time. All of these experiences and nursing practice were the dominating forces that gave her insight into nursing—what is it and what are its functions? A review of Henderson's educational preparation and nursing practice furnishes the basis on which to examine her definition of nursing.

EDUCATIONAL AND PRACTICE BACKGROUND

Henderson's interpretation of the nurse's function is the synthesis of many positive and negative influences.[4] A major influence was her basic nursing education in a general hospital affiliated with the Army School of Nursing. Her education emphasized learning by doing, speedy performance, technical competence, and successful mastery of nursing procedures, e.g., catheterization, making beds, dressing changes. As a result, an impersonal approach to care emerged and was interpreted as professional behavior. Although the importance of ethics in nursing and a compassionate attitude for humanity were stressed, these were not as high a priority as the nursing procedures.

Physician lectures were the major portion of classroom learning for the nursing students. The lectures used a cut-and-dried approach to learning and a simplified version of medical education. The focus was disease, diagnosis, and treatment regimens. Henderson was discontented with the regimentalized care based on medical teaching. She recognized this kind of nursing was merely an extension of medical practice.[5] Her dean, Annie W. Goodrich, agreed with this evaluation of nursing education.

Another educational concern for Henderson was a lack of an appropriate role model to emulate in giving nursing care. She yearned to observe patient care by either her teacher or graduate nurses. This was impossible since students staffed the hospital in return for their nursing education. Thus, clinical practice was viewed as a self-learned process while students cared for the sick and wounded soldiers. She perceived this atmosphere as one of indebtedness to the patients for having served the country in time of war. The nurse–patient relationship was described as warm and generous. The soldiers asked for little, and the nurses wanted to do all they could. This experience was believed to be unique and special since the opportunity to express indebtedness to military patients did not exist in a civilian hospital.

Her next educational experience, psychiatric nursing, was disappointing because the human relations skills that could have been learned in this setting failed to materialize. As in her previous experiences, the approach to psychiatric patient care continued to focus on disease entities and treatment. There was a lack of understanding about the nurse's role in the prevention of mental illness or in the curative aspects of care for the psychiatric patient. This experience resulted in a sense of failure as a nurse. The only value of the psychiatric affiliation was the opportunity to gain some appreciation of mental illness.

The pediatric nursing experience at the Boston Floating Hospital was more positive and introduced three concepts of care—patient-centered, continuity, and tender-loving care. The task-oriented and regimented approach to care was discarded in this setting. However, other shortcomings were identified, such as the failure to use family-centered care. Parents were not allowed to visit their sick child. Therefore the child was isolated from parental support when this was most needed. Furthermore, Henderson saw the lack of effort to assess the home environment to identify the needs of the child and family.

The final student experience at the Henry Street Visiting Nurse Agency in New York introduced her to community nursing care. The formal approach to patient care learned earlier was replaced with care that considered the sick person's life style. Henderson was concerned about discharging patients to the same environment that originally led them to hospitalization. She believed that the hospital care only served as a stopgap measure without getting to the cause of the problem. She recognized that this type of care failed to consider the person living outside the behavioral controls of the institutional setting.

As a graduate nurse, Henderson worked for several years at the Instructive Visiting Nursing Agency in Washington, D.C., since she deplored the hospital system of nursing. This experience was rewarding and offered the opportunity to try out her ideas about nursing.

Her next position was teaching nursing students at the Norfolk Protestant Hospital diploma program in Virginia. This five-year responsibility was accepted without further education. This situation was not uncommon since many diploma schools of this time did not require academic credentials for teaching. Despite this, she recognized the need for more knowledge and for clarification of the functions of nursing. Subsequently, she enrolled at Columbia University Teachers College to learn about the sciences and humanities relevant to nursing. These courses enabled Henderson to develop an inquiring and analytical approach to nursing.

After graduation, she briefly accepted the position of teaching supervisor at Strong Memorial Hospital's clinics in Rochester, New York. Next, she returned to Columbia where her distinguished teaching career continued until 1948. While at this university, Henderson implemented several ideas about nursing in her medical-surgical nursing courses. The concepts taught were patient-centered approach, nursing problem method replacing the medical model, field experience, family follow-up care, and chronic illness care. She also established nursing clinics and encouraged coordinated multidisciplinary care.

THE DEVELOPMENT OF HENDERSON'S DEFINITION OF NURSING

Two events are the basis for Henderson's development of a definition of nursing. First, she participated in the revision of a nursing textbook. Second, she was concerned that many states had no provision for nursing licensure to ensure safe and competent care for the consumer.

In the revision of the *Textbook of the Principles and Practice of Nursing,* coauthored with Bertha Harmer, a Canadian nurse, Henderson recognized the need to be clear about the functions of the nurse.[6a,6b] She believed a textbook that serves as a main learning source for nursing practice should present a sound and definitive description of nursing. Furthermore, the principles and practice of nursing must be built upon and derived from the definition of the profession.

—→ Henderson was committed to the process of regulating nursing practice through licensure by each state. In order to accomplish this she believed that nursing must be explicitly defined in Nurse Practice Acts. These Acts outline the legal parameters for the nurse's functions in caring for consumers and safeguard the public from unprepared and incompetent practitioners.

Although official statements on the nursing function were published by the American Nurses' Association (ANA) in 1932 and 1937, Henderson viewed these statements as nonspecific and unsatisfactory definitions of nursing practice.[7] Then, in 1955, the earlier ANA definition was modified to read:

> The practice of professional nursing means the performance for compensation of any act in the observation, care, and counsel of the ill, injured, or infirm, or in the maintenance of health or prevention of illness of others, or in the supervision and teaching of other personnel, or the administration of medications and treatment as prescribed by a licensed physician or dentist; requiring substantial specialized judgment and skill and based on knowledge and application of the principles of biological, physical, and social science. The foregoing shall not be deemed to include acts of diagnosis or prescription of therapeutic or corrective measures.[8]

This statement was seen as an improvement since nursing functions were identified but the definition still was thought to be very general and too vague. In the new statement, the nurse could observe, care for, and counsel the patient and could supervise other health personnel without herself or himself being supervised by the physician. The nurse was to give medications and do treatments ordered by the physician, but prohibited to diagnose, prescribe, or correct nursing care problems. Thus Henderson viewed the statement as another unsatisfactory definition of nursing.

Henderson's extensive experiences as a student, teacher, practitioner, author, and participant in conferences on the nurse's function contributed to the development of her definition of nursing. She regretted that publications of conference debates and investigations were not widely circulated. Only a few nurses were privy to the information published about the outcomes of these conferences.

In 1955, Henderson's first definition of nursing was published in Bertha Harmer's revised nursing textbook. It read:

Henderson's First (1955) Definition
Nursing is primarily assisting the individual (sick or well) in the performance of those activities contributing to health, or its recovery (or a peaceful death) that he would perform unaided if he had the necessary strength, will, or knowledge. It is likewise the unique contribution of nursing to help the individual to be independent of such assistance as soon as possible.[9a,9b]

This statement on nursing conveys the essence of her definition of nursing as it is known today. Since there was collaboration, it is instructive to compare Henderson's definition with Harmer's 1922 definition, which read as follows:

Harmer's 1922 Definition
Nursing is rooted in the needs of humanity and is founded on the ideal of service. Its object is not only to cure the sick and heal the wounded but to bring health and ease, rest and comfort to mind and body, to shelter, nourish, and protect and to minister to all those who are helpless or handicapped, young, aged or immature. Its object is to prevent disease and to preserve health. Nursing is, therefore, linked with every other social agency which strives for the prevention of disease and the preservation of health. The nurse finds herself not only concerned with the care of the individual but with the health of a people.[10a,10b]

Some similarities can be seen between the two definitions of nursing. Henderson's definition abbreviated and consolidated portions of Harmer's beliefs about nursing. Harmer's definition highlighted disease prevention, health preservation, and the need for linkages with other social agencies to strive for preventive care. Harmer stressed that nursing's role in society was oriented toward the community and wellness. Henderson placed more emphasis on the care of the sick and well individuals and did not mention nursing's concern for the health and welfare of the aggregate. However, a one-line statement in *Basic Principles of Nursing* acknowledges that some nurses do function with groups rather than individuals.[11]

Henderson's focus on individual care is evident in that she stressed assisting individuals with essential activities to maintain health, to recover, or to achieve peaceful death. She proposed fourteen components of basic nursing care to augment her definition.[12] The components are as follows:

1. Breathe normally.
2. Eat and drink adequately.
3. Eliminate body wastes.
4. Move and maintain desirable postures.
5. Sleep and rest.
6. Select suitable clothes—dress and undress.
7. Maintain body temperature within normal range by adjusting clothing and modifying the environment.
8. Keep the body clean and well groomed and protect the integument.
9. Avoid dangers in the environment and avoid injuring others.
10. Communicate with others in expressing emotions, needs, fears, or opinions.
11. Worship according to one's faith.
12. Work in such a way that there is a sense of accomplishment.
13. Play or participate in various forms of recreation.
14. Learn, discover, or satisfy the curiosity that leads to normal development and health and use the available health facilities.

In 1966, her ultimate statement on the definition of nursing was published in *The Nature of Nursing*. This statement was viewed as "the crystallization of my ideas."[13]

> The unique function of the nurse is to assist the individual, sick or well, in the performance of those activities contributing to health or its recovery (or to peaceful death) that he would perform unaided if he had the necessary strength, will or knowledge. And to do this in such a way as to help him gain independence as rapidly as possible.[13]

Except for slight wording changes, the 1955, 1966, and more recent 1978[14] definitions are quite similar, indicating that her definition of nursing, conceived earlier, remains intact. Henderson's definition of nursing in itself fails to fully explain her main ideas and views. To appreciate the breadth of her thoughts about nursing functions and the fourteen components of basic nursing care, it is necessary to study *Basic Principles of Nursing Care*, a publication of the International Council of Nurses. This text book eloquently describes each of the basic nursing care components so that they can be used as a guide to delineate the unique nursing functions. The definition of nursing and the fourteen components together outline the functions the nurse can initiate and control.

Henderson expects nurses to carry out the therapeutic plan of the physician as a member of the medical team. The nurse is the prime helper to the ill person in assuring that the medical prescriptions are instituted. This nursing function is believed to foster the therapeutic nurse–client relationship. As a member of an interdisciplinary health team, the nurse assists the individual to recovery or provides support in dying. The ideal situation for a nurse is full participation as a team member with no interference with the nurse's unique functions. The nurse serves as a substitute for whatever the patient lacks in order to make him or her "complete," "whole," or "independent," considering his or her available physical strength, will, or knowledge to attain good health.[15]

The nurse is cautioned about tasks that detract from the professional role and the need to give priority to the nurse's unique functions. However, Henderson encourages the nurse to assume the role and functions of other health workers if the need is apparent and the nurse has expertise. On a worldwide basis, nursing functions differ from country to country or even within countries. The ratio of nurses to physicians and to other health care providers affects what nurses do. Consequently, this creates confusion for the public about the nurse's role, particularly since the creation of nurse practitioners.

HENDERSON'S THEORY AND THE FOUR MAJOR CONCEPTS

In viewing the concept of the *human* or individual, Henderson considers the biological, psychological, sociological, and spiritual components. The fourteen components of nursing functions can be categorized in the following manner: The first nine components are physiological, the tenth and fourteenth are psychological aspects of communicating and learning; the eleventh component is spiritual and moral; and the twelfth and thirteenth components are sociologically oriented to occupation and recreation. She refers to humans as having basic needs that are included in the fourteen components. However, she goes on to state, "It is equally important to realize that these needs are satisfied by infinitely varied patterns of living, no two of which are alike."[16] Henderson also believes that mind and body are inseparable.[17] It is implied that the mind and body are interrelated.

Henderson emphasizes some aspects of the concept of *society/environment*. In her writing, she discusses primarily individuals. She sees individuals in relation to their families but minimally discusses the impact of the community on the individual and family. In the book co-authored with Harmer, she supports the tasks of private and public agencies in keeping people healthy.[18] She believes that society wants and expects the nurse's service of acting for individuals who are unable to function independently.[19] In return, she expects society to contribute to nursing education:

> the nurse needs the kind of education that, in our society, is available only in colleges and universities. Training programs operated on funds pinched from the budgets of service agencies cannot provide the preparation the nurse needs.[20]

This generalized education gives the nurse a better understanding of the consumers of nursing care and the various environmental factors that influence people.

Henderson's beliefs about health are related to human functioning. Her definition of health is based on the individual's ability to function independently as outlined in the fourteen components. Because good health is a challenging goal for individuals, she argues that it is difficult for the nurse to help the person reach it.[21] She also refers to nurses stressing promotion of health and prevention and cure of disease. [22] Henderson explains how the factors of age, cultural background, physical and intellectual capacities, and emotional balance affect one's health.[23] These conditions are always present and affect basic needs.

Henderson's concept of nursing is interesting from the perspective of time. She was one of the earlier leaders who believed nurses need a liberal education including knowledge of sciences, social sciences, and humanities. Aside from using the definition of nursing and the fourteen components of basic nursing care, the nurse is expected to carry out the physician's therapeutic plan. Individualized care is the result of the nurse's creativity in planning for care. Further, the nurse is expected to improve patient care using results of nursing research.

> The nurse who operates under a definition that specifies an area of independent practice, or an area of expertness, *must* assume responsibility for identifying problems, for continually validating her function, for improving the methods she uses, and for measuring the effect of nursing care. In this era research is the name we attach to the most reliable type of analysis.[24]

For Henderson, the nurse must be knowledgeable, have some base for practicing individualized and humane care, and be a scientific problem solver.

HENDERSON AND THE NURSING PROCESS

Henderson views the nursing process as "really the application of the logical approach to the solution of a problem. The steps are those of the scientific method."[25] With this approach, each person can receive individualized care. Likewise, with the nursing process, individualized care is the outcome.

In Henderson's more recent writings, she raises some issues regarding the nursing process. One of the issues asks if the problem-solving approach of the nursing process is peculiar to nursing. She compares the nursing process to the traditional steps of the medical processes: "the nursing history parallels the medical history; the nurse's health assessment, the physicians' medical examination; the nursing diagnosis corresponds to the physician's diagnosis; nursing orders to the plan of medical management; and nursing evaluation to medical evaluation."[26] It looks as if the language has been changed to fit nursing's purpose. Could other health care workers use the steps of the nursing process to fit their practice? If so, then what makes the nursing process peculiar to nursing?

Another issue Henderson raises also deals with problem solving. But now she asks if problem solving is all there is to nursing. Henderson states, " 'the' makes it so specific that activities outside those in the problem solving steps of the process cannot be peculiar to or characteristic of nursing."[27] She questions where intuition, experience, authority, and expert opinion fit into the nursing process since they are not stressed.[28] She further comments, "Expert opinion or authority is also, by implication, discredited as a basis for practice."[29] Does the 'the' in the nursing process make it too limiting for effective practice?

A third issue Henderson raises flows from the problem-solving approach. She asks where the art of nursing fits into the nursing process. If one views science as objective with little left undefined and art as subjective with some parts hard to define, then where does intuition fit? Henderson argues that "The nursing process now weighted so heavily on the scientific side, seems to belittle the intuitive, artistic side of nursing."[30] She also claims, "nursing process stresses the science of nursing rather than the mixture of science *and art* on which it seems effective health care service of any kind is based."[31] Does the nursing process disregard the subjective and intuitive qualities used in nursing?

The fourth concern Henderson raises about the nursing process deals with the lack of collaboration of health care workers, the patient, and the family. She states, "As currently defined, nursing process does not seem to suggest a collaborative approach on diagnosis, treatment, *or* care by health care workers, nor does it suggest the essential rights of patients and their families in all of these questions."[32] Henderson thinks nursing process stresses an independent function for the nurse rather than a collaborative one with other health professionals, the patient, and the patient's family.[33] Does the nursing process focus more on independent nursing functions rather than interdependent functions?

Perhaps it is semantics that are a problem with the nursing process. The real value of the nursing process depends on one's understanding, interpretation, integration, and utilization of it. The nursing process as discussed in Chapter 2 will be examined with Henderson's definition of nursing.

Even though Henderson's definition and explanation of nursing do not directly fit with the steps of the nursing process, a relationship between the two can be demonstrated. Although Henderson does not refer directly to assessment, she implies it in her description of the fourteen components of basic nursing care. The nurse uses the fourteen components to assess the individual's needs. For example, in assessing the first component, "breathe normally," the nurse gathers all pertinent data about the person's respiratory status. The nurse then moves to the next component and gathers data in that area. The gathering of data about the person continues until all components are assessed.

To complete the assessment phase of the nursing process, the nurse needs to analyze the data. According to Henderson, the nurse must have knowledge about what is normal in health and disease. Using this knowledge base, then, the nurse would compare the assessment data with what was known about that area. For example, if respirations were observed to be 40 per minute in an adult aged forty, the nurse would conclude that this person's respiratory rate is faster than normal. Or if a laboratory report showed that the urine was highly concentrated, the nurse would know this "means that the patient's fluid intake is inadequate, unless he is losing body fluids by other routes."[34] With a scientific knowledge base, the nurse can draw conclusions from the assessment data. Henderson states,

> The nursing needed by the individual is affected by age, cultural background, emotional balance, and his physical and intellectual capacities. All of these should be considered in the nurse's evaluation of the patient's needs for her help.[35]

Following the analysis of the data according to these factors, the nurse then determines the nursing diagnosis. Henderson does not specifically discuss nursing diagnoses. She believes the physician makes the diagnosis, and the nurse acts upon that diagnosis. However, if one looks at Henderson's definition, the nursing diagnosis deals with identifying the individual's ability to meet human needs with or without assistance, taking into account that person's strength, will, and knowledge. Based on the assessment data and the analysis of that data, the nurse *can* identify actual problems such as abnormal respirations. In addition, potential problems may be identified. For example, with component 11, about one's faith, a potential problem could develop because of hospitalization and a change in the person's normal activities of daily living. If, based on the nurse's assessment and analysis of the data, a person was unable to meet this need, then a nursing diagnosis regarding an actual problem would be made.

Once the nursing diagnosis is made, the nurse proceeds to the planning phase of the nursing process. Regarding the planning of care, Henderson states:

> All effective nursing care is planned to some extent. A written plan forces those who make it to give some thought to the individual's needs—unless they simply fit the person's regimen into the institution's routines.[36]

She also contends that *discharge planning* is influenced by the other members of the family.[36] Furthermore, plans need continuing modification, based on the individual's needs. Henderson advocates written nursing care plans so others giving nursing care can follow the planned sequence.[37] She emphasizes that "nursing care is always arranged around, or fitted into, the physician's therapeutic plan."[38] Henderson outlines the planning phase as making the plan fit the individual's needs, up-dating the plan as necessary based on those needs, being specific so others can implement it, and fitting with the physician's prescribed plan. Written nursing care plans, in essence, identify the nursing needs of the person. Even though Henderson does not apply the current terminology about nursing plans, she uses the same ideas.

Implementation follows the planning of nursing care. For Henderson, nursing implementation is based on helping the patient meet the fourteen components. For example, in helping the individual with sleep and rest, the nurse tries known methods of inducing sleep and rest before giving drugs. She summarizes, "I see nursing as primarily complementing the patient by supplying what he needs in knowledge, will, or strength to perform his daily activities and to carry out the treatment prescribed for him by the physician."[39] Henderson also states, "This primary function of the practicing nurse, of course, must be performed in such a way that it promotes the physician's therapeutic plan."[40] So the nurse needs to carry out the physician's orders of treatment with her nursing care.

Another important aspect of implementation that Henderson discusses is the relationship between nurse and patient. The nurse gets "inside the skin" to better understand the patient's needs and carry out measures to meet those needs.[41] Henderson also speaks about the quality of nursing care:

> The danger of turning over the physical care of the patient to relatively unqualified nurses is two-fold. They may fail to assess the patient's needs adequately but, perhaps more important, the qualified nurse, being deprived of the opportunity while giving physical care to assess his needs, may not find any other chance to do so. In this connection it should also be pointed out that it is easier for any person to develop an emotional supportive role with another if he can perform a tangible service.[42]

This statement clearly supports that the competent nurse uses both the interpersonal process and assessment while giving care.

Henderson bases the evaluation of each person "according to the speed with which, or the degree to which, he performs independently the activities that make, for him, a normal day."[43] This notion is outlined in the definition and the unique function of the nurse. For evaluation purposes, changes in a person's level of functioning need to be observed and recorded. A comparison of the data about the person's functional abilities is done pre- and post-nursing care. All changes would be noted for evaluation.

To summarize the stages of the nursing process as applied to Henderson's definition of nursing and to the fourteen components of basic nursing care, refer to Table 5–1.

TABLE 5–1. A SUMMARY OF THE NURSING PROCESS AND OF HENDERSON'S FOURTEEN COMPONENTS AND DEFINITION OF NURSING

Nursing Process	Henderson's Fourteen Components and Definition of Nursing
Nursing assessment	Assess needs of human being based on the fourteen components of basic nursing care:
	1. Breathing normally
	2. Eat and drink adequately
	3. Elimination of body wastes
	4. Move and maintain posture
	5. Sleep and rest
	6. Suitable clothing dress or undress
	7. Maintain body temperature
	8. Keep body clean and well-groomed
	9. Avoid dangers in environment
	10. Communication
	11. Worship according to one's faith
	12. Work accomplishment
	13. Recreation
	14. Learn, discover, or satisfy curiosity
	Analysis: Compare data to knowledge base of health and disease.
Nursing diagnosis	Identify individual's ability to meet own needs with or without assistance, taking into consideration strength, will, or knowledge.
Nursing plan	Document how the nurse can assist the individual, sick or well.
Nursing implementation	Assist the sick or well individual in the performance of activities in meeting human needs to maintain health, recover from illness, or to aid in peaceful death. Implementation based on physiological principles, age, cultural background, emotional balance, and physical and intellectual capacities. Carry out treatment prescribed by the physician.
Nursing evaluation	Use the acceptable definition of nursing and appropriate laws related to the practice of nursing. The quality of care is drastically affected by the preparation and native ability of the nursing personnel rather than the amount of hours of care. Successful outcomes of nursing care are based on the speed with which or degree to which the patient performs independently the activities of daily living.

HENDERSON'S WORK AND THE CHARACTERISTICS OF A THEORY

Henderson wrote her definition of nursing prior to the development of concepts and theories about nursing. Her intent was to identify the specific functions the nurse performs rather than to describe the theoretical basis for nursing practice. Nevertheless, some characteristics of a theory discussed in Chapter 1 can be applied to Henderson's work.

1. Theories can interrelate concepts in such a way as to create a different way of looking at a particular phenomenon. Henderson uses the concepts of fundamental human needs, biophysiology, culture, and interaction–communication. These concepts are borrowed from other disciplines rather than being unique to nursing. In a way, one might view the collection of these concepts as middle-level theory since delineating nursing practice was a major goal of Henderson's.

Maslow's hierarchy of human needs fits well with the fourteen basic components.[44] The first nine components are physiological and safety needs. The remaining five components deal with the love and belonging, social esteem, and self-actualization needs. Henderson uses the biophysiological concept when she stresses the importance of physiology and physiological balances in making decisions about nursing care. The concept of culture as it affects human needs is learned from the family and other social groups. Because of this, Henderson suggests that a nurse is unable to fully interpret or supply all the requirements for the individual's well-being. At best the nurse can merely assist the individual in meeting human needs.

The concept of interaction–communication can be seen in Henderson's writings. She believes sensitivity to nonverbal communication is essential to encourage the expression of feelings.[45] Furthermore a prerequisite to validate patient's needs is a constructive nurse–patient relationship. As mentioned earlier, several concepts can be identified from the definition of nursing and the fourteen components of care. Each of the concepts can be interrelated to describe nursing as it is viewed by Henderson. Thus, she created a new way of understanding the relationships of several concepts in her definition of nursing. How the concepts interrelate remains to be tested.

2. Theories must be logical in nature. Henderson's definition and components are logical. The nurse assists the individual to perform those activities contributing to health, its recovery, or peaceful death and encourages independence as quickly as possible. The fourteen components are a guide for the individual and nurse in reaching the chosen goal. The components start with physiological functioning and move to the psychosocial aspects which may convey that bodily operation is a priority to emotional or cognitive status.

3. Theories should be relatively simple yet generalizable. Henderson's work is relatively simple yet generalizable with some limitations. Her work can be applied to the health of individuals of all ages. Nurses functioning at various levels and in various cultures have used Henderson's definition and components in their practice. An important shortcoming is the lack of empirical testing to determine the generalizability of the definition and the fourteen components.

4. Theories can be the bases for hypotheses that can be tested. Henderson's definition of nursing cannot be viewed as a theory, therefore, it is impossible to generate testable hypotheses. However, some questions to investigate the definition of nursing and the fourteen components may be useful. Some examples of these questions are:

1. Is the sequence of the fourteen components followed by nurses in the United States and other countries?
2. What priorities are evident in the use of the basic nursing functions?
3. Do nurses give care to presenting medical problems initially and then use the unique functions?
4. Which clinical specialty areas of nursing practice include or exclude components ten through fourteen?

Henderson is an advocate for conducting research in nursing. She favors studies directed to improve practice rather than those conducted as an academic or theoretical endeavor.[46]

5. Theories contribute to and assist in increasing the general body of knowledge within the discipline through the research implemented to validate them. Henderson's ideas of nursing practice are well accepted throughout the world as a basis for nursing care. However, the impact of the definition and components have not been established through research. Well-designed empirical studies are needed to determine Henderson's contribution to worldwide knowledge about nursing practice and patient outcomes. This would help validate Henderson's beliefs about the unique function of nursing.

6. Theories can be utilized by practitioners to guide and improve their practice. Ideally, the nurse would improve nursing practice by using Henderson's definition and fourteen components to improve the health of individuals and thus reduce illness. The final desirable outcome would be a measure of recovery rate, health promotion and maintenance, or peaceful death.

7. Theories must be consistent with other validated theories, laws, and principles but will leave open unanswered questions that need to be investigated. There is a potential for comparison for Henderson's definition and components with validated theories, laws, and principles. The concepts of fundamental human needs, culture, independence, and inter-action—communication are widely investigated by nurse researchers as well as those in the social and psychological disciplines. In the 1980s, Henderson writes that nursing must accept the responsibility to conduct investigations on nursing practice. Furthermore, focus ought to be on measures of consumer welfare, satisfaction, and cost-effectiveness.[47]

LIMITATIONS

Henderson based her ideas about nursing care on fundamental human needs and the physical and emotional aspects of the individual. A major shortcoming in her work is the lack of a conceptual linkage between physiological and other human characteristics. The concept of the holistic nature of human beings does not clearly emerge from her publications. However, the reader must keep in mind that Henderson wrote her ideas about nursing before the emergence of the holism concept. If the assumption is made that the fourteen components are prioritized, the relationship among the components is unclear. Each component does affect the next one on the list. More recently, Henderson has stated some beliefs about the acceptance of the holistic approach to nursing.[48]

If priority according to individual needs is implied in the listing of the components, does a presenting emotional problem take a back seat to physical care? Is the emotional area of care deferred until the physiological needs have been given proper attention? Henderson specifies that the nurse must consider such factors as age, temperament, social or cultural status, and physical and intellectual capacity in the use of the components, thus emphasizing differences among individuals. How these factors interrelate and influence nursing care is vague, except individualized care must emerge when all factors of a person are taken into account in the process of nursing.

In fairness to Henderson, her effort to define nursing evolved before the discussions of a theoretical basis for the profession emerged. Therefore, the lack of theory in her definition of nursing should not lessen her contribution to nurses and nursing. Her pioneering spirit to lead nursing toward a profession and accountability to the public for competent care were enormous contributions to society as well as to nursing.

Lastly, in assisting the individual in the dying process, Henderson contends that the nurse helps, but there is little explanation of what the nurse does. In her definition of nursing, the placing of a parenthesis around the words "peaceful death" is curious. It leads one to wonder why this treatment was chosen or if it was merely to single out this event as an important one in which nursing has a significant role.

CONCLUSIONS

The concept of nursing formulated by Henderson in her definition of nursing and the fourteen components of basic nursing care is uncomplicated and self-explanatory. Therefore, it could be used as a guide for nursing practice by most without difficulties. Many of the ideas she presented continue to be used worldwide in both developed and undeveloped countries to guide nursing curricula and practice. This is validated by the demand for her ICN publication, which in 1972 was in its seventh printing.

If a suggestion can be made to improve Henderson's concept of nursing, it is the incorporation of theory. For example, it would be interesting to see how holism or general system theory might explain the relationship of the components of basic nursing care. Confirmation of whether or not the list of components are prioritized is needed to clarify what the nurse ought to do if the presenting problem is other than a physical one.

In view of the time in which Henderson published her definition of nursing, she deserves much credit as a leader in the development of nursing practice, education, and licensure. Her work ought to be considered a beginning and impetus for nurses to pursue the highest academic degree. This is critical for analyses of nursing practice and to identify and test the theoretical bases for patient care.

SUMMARY

In conclusion, Henderson provides the essence of what she believes is a definition of nursing. She states:

> I believe that the function the nurse performs is primarily an independent one—that of acting for the patient when he lacks knowledge, physical strength, or the will to act for himself as he would ordinarily act in health, or in carrying out prescribed therapy. This function is seen as complex and creative, as offering unlimited opportunity for the application of the physical, biological, and social sciences, and the development of skills based on them.[49]

REFERENCES

1.(a) Henderson, V. *The Nature of Nursing*, New York: The Macmillan Co., 1966.

1.(b) Henderson, V. *Basic Principles of Nursing Care*, Geneva: International Council of Nurses, 1960.

2.(a) Henderson, V. Preserving the Essence of Nursing in a Technological Age, Part I, *Nursing Times*, 1979, 75, 2012–13.

2.(b) Preserving the Essence of Nursing in a Technological Age, Part II, *Nursing Times*, 1979, 75, 2056–58.

2.(c) Henderson, V. The Concept of Nursing, *Journal of Advanced Nursing*, 1978, 3, 16–17.

2.(d) Henderson, V. The Nursing Process—Is the Title Right? *Journal of Advanced Nursing*, 1982, 7, 103–9.

2.(e) Henderson, V. The Essence of Nursing in High Technology, *Nursing Administration Quarterly*, 1985, 9, 1–9.

2.(f) Henderson, V. Nursing Process—A Critique, *Holistic Nursing Practice*, 1987, 1, 7–18.

3.   Henderson, *The Nature of Nursing*, p. 1.

4.   Ibid, 6.

5.   Ibid, 7.

6.(a) Harmer, B., & Henderson, V. *Textbook of the Principles and Practice of Nursing* (4th ed.), New York: The Macmillan Co., Inc., 1939.

6.(b) Safier, G. *Contemporary American Leaders in Nursing*, New York: McGraw-Hill, 1977, p. 119.

7. Henderson, *The Nature of Nursing*, p. 3.

8. ANA Statement on Auxiliary Personnel in Nursing Service, *The American Journal of Nursing*, 1962, *62*, 7.

9.(a) Harmer, B., & Henderson, V. *Textbook of the Principles and Practice of Nursing* (5th ed.), New York: Macmillan, 1955, p. 4.

9.(b) Nursing Development Conference Group, *Concept Formalization in Nursing: Process and Product*, Boston: Little, Brown, 1973, pp. 41–42.

10.(a) Harmer, B. *Textbook of the Principles and Practice of Nursing*, New York: Macmillan, 1922, p. 3.

10.(b) Nursing Development Conference Group, *Concept Formalization*, p. 40.

11. Henderson, *Basic Principles*, p. 5.

12. Henderson, *The Nature of Nursing*, pp. 16–17.

13. Ibid, 15.

14. Henderson, V., & Nite, G. *Principles and Practice of Nursing* (6th ed.), New York: Macmillan, 1978.

15. Henderson, *The Nature of Nursing*, p. 16.

16. Henderson, *Basic Principles*, p. 3.

17. Henderson, *The Nature of Nursing*, p. 11.

18. Harmer & Henderson, *Textbook of the Principles* (5th ed.), p. 33.

19. Henderson, *The Nature of Nursing*, pp. 68–69.

20. Ibid, 69.

21. Henderson, *Basic Principles*, p. 4.

22. Henderson, *The Nature of Nursing*, pp. 20–21.

23. Henderson, *Basic Principles*, p. 7.

24. Henderson, *The Nature of Nursing*, p. 38.

25. Henderson, V. Nursing—Yesterday and Tomorrow, *Nursing Times*, 1980, *76*, 905–7.

26. Ibid, 107.

27. Henderson, Nursing Process—A Critique, p. 8.

28. Ibid, 14.

29. Henderson, The Nursing Process—Is the Title Right? p. 108.

30. Henderson, Nursing Process—A Critique, p. 8.

31. Ibid, 9.

32. Henderson, The Nursing Process—Is the Title Right? p. 109.

33. Henderson, Nursing Process—A Critique, p. 8.

34. Henderson, *Basic Principles*, p. 19.

35. Ibid, 7.

36. Ibid, 11.

37. Ibid, 11, 42.

38. Ibid, 11.

39. Henderson, *The Nature of Nursing*, p. 21.

40. Ibid, 27.

41. Ibid, 16.

42. Henderson, *Basic Principles*, pp. 10–11.

43. Henderson, *The Nature of Nursing*, p. 27.

44. Maslow, A. *Motivation and Personality* (2nd ed), New York: Harper & Row, 1970.

45. Henderson, *The Nature of Nursing*, p. 24.
46. Henderson, V. We've Come a Long Way But What of the Direction? *Nursing Research*, 1977, *26*, 163–64.
47. Henderson, V. speech at History of Nursing Museum, Philadelphia, May, 1982.
48. Henderson, The Essence of Nursing in High Technology, pp. 1–9.
49. Henderson, *The Nature of Nursing*, p. 68.

BIBLIOGRAPHY

Campbell, C., Virginia Henderson: The Definitive Nurse, *Nursing Mirror*, 1985, *160*, 12.

Henderson, V., Health Records and Nursing, *Connecticut Nursing News*, 1985, *54*, 1, 4.

Henderson, V., Is the Study of History Rewarding for Nurses? *Society for Nursing History Gazette*, 1982, *2*, 1–2.

Henderson, V., Some Observations on Health Care by Health Services or Health Industries (Editorial), *Journal of Advanced Nursing*, 1986, *1*, 1–2.

Henderson, V. & Watt, S., Epidermolysis Bullosa, *Nursing Times*, 1983, *79*, 43–46.

Henderson, V. & Watt, S., 70+ and Going Strong, Virginia Henderson, A Nurse for All Ages, *Geriatric Nursing*, 1983, *4*, 58–59.

Henderson, V., and others, *Reference Resource for Research and Continuing Education in Nursing*. Kansas City, Mo.: American Nurses' Association Publication No. 6125, 1977.

McCarty, P. How Can Nurses Prepare for Year 2000? (A response from Virginia Henderson), *The American Nurse*, 1987, *19*, 3, 6.

Shamansky, S.L. CHN Revisited: A Conversation with Virginia Henderson, *Public Health Nursing*, 1964, *1*, 193–201.

Shamanski, S., Virginia Henderson: A National Treasure, *Focus Critical Care*, 1984, *11*, 60–61.

CHAPTER 6
Lydia E. Hall
Julia B. George*

Lydia E. Hall received her basic nursing education at York Hospital School of Nursing in York, Pennsylvania. Both her BS in Public Health Nursing and MA in teaching Natural Sciences are from Teachers College, Columbia University, New York.

Lydia Hall was the first director of the Loeb Center for Nursing and Rehabilitation and continued in that position until her death in 1969. Her experience in nursing spans the clinical, educational, research, and supervisory components. Her publications include several articles on the definition of nursing and quality of care. Lydia Hall put forth what she considered a basic philosophy of nursing upon which the nurse may base patient care. This philosophy is still used as a working reality at the Loeb Center for Nursing.

LOEB CENTER FOR NURSING AND REHABILITATION

Lydia Hall originated the philosophy of care of Loeb Center at Montefiore Hospital, Bronx, New York. Loeb Center opened in January 1963 to provide professional nursing care to persons who are past the acute stage of illness. The center's functioning concept is that the need for professional nursing care increases as the need for medical care decreases.

Those in need of continued professional care who are sixteen years of age or older and are no longer experiencing an acute biological disturbance are transferred from the acute care hospital to Loeb Center. Good candidates for care at Loeb are those who have a desire to come to Loeb, are recommended by their physicians, and possess a favorable potential for recovery and return to the community.

Physically, Loeb Center has a capacity of eighty beds and is attached to Montefiore Hospital. The rooms are arranged with patient comfort and maneuverability as first priority. The patients also have access to a large communal dining room. The primary care givers are registered professional

---

*Gratitude is expressed to Kathleen Hale for her contributions to this chapter in the first edition.

nurses. Nonpatient care activities are supplied by messenger–attendants and ward secretaries.

> Loeb's primary purpose was and is to demonstrate that high quality nursing care given by registered nurses, in a non-directive setting, offers a supportive setting to people in the post-acute phase of their illness that enables them to recover sooner, and to leave the center able to cope with themselves and what they must face in the future.[1]

To create a nondirective setting, there are very few rules or routines, no schedules, and no dictated mealtimes or specified visiting hours.[2] The nurses at Loeb strive to help the patient determine and clarify goals and, with the patient, work out ways to achieve the goals at the individual's pace, consistent with the medical treatment plan and congruent with the patient's sense of self.[3]

LYDIA HALL'S THEORY OF NURSING

Lydia Hall presents her theory of nursing visually by drawing three interlocking circles, each circle presenting a particular aspect of nursing. The circles represent *care, core,* and *cure.*

The Care Circle
The care circle (Fig. 6–1) represents the nurturing component of nursing and is exclusive to nursing. Nurturing involves using the factors that make up the concept of mothering (care and comfort of the person) and provide for teaching–learning activities.

The professional nurse provides bodily care for the patient and helps

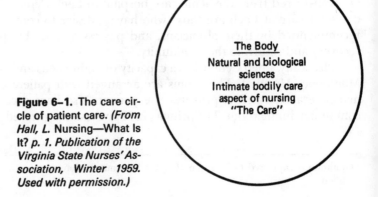

Figure 6–1. The care circle of patient care. *(From Hall, L. Nursing—What Is It? p. 1. Publication of the Virginia State Nurses' Association, Winter 1959. Used with permission.)*

The Body
Natural and biological sciences
Intimate bodily care aspect of nursing
"The Care"

complete such basic daily biological functions as eating, bathing, and dressing. When providing this care, the nurse's goal is the comfort of the patient.

Providing care for a patient at the basic needs level presents the nurse and patient with an opportunity for closeness. When this is developed to the fullest, the patient can share and explore feelings with the nurse. This opportunity to explore feelings represents the teaching–learning aspect of nurturing.

When functioning in the care circle, the nurse applies knowledge of the natural and biological sciences to provide a strong theoretical base for nursing implementations. In interactions with the patient the nurse's role needs to be clearly defined. A strong theory base allows the nurse to maintain a professional status rather than a mothering status, while at the same time incorporating closeness and nurturance in giving care. The patient views the nurse as a potential comforter, one who provides care and comfort through the laying on of hands.

The Core Circle

The core circle (Fig. 6–2) of patient care involves the therapeutic use of self and is shared with other members of the health team. The professional nurse, by developing an interpersonal relationship with the patient, is able to help the patient verbally express feelings regarding the disease process. Through such expression the patient is able to gain self-identity and further develop toward maturity.

The professional nurse, by use of the reflective technique (acting as a mirror for the patient), helps the patient look at and explore feelings regarding his or her current health status and related potential changes in life style. The nurse uses a freely offered closeness to help the patient bring into awareness the verbal and nonverbal messages being sent to others. Motivations are discovered through the process of bringing into awareness

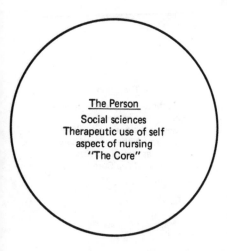

The Person
Social sciences
Therapeutic use of self
aspect of nursing
"The Core"

Figure 6–2. The core circle of patient care. *(From Hall, L. Nursing—What Is It? p. 1. Used with permission.)*

the feelings being experienced. The patient is now able to make conscious decisions based on understood and accepted feelings and motivations. The motivation and energy necessary for healing exist within the patient rather than the health care team.

> To look at and listen to self is often too difficult without the help of a significant figure (nurturer) who has learned how to hold up a mirror and sounding board to invite the behaver to look and listen to himself. If he accepts the invitation, he will explore the concerns in his acts and as he listens to his exploration through the reflection of the nurse, he may uncover in sequence his difficulties, the problem area, his problem and eventually the threat which is dictating his out-of-control behavior.[4]

The Cure Circle

The cure circle of patient care (Fig. 6–3) is based in the pathological and therapeutic sciences and is shared with other members of the health team. The professional nurse helps the patient and family through the medical, surgical, and rehabilitative prescriptions made by the physician. During this aspect of nursing care the nurse is an active advocate of the patient.

The nurse's role during the cure aspect is different from the care circle since many of the nurse's actions take on a negative quality of avoidance of pain rather than a positive quality of comforting. This is negative in the sense that the patient views the nurse as a potential cause of pain, involved in such actions as administering injections, versus the potential comforter who provided care and comfort.

Interaction of the Three Aspects of Nursing

Since Hall emphasizes the importance of a total person approach, it is important that the three aspects of nursing (see Fig. 6–4) are not viewed as functioning independently but rather as interrelated. The three aspects

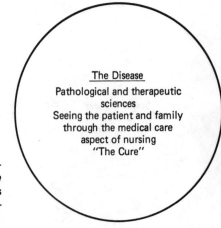

The Disease
Pathological and therapeutic sciences
Seeing the patient and family through the medical care aspect of nursing
"The Cure"

Figure 6–3. The cure circle of patient care. *(From Hall, L. Nursing—What Is It? p. 1. Used with permission.)*

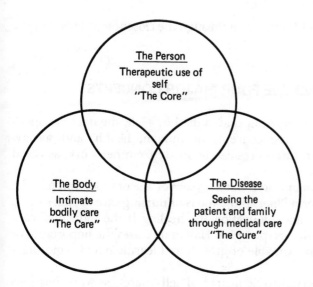

Figure 6–4. Hall's three aspects of nursing.

interact and the circles representing them change size depending on the patient's total course of progress.

In the philosophy of Loeb Center, the professional nurse functions most therapeutically when patients have entered the second stage of their hospital stay (i.e., they are recuperating and are past the acute stage of illness).

During this recuperation stage, the care and core aspects are the most prominent, and the cure aspect is less prominent (see Fig. 6–5). The size of the circles represents the degree to which the patient is progressing in each of the three areas. The professional nurse at this time is able to help the

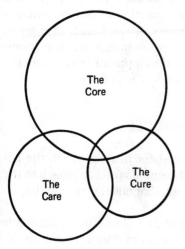

Figure 6–5. Care and core predominate.

patient reach the core of his problem through the closeness provided by the care aspect of nursing.

HALL'S THEORY AND THE FOUR MAJOR CONCEPTS

Although the concept of nursing is identified by Hall, she does not speak directly to the other three concepts of human, health, and society-environment. However, inferences can be made from her work, as noted below.

The *individual* human who is sixteen years of age or older and past the acute stage of a long-term illness is the focus of nursing care in Hall's work. The source of energy and motivation for healing is the individual care recipient, not the health care provider. Hall emphasizes the importance of the individual as unique, capable of growth and learning, and requiring a total person approach.

Health can be inferred to be a state of self-awareness with conscious selection of behaviors that are optimal for that individual. Hall stresses the need to help the person explore the meaning of his or her behavior to identify and overcome problems through developing self-identity and maturity.

The concept of *society/environment* is dealt with in relation to the individual. Hall is credited with developing the concept of Loeb Center because she assumed the hospital environment during treatment of acute illness creates a difficult psychological experience for the ill individual.[5] Loeb Center focuses on providing an environment that is conducive to self-development. The focus of the action of nurses is the individual, so that any actions taken in relation to society or environment would be for the purpose of assisting the individual in attaining a personal goal.

Nursing is identified as consisting of participation in the care, core, and cure aspects of patient care. Care is the sole function of nurses, whereas core and cure are shared with other members of the health care team. However, the major purpose of care is to achieve an interpersonal relationship with the individual that will facilitate the development of core, i.e., the development of self-identity and self-direction by the patient.

HALL'S THEORY AND THE NURSING PROCESS

Hall places the motivation and energy needed for healing within the patient. This aspect of her theory influences the nurse's total approach to the five phases of the nursing process: assessment, diagnosis, planning, implementation, and evaluation.

The *assessment* phase involves collection of data about the health status of the individual. According to Hall, the process of data collection is directed for the benefit of the patient rather than for the benefit of the nurse. Data collection should be directed toward increasing the patient's self-awareness. Through use of observation and reflection, the nurse is able to assist the patient in becoming aware of both verbal and nonverbal behaviors. In the individual, increased awareness of feelings and needs in relation to health status increases his or her ability for self-healing.

The assessment phase also pertains to guiding the patient through the cure aspect of nursing. The health team collects biological data (physical and laboratory) to help the patient and family understand and progress through the medical regimen.

The second phase is the *nursing diagnosis,* or statement of the patient's need or problem area. How a nurse envisions the nursing role will influence the interpretation of assessment data and conclusions reached. Viewing the patient as the power for self-healing will direct conclusions differently than if the healing power rests in the physician or nurse. The patient will be the one in control.

Planning involves setting priorities and mutually establishing patient-centered goals. The patient will decide what is of highest priority and also what goals are desirable.

The core is involved in planning. The role of the nurse is to use reflection to help the patient become aware of and understand needs, feelings, and motivations. Once motivations are clarified, Hall indicates the patient is the best person to set goals and arrange priorities. The nurse seeks to increase patient awareness and to support decision making based on the patient's new level of awareness. The nurse works with the patient to help keep the goals consistent with the medical prescription. The nurse needs to draw on a knowledge base in the social and scientific areas to present the patient with creative alternatives from which to choose.

Implementation involves the actual institution of the plan of care. This phase is the actual giving of nursing care. In the care circle, the nurse works *with* the patient, helping with bathing, dressing, eating, and other care and comfort needs.

The nurse also helps the patient and family through the cure aspect of nursing. He or she works with the patient and family to help them understand and implement the medical plan.

The professional nurse uses a "permissive non-directive teaching–learning approach" to implement nursing care, thus helping the patient reach the established goals.[5] This includes "helping the patient with his feelings, providing requested information and supporting patient-made decisions."[6]

Evaluation is the process of assessing the patient's progress toward the health goals. The evaluation phase of the process is directed toward deciding whether or not the patient is successful in reaching the established goals. The following questions would apply to the use of Hall's theory in the evaluation phase:

1. Is the patient learning "who he is, where he wants to go, and how he wants to get there?"[7]
2. Is the patient learning to understand and explore the feelings that underlie behavior?
3. Is the nurse helping the patient see motivations more clearly?
4. Are the patient's goals congruent with the medical regime? Is the patient successful in meeting the goals?
5. Is the patient physically more comfortable?

Whether or not a person is growing in self-awareness regarding his or her feelings and motivations can be recognized through changes in his or her outward behavior.

HALL'S WORK AND THE CHARACTERISTICS OF A THEORY

Hall's work can be compared to the characteristics of a theory as presented in Chapter 1.

1. Theories can interrelate concepts in such a way as to create a different way of looking at a particular phenomenon. The use of the terms *care, core,* and *cure* is unique to Hall. She interrelated these concepts and, in 1963, provided a different way of looking at the phenomenon of care of the individual with a long-term illness, which was an acute social problem of the time. Although other developments in health care have altered the need to some extent, her ideas are still relevant and useful, particularly if some of the limitations she imposed are removed. For example, care, core, and cure needs exist in acute and ambulatory settings and in individuals younger than sixteen.

2. Theories must be logical in nature. On first reading, Hall's work appears to be completely and simply logical. However, closer scrutiny reveals that although Hall indicates that care, the bodily laying on of hands, is the only aspect that is solely nursing—implying that it is the major focus for nursing, her major emphasis is on core. The care aspect is a means to achieving core rather than an end in itself.[8] Although this is not illogical, the initial impression is not the true logic of the work.

3. Theories should be relatively simple yet generalizable. Hall's work is simple in its presentation. However, the openness and flexibility required for its application may not be so simple for nurses whose personality, educational preparation, and experience have not prepared them to function with minimal structure. This and the self-imposed age and illness requirements limit the generalizability. Although the need for structure is a personal characteristic of the nurse, the limitations of age and stage of illness do not necessarily apply outside of Loeb Center.

4. Theories are the bases for hypotheses that can be tested, and **5. Theories contribute to and assist in increasing the general body of knowl-**

edge within the discipline through the research implemented to validate them. These two characteristics are certainly true for Hall's work and have been demonstrated in the research conducted to evaluate the effectiveness of Loeb Center. This research was conducted at Mrs. Hall's insistence, in spite of the enthusiastic acceptance of Hall's philosophy by those in the Montefiore health care community.[9] This research is evidence that hypotheses can be developed and tested. In addition, the sharing of a report about the Loeb Center in a Congressional hearing is evidence of an increase in the general body of knowledge.[10]

6. Theories can be utilized by practitioners to guide and improve their practice. If no other characteristic of a theory was met by Hall's work, Loeb Center is an ideal demonstration of this characteristic. Hall's work was designed for practice and has been implemented by practitioners successfully for over two decades.

7. Theories must be consistent with other validated theories, laws, and principles but will leave open unanswered questions that need to be investigated. Hall recognized the importance of knowledge of validated theories, laws, and principles. She indicated the theoretical base for each of the aspects of patient care. The care aspect is based in the natural and biological sciences, core in the social sciences, and cure in the pathological and therapeutic sciences. The specific applications of these sciences provide a source of unanswered questions to be investigated.

Hall's work presents interrelated concepts in a way that provides a new view of a particular phenomenon. It is logical in nature, simpler in presentation than application but capable of being generalized, can be the basis of testable hypotheses, has led to research, is used by practitioners to guide practice, and is consistent with other validated theories, laws, and principles. Thus her work may be considered a theory.

APPLICATION AND LIMITATIONS OF THE THEORY

In reviewing Hall's theory of nursing there are several areas that limit its application to patient care.

The first of these areas is the stage of illness. Hall applies her ideas of nursing to a patient who has passed the acute stage of biological stress; i.e., the patient who is experiencing the acute stage of illness is not included in Hall's approach to nursing care. However, it is possible to apply the care, core, and cure ideas to the care of those who are acutely ill. The acutely ill individual often needs care in relation to basic needs; he or she also needs core awareness of what is going on and cure understanding of the plan of medical care.

A second limiting factor is age. Hall refers only to adult patients in the second stage of their illness. This eliminates all younger patients. Based on this theory, Loeb Center admits only patients sixteen years of age and older.

However, it would be possible to apply Hall's theory with younger individuals. Certainly adolescents younger than sixteen are capable of seeking self-identity.

A third limiting factor is the description of how to help a person toward self-awareness. The only tool of therapeutic communication discussed is reflection. By inference, all other techniques of therapeutic communication are eliminated. This emphasis on reflection arises from the belief that both the problem and the solution lie in the individual, and the nurse's function is to help the individual find them. But reflection is not always the most effective technique to be used. Other techniques such as active listening and nonverbal support may be used to facilitate the development of self-identity.

Fourth, the family is mentioned only in the cure circle. This means the nursing contact with families is used only in regard to the patient's own medical care. It does not allow for helping a family increase awareness of the family's self.

Finally, Hall's theory relates only to those who are ill. This would indicate no nursing contact with healthy individuals, families, or communities, and it negates the concept of health maintenance and health care to prevent illness.

Basically, Hall's theory can be readily applied within the confines of the definition of adults past the acute stage of illness. However, this is too confining for a total view of nursing, which includes working with individuals, families, and communities throughout the life cycle and in varying states of health.

However, it should be noted that the nurse who uses Hall's theory will function in a manner similar to the method of assignment known as *primary nursing*. Considering that Hall instituted Loeb Center in the early 1960s, her ideas certainly provided leadership and innovation in nursing practice. She is also deserving of praise for having the courage to create a new environment in which to put her ideas into practice.

SUMMARY

Although Lydia Hall first presented her theory of nursing during the late 1950s and early 1960s, Loeb Center for Nursing and Rehabilitation is still using Hall's theory to provide patient care today.

Hall's theory of nursing involves three interlocking circles, each representing one aspect of nursing. The care aspect represents intimate bodily care of the patient. The core aspect deals with the innermost feelings and motivations of the patient. The cure aspect tells how the nurse helps the patient and family through the medical aspect of care. The main tool the nurse uses to help the patient realize his or her motivations and to grow in self-awareness is that of reflection.

Of the major concepts, only nursing is defined as the function necessary to carry out care, core, and cure. Hall presents a philosophical view of humans as having the energy and motivation for self-awareness and growth. Definitions of health and society or environment must be inferred.

Her work may be considered a theory since it meets each of the characteristics of theories presented in Chapter 1.

Lydia Hall's theory may be used in the nursing process. The core, care, and cure aspects are all applicable to each phase of the nursing process. The limitations of Hall's theory—illness orientation, age, family contact restrictions, and use of reflection only—can be overcome by taking a broader view of care, core, and cure and by emphasizing the aspect that is most appropriate for a particular situation.

REFERENCES

1. Bowar-Ferres, S. Loeb Center and Its Philosophy of Nursing, *The American Journal of Nursing*, 1975, *75*, 810.
2. Ibid, 814.
3. Ibid, 813.
4. Hall, L. Another View of Nursing Care and Quality, address given at Catholic University Workshop, Washington, D.C., 1965.
5. Bowar-Ferres, Loeb Center and its Philosophy of Nursing, p. 813.
6. Brown, E.L. *Nursing Reconsidered: A Study of Change, Part I: The Professional Role in Institutional Nursing*, Philadelphia: Lippincott, 1970, p. 159.
7. Bowar-Ferres, Loeb Center and Its Philosophy of Nursing, p. 813.
8. Stevens, B.J. *Nursing Theory*, Boston: Little, Brown, 1979, pp. 19–28.
9. Brown, *Nursing Reconsidered*, pp. 164–165.
10. Loeb Center for Nursing and Rehabilitation Project Report, *Congressional Record*, May–June 1963, pp. 1515–62.

BIBLIOGRAPHY

Alfano, G., Administration Means Working with Nurses, *The American Journal of Nursing*, 1964, *64*, 83–85.

Alfano, G., Loeb Center, *Nursing Clinics of North America*, 1969, *4*, 3.

Bernardin, E., Loeb Center—As the Staff Nurse Sees It, *The American Journal of Nursing*, 1964, *64*, 85–86.

Englert, B., How a Staff Nurse Perceives Her Role at Loeb Center, *Nursing Clinics of North America*, 1978, *6*.

Hall, L., Quality of Nursing Care, *Public Health News*, New Jersey State Department of Health, June 1955, *36* (6), 212–215.

Hall, L., *Nursing—What Is It?* Publication of the Virginia State Nurses Assn., Winter 1959.

Hall, L., A Center for Nursing, *Nursing Outlook*, 1963, *2*, (1), 805–806.

Hall, L., Can Nursing Care Hasten Recovery? *The American Journal of Nursing*, 1964, *64*, 6.

Hall, L., The Loeb Center for Nursing and Rehabilitation at Montefiore Hospital and Medical Center, *International Journal of Nursing Studies*, 1969, *6*, 81–95.

Isler, C., New Concepts in Nursing Therapy, More Care as the Patient Improves, *R.N.*, 1964, *27*, 58–70.

CHAPTER 7

Dorothea E. Orem

Peggy Coldwell Foster
Nancy P. Janssens

Dorothea E. Orem, MSNEd, DSc, RN, began her nursing education at Providence Hospital School of Nursing in Washington, D.C. After graduating in the early 1930s, she obtained her Bachelor of Science in nursing education in 1939 and her Master of Science in nursing education in 1945 from the Catholic University of America. During her professional nursing career, she has worked as a staff nurse, private duty nurse, nurse educator and administrator, and nurse consultant.

Since 1970, Orem has worked as a consultant in nursing and nursing education with the firm of Orem and Shields in Chevy Chase, Md. She has received several national awards including an honorary Doctor of Science degree from Georgetown University, Washington, D.C. in 1976, and the Catholic University of America's Alumni Achievement Award for Nursing Theory in 1980.

> *If you give a man a fish he will have a single meal;*
> *If you teach him how to fish he will eat all his life.*
> *—Kuan Tzer*

During 1958–59, as a consultant to the Office of Education, Department of Health, Education, and Welfare, Dorothea E. Orem participated in a project to improve practical (vocational) nurse training. This work stimulated her to consider the question, "What condition exists in a person when that person or others determine that that person should be under nursing care?" Her answer encompassed the idea that a nurse is "another self." This evolved into her nursing concept of "self-care."[1] That is, when able, individuals care for themselves. When the person is unable to provide self-care, then the nurse provides assistance.

In 1959, Orem's concept of nursing as the provision of self-care was first published.[2] In 1965, she joined with several faculty members from the Catholic University of America to form a Nursing Model Committee. In 1968, a portion of the Nursing Model Committee, including Orem, continued their work through the Nursing Development Conference Group (NDCG). This group was formed to produce a conceptual framework for nursing and to establish the discipline of nursing. The NDCG published *Concept Formalization in Nursing: Process and Product* in 1973 and 1979.[3a,3b]

Orem further developed her nursing concepts of "self-care" and in 1971 published *Nursing: Concepts of Practice*.[4] The second and third editions of this book were published in 1980 and 1985. The first edition focused on the individual. The second edition was expanded to include multiperson units (families, groups, and communities). The third edition has evolved to present Orem's general theory of nursing which is constituted from three related theoretical constructs: (1) the theory of self-care, (2) the theory of self-care deficits, and (3) the theory of nursing systems.[5]

OREM'S GENERAL THEORY OF NURSING

According to Orem, "nursing has as its special concern *the individual's need for self-care action and the provision and management of it on a continuous basis in order to sustain life and health, recover from disease or injury, and cope with their effects*."[6] In her third edition of *Nursing: Concepts of Practice*, Orem develops her general theory of nursing in three related parts. These parts are: (1) self-care, (2) self-care deficit, and (3) nursing systems.

The Theory of Self-Care
The theory of self-care includes self-care, self-care agency, and therapeutic self-care demand as well as self-care requisites. *Self-care* is the "practice of activities that individuals initiate and perform on their own behalf in maintaining life, health, and well-being."[7] "Self-care . . . effectively performed contributes in specific ways to human structural integrity, human functioning, and human development."[8] *Self-care agency* is a human ability which is "the ability for engaging in self-care."[9]

"The individual's abilities to engage in self-care . . . are conditioned by age, developmental state, life experience, sociocultural orientation, health, and available resources."[10] "Normally, adults voluntarily care for themselves. Infants, children, the aged, the ill, and the disabled require complete care or assistance with self-care activities."[11] The *therapeutic self-care demand* is the "totality of self-care actions to be performed for some duration in order to meet self-care requisites by using valid methods and related sets of operations and actions."[12]

Orem presents three categories of *self-care requisites* or requirements as: (1) universal, (2) developmental, and (3) health deviation. Self-care requisites can be defined as actions directed toward the provision of self-care. *Universal self-care requisites* are associated with life processes and the maintenance of the integrity of human structure and functioning. They are common to all human beings during all stages of the life cycle and should be viewed as interrelated factors, each affecting the others. A common term for these requisites are the activities of daily living. Orem identifies self-care requisites as[13]:

1. The maintenance of a sufficient intake of air.
2. The maintenance of a sufficient intake of water.
3. The maintenance of a sufficient intake of food.
4. The provision of care associated with elimination processes and excrements.
5. The maintenance of a balance between activity and rest.
6. The maintenance of a balance between solitude and social interaction.
7. The prevention of hazards to human life, human functioning, and human well-being.
8. The promotion of human functioning and development within social groups in accord with human potential, known human limitations, and the human desire to be normal. *Normalcy* is used in the sense of that which is essentially human and that which is in accord with the genetic and constitutional characteristics and the talents of individuals.

Developmental self-care requisites are "either specialized expressions of universal self-care requisites that have been particularized for developmental processes or they are new requisites derived from a condition . . . or associated with an event."[14a] Examples of this would be adjusting to the loss of a significant other, adjusting to a new job, or adjusting to body changes such as facial lines or gray hair.

Health deviation self-care is required in conditions of illness, injury, or disease or may result from medical measures required to diagnose and correct the condition (e.g., right upper quadrant abdominal pain when greasy foods are eaten, or learning to walk using crutches following the casting of a fractured leg.) The health deviation self-care requisites are[14b]:

1. Seeking and securing appropriate medical assistance . . .
2. Being aware of and attending to the effects and results of pathologic conditions and states . . .
3. Effectively carrying out medically prescribed . . . measures . . .
4. Being aware of and attending to or regulating the discomforting or deleterious effects of prescribed medical care measures . . .
5. Modifying the self-concept (and self-image) in accepting oneself as being in a particular state of health and in need of specific forms of health care
6. Learning to live with the effects of pathological conditions and states and the effects of medical diagnostic and treatment measures in a lifestyle that promotes continued personal development.

In the theory of self-care, Orem explains *what* is meant by self-care and lists the various factors that affect its provision. In the self-care deficit theory, she specifies *when* nursing is needed to assist the individual in the provision of self-care.

The Theory of Self-Care Deficit
The theory of self-care deficit is the core of Orem's general theory of nursing because it delineates when nursing is needed. Nursing is required

when an adult (or in the case of a dependent, the parent or guardian) is incapable or limited in the provision of continuous effective self-care. Nursing may be provided if the "care abilities are less than those required for meeting a known self-care demand . . . [or] self-care or dependent-care abilities exceed or are equal to those required for meeting the current self-care demand but a future deficit relationship can be foreseen because of predictable decreases in care abilities, qualitative or quantitative increases in the care demand, or both"[15]; when individuals need "to incorporate newly prescribed, complex self-care measures into their self-care systems, the performance of which requires specialized knowledge and skills to be acquired through training and experience"[16]; or the individual needs help "in recovering from disease or injury, or in coping with their effects."[17] It is important to note that the first category includes universal, developmental, and health-deviation self-care needs while the other categories focus on health-deviation self-care.

Orem identifies five methods of helping. These are[18]:

1. Acting for or doing for another
2. Guiding another
3. Supporting another (physically or psychologically)
4. Providing an environment that promotes personal development in relation to becoming able to meet present or future demands for action
5. Teaching another

The nurse may help the individual by using any or all of these methods to provide assistance with self-care.

Orem presents a model to show the relationship between her concepts (Fig. 7–1). From this model, it can be seen that at a given time an individual has specific self-care abilities as well as therapeutic self-care demands. If there are more demands than abilities, nursing is needed. The activities in which nurses engage when they provide nursing care can be used to describe the domain of nursing. Orem has identified five areas of activity for nursing practice[19]:

1. Entering into and maintaining nurse–patient relationships with individuals, families, or groups until patients can legitimately be discharged from nursing
2. Determining if and how patients can be helped through nursing
3. Responding to patients' requests, desires, and needs for nurse contacts and assistance
4. Prescribing, providing, and regulating direct help to patients and their significant others in the form of nursing
5. Coordinating and integrating nursing with the patient's daily living, other health care needed or being received, and social and educational services needed or being received

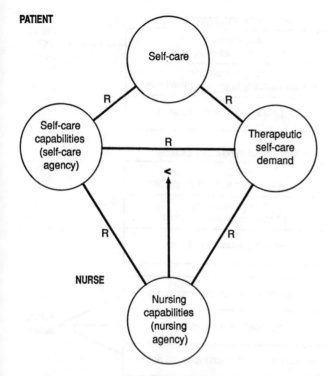

Figure 7–1. A conceptual framework for nursing (R = relationship; < = deficit relationship, current or projected). *(Used with permission from Orem, D.E. Nursing: Concepts of Practice (2nd ed.), New York: McGraw-Hill, p. 32.)*

Self-care has been defined and the need for nursing explained in the first and second theories. In Orem's third theory of nursing systems, she outlines *how* the patient's self-care needs will be met by the nurse, the patient, or both.

The Theory of Nursing Systems

The nursing system, designed by the nurse, is based on the self-care needs and abilities of the patient to perform self-care activities. Orem has identified three classifications of nursing systems to meet the self-care requisites of the patient (see Fig. 7–2). These systems are: the wholly compensatory system, the partly compensatory system, and the supportive–educative system.

The design and elements of the nursing system define "(1) the scope of the nursing responsibility in health care situations, (2) the general and specific roles of nurses and patients, (3) reasons for nurses' relationships with patients, and (4) the kinds of actions to be performed and the performance patterns and nurses' and patients actions in regulating patients' self-care agency and in meeting their therapeutic self-care demand."[20]

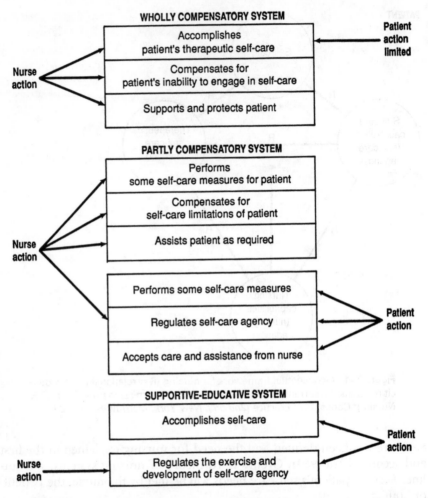

Figure 7–2. Basic nursing systems. *(Adapted with permission from Orem, D.E.* Nursing: Concepts of Practice *(3rd ed.), New York: McGraw-Hill, 1985, p. 153.)*

The *wholly compensatory nursing system* is represented by a situation in which the individual is unable "to engage in those self-care actions requiring self-directed and controlled ambulation and manipulative movement or the medical prescription to refrain from such activity . . . Persons with these limitations are socially dependent on others for their continued existence and well-being."[21] Subtypes of the wholly compensatory system are nursing systems for people who are: "1) unable to engage in any form of deliberate action, for example, persons in coma 2) . . . aware and who may be able to make observations, judgments, and decisions about self-care and other matters but cannot or should not perform actions requiring ambulation or manipulative movements 3) . . . unable to attend to themselves and make reasoned judgments and decisions about self-care and other matters but who can be ambulatory and may be able to perform some measures of self-care with continuous guidance and supervision."[21] Examples of persons in the second subtype could include those with C3–C4 vertebral fractures and, the third subtype, persons with advanced senility or some forms of mental retardation.

The *partly compensatory nursing system* is represented by a situation in which "both nurse and patient perform care measures or other actions involving manipulative tasks or ambulation . . . [Either] the patient or the nurse may have the major role in the performance of care measures."[22] An example of a person needing nursing care in the partly compensatory system would be an individual who has had recent abdominal surgery. This patient might be able to wash his or her face and brush his or her teeth but needs the nurse for help in ambulating and in changing the surgical dressing.

The third nursing system is the *supportive–educative system*. In this system, the person "is able to perform or can and should learn to perform required measures of externally or internally oriented therapeutic self-care but cannot do so without assistance."[22] This is also known as a supportive–developmental system.[22] In this system the patient is doing all of his self-care. The "patient's requirements for help are confined to decision making, behavior control, and acquiring knowledge and skills."[22] The nurse's role, then, is to promote the patient as a self-care agent. An example of a person in this system would be a sixteen-year-old who is requesting birth control information.

Orem states that "one or more of the three types (of systems) may be used with a single patient."[23] For example, a woman in labor may move from a supportive–educative system in early labor to a partly compensatory system as her labor advances. If she requires a cesarean delivery, her care might require her to be in a wholly compensatory system. She would then progress to a partly compensatory system as she recovers from the anesthetic. Later, as she prepares to go home, a supportive–educative system would again be appropriate.

OREM'S THEORY AND THE FOUR MAJOR CONCEPTS

Orem discusses each of the four major concepts of human beings, health, society, and nursing in her work. *"Human beings* are distinguished from other living things by their capacity (1) to reflect upon themselves and their environment, (2) to symbolize what they experience, and (3) to use symbolic creations (ideas, words) in thinking, in communicating, and in guiding efforts to do and to make things that are beneficial for themselves or others."[24] Integrated human functioning includes physical, psychological, interpersonal, and social aspects. Orem believes that individuals have the potential for learning and development. The way an individual meets his or her self-care needs is not instinctual but is a learned behavior. Factors that affect learning include: age, mental capacity, culture, society, and the emotional state of the individual. If the individual cannot learn self-care measures, others must learn the care and provide it.

In the third edition of *Nursing: Concepts of Practice,* Orem considers human beings from two different perspectives. The first is as persons viewed as moving "toward maturation and achievement of the individual's human potential . . . *Self-realization* and *personality* are terms used at times to refer to the process of personalization."[25] The second perspective "focuses on structural and functional differentiation within the unity that is a human being . . . developed by various human and life sciences . . . [including] biochemistry, biophysics, human anatomy and human physiology, . . . psychology, psychophysiology and social psychology."[25] She emphasizes, however, that both perspectives need to be integrated for effective nursing.

Orem supports the World Health Organization's definition of *health* as the state of physical, mental, and social well-being and not merely the absence of disease or infirmity. She states that "the physical, psychological, interpersonal and social aspects of health are inseparable in the individual."[26] Orem also presents health based on the concept of preventive health care. This health care includes the promotion and maintenance of health (primary prevention), the treatment of disease or injury (secondary prevention), and the prevention of complications (tertiary prevention).

About *nursing,* Orem states:

> In modern society, adults are expected to be self-reliant and responsible for themselves and for the well-being of their dependents. Most social groups further accept that persons who are helpless, sick, aged, handicapped, or otherwise deprived should be helped to attain or regain responsibility within their existing capacities. Thus, both self-help and help to others are valued by society as desirable activities. Nursing as a specific type of human service is based on both values. In most communities people see nursing as a desirable and necessary service.[27]

Orem speaks to several factors related to the concept of nursing. These are the art and prudence of nursing, nursing as a service, role theory related to nursing, and technologies in nursing. The art of nursing includes "making a comprehensive determination of the reasons why people can be helped through nursing."[28] These decisions require a theoretical base in nursing disciplines and in the sciences, arts, and humanities. This base directs decisions when designing nursing systems within the nursing process. "*Nursing prudence* is the quality of nurses that enables them (1) to seek and take counsel in new or difficult nursing situations, (2) to make correct judgments. . . , (3) to decide to act in a particular way, and (4) to take action."[29] The development of the individual nurse's art and prudence is affected by unique life and nursing experiences.

Orem further defines nursing as "human service . . . a mode of helping men, women, and children and not a tangible commodity."[30] "Nursing
is deliberate action, . . . a function of the practical intelligence of nurses, . . .
to bring about humanely desirable conditions in persons and their environments . . . Nursing is distinguished from other human services . . . by the
way in which it focuses on human beings."[31] The "specialized abilities that
enable [nurses] to provide [nursing] care to individuals or multiperson
units, when conceptualized as a unit, is termed nursing agency."[32]

The nurse's and the patient's roles define the expected behaviors for
each in the specific nursing situation. Various factors that influence the
expected role behaviors are culture, environment, age, sex, the health setting, and finances. The roles of nurse and patient are complementary. That
is, a certain behavior of the patient elicits a certain response in the nurse,
and vice versa. Both work together to accomplish the goal of self-care.

In the nurse–patient relationship, the nurse or patient may experience role conflict since each is performing concurrent roles; for example,
the patient also has expected behaviors from his roles as father, husband,
cub scout leader, soccer coach, and librarian. Thus, the conflict in the
behaviors required for the various roles may affect the performance of
self-care.

It is important to note that although Orem recognizes that specialized
technologies are usually developed by members of the health professions,
she emphasizes the need for social and interpersonal dimensions in nursing. She states:

> A technology is systematized information about a process or a method for
> affecting some desired result through deliberate practical endeavor, with
> or without the use of materials or instruments.[33]

Two categories of technologies used in nursing are social or interpersonal
technologies and regulatory technologies.

> *Social and interpersonal technologies* include: (1) communication adjusted to
> age and developmental state, to health state, and to sociocultural orienta-
> tion; (2) bringing about and maintaining interpersonal, intragroup, or
> intergroup relations for coordination of effort; (3) bringing about and
> maintaining therapeutic relations in light of psychosocial modes of func-
> tioning in health and disease; and (4) giving human assistance adapted to
> human needs and action abilities and limitations. *Regulatory technologies*
> include: (1) maintaining and promoting life processes, (2) regulating psy-
> chophysiological modes of functioning in health and disease, (3) promot-
> ing human growth and development, and (4) regulating position and
> movement in space.[33]

The effective integration of social and interpersonal technologies with regulatory technologies promotes quality professional nursing.

OREM'S THEORY AND THE NURSING PROCESS

Orem's approach to the nursing process presents a method to determine the self-care deficits and then to define the roles of the person or nurse to meet the self-care demands. Table 7–1 compares the nursing process presented in Chapter 2 with Orem's nursing process.

The steps of Orem's nursing process may be summarized as follows[34]:

Step 1: The initial and continuing determination of why a person should be under nursing care.
Step 2: The designing of a system of nursing . . . [and] planning for the delivery of nursing according to the designed system . . .
Step 3: The initiation, conduction, and control of assisting actions to: (1) compensate for the patient's self-care limitations . . . (2) overcome when possible self-care limitations . . . and (3) foster and protect the patient's self-care abilities.

These three steps are considered by Orem to be the technical component of the nursing process. Orem emphasizes that the technological component "must be coordinated with interpersonal and social processes within nursing situations."[34]

The following example will demonstrate the use of Orem's model and the nursing process (see Tables 7–2 and 7–3):

Situation. Ms. M, a well-groomed university faculty member of Italian Catholic descent, is 48 years old, 5 feet 2 inches, and weighs 175 pounds She smokes one and a half packs of cigarettes per day. She was very happily married for 25 years and has been widowed for six months. She and her husband enjoyed social activities, including playing bridge, gourmet cooking, and collecting antiques. She has not participated in any of these activities since her husband's death because of lack of interest and energy. Currently, she engages in no regular exercise, eats mainly fast-foods during her 12-hour working day, and eats a late evening meal before retiring.

TABLE 7–1. COMPARISON OF OREM'S NURSING PROCESS AND THE NURSING PROCESS

Nursing Process[a]	Orem's Nursing Process
1. Assessment	Step 1. Diagnosis and prescription; Determine why nursing
2. Nursing diagnosis	is needed. Analyze and interpret—make judgments
3. Plans with	regarding care.
scientific rationale	Step 2. Design of a nursing system and plan for delivery of
4. Implementation	care.
5. Evaluation	Step 3. Production and management of nursing systems.

[a]Five-step process outlined in Chapter 2 of this text.

Ms. M's mother died of a stroke and her father had a heart attack at age 50. During her annual physical two weeks ago, her vital signs were 138/86, P 92, R 30, T 98.4. Her laboratory values were all within normal limits except a blood cholesterol of 280 mg. Her physician advised her to lose 40 pounds, but recognizes that she has inadequate knowledge of basic nutrition and has not been motivated to lose weight. He foresees potential problems related to cardiovascular disease.

Step 1. Orem defines Step 1 as the diagnosis and prescription phase, determining if nursing is needed. In this assessment phase, the nurse would collect data in six areas:

1. The person's health status
2. The physician's perspective of the person's health
3. The person's perspective of his or her health
4. The health goals within the context of life history, life style, and health status
5. The person's requirements for self-care
6. The person's capacity to perform self-care

Specific data are gathered in the areas of the individual's universal, developmental, and health-deviation self-care needs and their interrelationship. Data are also collected about the individual's knowledge, skills, motivation, and orientation.

Within Step 1, the nurse would seek answers to the following questions[35]:

1. What is the patient's therapeutic care demand? Now? At a future time?
2. Does the patient have a deficit for engaging in self-care to meet the therapeutic self-care demand?
3. If so, what is its nature and the reasons for its existence?
4. Should the patient be helped to refrain from engagement in self-care or to protect already developed self-care capabilities for therapeutic purposes?
5. What is the patient's potential for engaging in self-care at a future time period? Increasing or deepening self-care knowledge? Learning techniques of self-care? Fostering willingness to engage in self-care? Effectively and consistently incorporating essential self-care measures (including new ones) into the systems of self-care and daily living?

Once the assessment data have been gathered, they must be analyzed. Analyzing Ms. M's data: In the category of universal self-care needs, Ms. M demonstrates a deficit in adequate air, water, and food intake since she is 5'2", weighs 175 pounds, consumes excessive calories and cholesterol from fast food and late night meals. Ms. M shows an imbalance between activity and rest since she has minimal exercise. There is also an imbalance between

TABLE 7-2. APPLICATION OF OREM'S THEORY TO NURSING PROCESS

	Assessment				
Personal Factors	Universal Self-Care	Developmental Self-Care	Health Deviations	Medical Problem and Plan	Self-Care Deficits
Age	Air, water, food	Specialized needs for developmental process	Conditions of illness or injury	Physician's perspective of condition	Difference between self-care needs and self-care capabilities
Sex	Excrements	New requisites from a condition	Treatments to correct the condition	Medical diagnosis	
Height	Activity and rest	Requisites associated with an event		Medical treatment	
Weight	Solitude and social interaction				
Culture	Hazards to life and well-being				
Race	Promotion of human functioning and development				
Marital Status					
Religion					
Occupation					

(Continued)

Nursing Diagnosis	Plan	Implementation	Evaluation
Based on self-care deficits	Nursing goals and objectives: a. Congruent with nursing diagnosis b. Based on self-care demands c. Promote patient as self-care agent Designing the Nursing System: a. Wholly compensatory b. Partly compensatory c. Supportive–educative Appropriate methods of helping: a. Guidance b. Support c. Teaching d. Acting or doing for e. Providing developmental environment	Nurse–patient actions to: a. Promote patient as self-care agent b. Meet self-care needs c. Decrease self-care deficits	Effectiveness of nurse–patient actions to: a. Promote patient as self-care agent b. Meet self-care needs c. Decrease self-care deficits

Adapted from Pinnell, N. N. & de Meneses, M. *The Nursing Process—Theory, Application and Related Processes,* Norwalk, Conn.: Appleton-Century-Crofts, 1986, p. 66. Used with permission.

TABLE 7-3. APPLICATION OF OREM'S THEORY USING MS. M.'S CASE STUDY WITHIN THE NURSING PROCESS

Personal Factors	Universal Self-Care	Developmental Self-Care	Health Deviation	Medical Problem and Plan	Self-Care Deficits
48 yr	Smokes 1.5 ppd	Loss of husband	Potential for cardiac disease related to obesity, smoking, cholesterol, lack of exercise, family history	Diagnoses of obesity with potential for cardiac disease and low motivation for weight loss	Difference between Ms. M.'s knowledge base and life style which increases risk for heart attack or stroke
Female	Fast foods	Loss of social activity			
5'2"	Late PM meal			Prescription to:	
175 lb	No data			Monitor cholesterol levels and vital signs	
Italian	No exercise			Decrease cholesterol intake	
White	Decreased social interaction × 6 mo			Increase exercise	
Widowed					
Catholic	Family history:				
University faculty	F—heart attack age 50				
	M—stroke				
	Cholesterol 280 mg				
	High fat diet				
	Lacks knowledge of risk factors and cardiovascular functioning				
	T = 98.4				
	138/96				
	P = 92				
	R = 30				
	Works 12 hour days				
	Well groomed				

(Continued)

Nursing Diagnosis	Plan	Implementation	Evaluation
Potential for impaired cardio-vascular functioning related to her lack of knowledge about relationship between current life style and risk of heart attack or stroke	Nursing goals and objectives: *Goal:* To decrease risk for cardiac impairment *Objective:* Ms. M. will state that high cholesterol levels increase her risk for cardiac impairment Design of Nursing System: Supportive–educative Methods of helping: Guidance, support, teaching, and provision of a developmental environment	Jointly develop contract related to goal of cholesterol reduction Ms. M. will keep a 3-day food diary Ms. M. will learn about cholesterol and its effect on cardiovascular functioning Ms. M. will request or obtain cholesterol content of fast foods Ms. M. will learn about low cholesterol foods, foods which decrease cholesterol, and restaurants which serve low cholesterol foods Jointly analyze food diary and decide how to decrease cholesterol intake Jointly determine Italian foods which are low in cholesterol, or recipes which may be adapted Ms. M.'s accomplishments will be reinforced	Does Ms. M. understand that with her present life style her risk of heart attack or stroke is high? Did Ms. M. select low cholesterol foods? Is Ms. M.'s cholesterol level lower? Did Ms. M.'s self-care deficit decrease? Was the supportive–educative system effective in promoting Ms. M. as a self-care agent?

105

her solitude and social interaction since her husband's death. This represents a significant loss for her in the mid-life developmental needs category. Ms. M.'s elevated cholesterol levels when interrelated with her family history of stroke and heart attack present a hazard to her life, functioning, and well-being. The physician's perspective is that Ms. M. needs to lose 40 pounds because of her family history and elevated blood cholesterol but has limited nutritional knowledge. However, Ms. M. has a motivational deficit to lose weight because her Italian cultural tradition associates food with family and love.

Based on the analysis of Ms. M's data, she has potential hazards to her health related to obesity, high cholesterol, smoking, social isolation, and decreased exercise. The analysis of the collected data leads to the nursing diagnosis, enabling the nurse to prioritize self-care deficits. The nursing diagnosis must include the response and etiology pattern. Within Orem's framework, the nursing diagnosis would be stated as: an inability to meet the self-care demand (the response) related to the self-care deficit (etiology).[36] For Ms. M. the response pattern would be: "potential for impaired cardiovascular functioning," and the etiology would be "lack of knowledge about how her current life style increases her risk for heart attack and stroke." Therefore, for Ms. M., the nursing diagnosis could be stated: "Potential for impaired cardiovascular functioning related to lack of knowledge about how her current life style increases her risk for heart attack and stroke."

Step 2. Orem defines Step 2 as designing of the nursing systems and planning for the delivery of nursing. The nurse designs a system that is wholly compensatory, partly compensatory, or supportive–educative. The two actions involved in the design of the nursing systems would be: (1) "bringing about a good organization of the components of patients' therapeutic self-care demands," and (2) "selection of the combination of ways of helping that will be both effective and efficient in compensating for or overcoming patients' self-care deficits."[37]

Using Orem's model, the goals are congruent with the nursing diagnosis enabling the patient to become an effective self-care agent. Goals are directed by the response statement of the nursing diagnosis and are health focused. The goal for Ms. M. would be: Decrease her risk of cardiovascular impairment.

Once the goals have been determined, the objectives can be stated. An example of an objective for Ms. M. would be: Ms. M. will state that high cholesterol levels increase her risk for cardiac impairment. Other objectives might relate to the risk factors of obesity, lack of exercise, smoking, and family history. The designed nursing system for Ms. M. would be the supportive–educative nursing system.

Step 3. Within Orem's nursing process, Step 3 includes the production and management of the nursing system. In this step, the nurse assists "the patient (or family), . . . in self-care matters to achieve identified and described health and health-related results, . . . collecting evidence to describe the results of care and . . . using this evidence in evaluating results achieved against results specified in the nursing system design."[38]

The nurse and patient actions are directed by the etiology component of the nursing diagnosis. "Lack of knowledge about how her current life style increases her risk for heart attack and stroke" is the etiology component of Ms. M.'s nursing diagnosis. When the nurse and patient implement this supportive–educative system, each has specific roles. Examples of these roles might be: Together they would develop a contract that would relate to the goal of cholesterol reduction. Ms. M. would keep a three-day food diary. The nurse would provide information about cholesterol and its effects on cardiovascular function. Ms. M. would request and obtain the cholesterol content of the fast-food menu items from the restaurants she frequents. The nurse would provide information about specific foods that are low in cholesterol, those food items that help reduce cholesterol, and a list of fast-food restaurants that offer low cholesterol food items. Together they will analyze the three-day food diary and decide how Ms. M. might modify her diet to reduce her cholesterol intake. They will determine which Italian dishes are low in cholesterol or how these recipes can be adapted. As the cholesterol levels decrease, Ms. M. will be praised for her accomplishments. During this implementation, the nurse teaches, guides, and supports Ms. M. while providing a developmental environment.

Step 3 includes evaluation. The nurse and patient together do the evaluation. Questions they might ask are: When evaluating some of Ms. M's plans, does she understand that her present life style may increase her risk of developing a heart attack or stroke? Did she select low cholesterol fast foods? Did she attain her goal of reducing her cholesterol levels? Were the plans effective in decreasing the self-care deficit? Was the nursing system effective in promoting the patient as a self-care agent?

Evaluation is an ongoing process. Is it essential that the nurse and patient continually evaluate any changes in the data that would affect the self-care deficit, the self-care agent, and the nursing system.

OREM'S WORK AND THE CHARACTERISTICS OF A THEORY

Orem identified her work as a framework of "concepts of practice" in the first and second editions of her book *Nursing: Concepts of Practice*. In the third edition, however, she refers to her work as a general, comprehensive theory of nursing constituted from three related theoretical constructs.[39] Orem's theory will be compared with the characteristics of a theory from Chapter 1 of this text.

1. Theories can interrelate concepts in such a way as to create a

different way of looking at a particular phenomenon. Orem's theoretical constructs of self-care, self-care deficits, and nursing systems are interrelated in her general comprehensive theory of nursing. This interrelationship provides a view of the practice of nursing (a particular phenomenon) that is unique.

2. Theories must be logical in nature. Orem's theory follows a logical thought process. She states her general theory, presents the constructs of her theory, supports the constructs with propositions, and then supports the propositions. With her construct of self-care deficit, she presents the propositions of self-care agency and delineates when nursing is needed.[40] These propositions are supported by the presupposition that self-care requires self-management and rests on the cultural attainments of social groups.

3. Theories should be relatively simple yet generalizable. Orem's theory is used by several schools of nursing as a theory base for a student's basic preparation for practice. Orem's concept of self-care with its proposition of universal self-care needs is easily understood by beginning and advanced nursing practitioners as the activities of daily living. The constructs of self-care deficits and nursing systems can be comprehended and applied to all individual patients and with further adaptation to multiperson units. One group has applied Orem's theory to women's health care.[41]

4. Theories are the bases for hypotheses that can be tested. Orem's theory of self-care has been used to generate testable hypotheses. Several researchers have tested Orem's theory in the area of self-care agency, with a number of these studies focused on the development of tools to measure aspects of self-care.[42a,42b]

5. Theories contribute to and assist in increasing the general body of knowledge within the discipline through the research implemented to validate them. Orem focuses on nursing as a helping art, assisting the individual to meet self-care needs, as the foundation for nursing practice. Research on self-care needs, and the assistance to meet them, adds to nursing's body of knowledge. Orem's theory is being tested by several nursing researchers.[43a–43c]

6. Theories can be used by the practitioners to guide and improve their practice. Orem's theory is used by an independent practitioner and by practitioners in clinical settings who have published information about their practices. Kinlein has adapted Orem's theory for her use as an independent nursing practitioner.[44] Knust and Quarn have used Orem's theory in rehabilitative nursing.[45]

7. Theories must be consistent with other validated theories, laws, and principles. Orem's theory is consistent with role theory, need theory, field theory, and preventive health concepts. For example, she discusses the importance of an understanding of the roles of nurse and patient. Self-care is based upon needs.

STRENGTHS AND LIMITATIONS

Dorothea E. Orem's theory of nursing provides a comprehensive base for nursing practice. It has utility for professional nursing in the areas of nursing education curricula, clinical nursing practice, nursing administration, and nursing research. A major strength of Orem's theory is that she specifies when nursing is needed. She also includes continuing education as part of the professional component of nursing education.[46]

Orem promotes the concept of professional nursing. She defines the roles of vocational, technical, and professional nurses and recognizes the importance of each.[47] Orem emphasizes that nurses are educated, not trained. In the process of that education, nurses learn to "think nursing" as an action distinct from the "skilled performance of standardized sets of operations or skilled performance of tasks."[48]

Her self-care premise is contemporary with the concepts of health promotion and health maintenance. Self-care in Orem's theory is comparable to holistic health in that both promote the individual's responsibility for health care. This is especially relevant with today's emphasis on early hospital discharge, home care, and outpatient services.

Orem has expanded her focus of individual self-care to include multiperson units (families, groups, and communities). Although most of her third edition still focuses on the individual, she recognizes the value of family members and significant others for the individual's provision of self-care. However, she suggests that "it is advisable at this stage of the development of nursing knowledge to confine the use of the three nursing systems to situations where individuals are the units of care or service."[49]

According to Orem, "nurses should select the type of nursing system or sequential combination of nursing systems that will have the optimum effect in achieving the desired regulation of patients' self-care agency and the meeting of their self-care requisites."[50] Some practitioners have found Orem's theory to be more clinically applicable when more than one system is used concurrently.[51]

Orem recognizes the term "client" as a regular seeker of services but prefers the term "patient" for one who is "under the care of nurses, physicians, or other direct health care providers."[52]

Orem's use of the term, system, is different than that used in general system theory. She defines a system as a "single, whole thing."[53] In general system theory, a system is viewed as a dynamic flowing process.

Health is often viewed as dynamic and everchanging. Orem's visual presentation of the boxed nursing systems (see Fig. 7–2) implies three static conditions of health. Another impression from the diagram of nursing systems is that the major determining factor for placement of a patient in a system is the individual's capacity for physical movement. Throughout her work there is limited acknowledgment of the emotional needs of humans.

Orem has organized her third edition into the three broad divisions of an introduction, theoretical development, and application in nursing practice. Within this edition she has further defined the terms used within her theory, i.e., nursing agency and self-care agency. However, some terms need more clarification, i.e., diagnosis, prescription, technologies, and therapeutic self-care demands. The term self-care is used with numerous connotations. This multitude of terms, such as self-care agency, self-care demand, self-care premise, self-care deficit, and universal self-care, can be confusing to the reader.

A limitation is found in her references. While Orem's third edition was published in 1985, some of her references could be considered outdated relative to contemporary nursing. For example, many of the journal articles in her lists of selected readings are from the 1960s and are not accompanied by companion, or comparison, articles from the 1980s.

SUMMARY

Orem presents her general theory of nursing, which is composed of three interrelated theories or constructs, self-care, self-care deficit, and nursing system. Within these constructs are the universal, developmental, and health-deviation self-care requisites. The self-care deficit construct delineates when nursing is needed, that is, when the self-care demands are greater than the self-care abilities.

Orem's construct of nursing systems is designed by the nurse when it has been determined that nursing is needed. The systems of wholly compensatory, partly compensatory, and supportive–educative specify the roles of the nurse and the patient.

Throughout Orem's work, she interprets the concepts of human beings, health, nursing, and society. She defines the three steps of the nursing process as: (1) diagnosis and prescription, (2) design of a nursing system and planning for the delivery of care, and (3) production and management of nursing systems. This closely parallels the nursing process of assessment, diagnosis, planning, implementation, and evaluation.

Orem's concept of self-care has pragmatic application in nursing practice. Documented use of Orem's theory in clinical settings includes self-care of clients with enterostomal therapy,[54] diabetes,[55] in psychiatric settings,[56] in public health,[57] with the elderly,[58a,58b] and with the terminally ill.[59]

Orem's theory offers a unique way of looking at the phenomenon of nursing. Her work contributes significantly to the development of nursing theories.

REFERENCES

1.   Orem, D.E. *Nursing: Concepts of Practice* (3rd ed.), New York: McGraw-Hill, 1985, p. 19.

2.   Orem, D.E. *Guides for Developing Curricula for the Education of Practical Nurses,* Washington, D.C.: Government Printing Office, 1959.

3.(a) Nursing Development Conference Group, *Concept Formalization in Nursing: Process and Product,* Boston: Little, Brown, 1973.

3.(b) Nursing Development Conference Group, *Concept Formalization in Nursing: Process and Product* (2nd ed.), Boston: Little, Brown, 1979.

4.   Orem, D.E. *Nursing: Concepts of Practice,* New York: McGraw-Hill, 1971.

5.   Orem, *Nursing,* 3rd ed., pp. 34–37.

6.   Ibid, 54.

7.   Ibid, 84.

8.   Ibid, 85.

9.   Ibid, 106.

10.   Ibid, 35.

11.   Ibid, 84.

12.   Ibid, 88.

13.   Ibid, 90–91.

14.(a) Ibid, 95.

14.(b) Ibid, 99.

15.   Ibid, 35.

16.   Ibid, 130.

17.   Ibid, 55.

18.   Ibid, 138.

19.   Ibid, 80–81.

20.   Ibid, 150.

21.   Ibid, 154.

22.   Ibid, 156.

23.   Ibid, 157.

24.   Ibid, 174.

25.   Ibid, 180.

26.   Ibid, 174.

27.   Ibid, 54.

28.   Ibid, 107.

29.   Ibid, 144.

30.   Ibid, 53.

31.   Ibid, 15.

32.   Ibid, 143.

33.   Ibid, 146.

34.   Ibid, 224.

35.   Ibid, 225–226.

36.   Ziegler, S.M., Vaughn-Wrobel, B.C., & Erlen, J.A. *Nursing Process, Nursing Diagnosis, Nursing Knowledge—Avenues to Autonomy,* Conn.: Appleton-Century-Crofts, 1986, pp. 77–78.

37.   Orem, *Nursing,* 3rd ed., p. 232.

38.   Ibid, 223.

39.   Ibid, 34.

40.   Ibid, 35–38.

41.   Webster, D., Leslie, L., McElmurray, B.J., Dan, A., et al; Nursing Practice in Women's Health—Concept Paper, *Nursing Research,* 1968, *35,* 143.

42.(a) Weaver, M.T., Perceived Self-Care Agency: A Lisrel Factor Analysis of Bickel and Hanson's Questionnaire, *Nursing Research*, 1987, *36*, 381–387.

42.(b) Kearney, B. & Fleischer, B.L. Development of an Instrument to Measure Exercise of Self-Care Agency, *Research in Nursing and Health*, 2, 25–34.

43.(a) Horn, B.J. & Swain, M.A. *Development of Criterion Measures for Nursing Care*, *Vols. 1 and 2*, University of Michigan and National Center for Health Services Research, U.S. Dept. of Commerce, National Technical Information Service, Springfield, Va., 1977, Publication nos. 267-004 and 267-005.

43.(b) Gulick, E.F. Parsimony and Model Confirmation of the ADL Self-Care Scale for Multiple Sclerosis Persons, *Nursing Research*, 1987, *36*, 278–283.

43.(c) Denyes, M.J. Measurement of Self-Care Agency in Adolescents, *Nursing Research*, 1982, *31*, 63.

44.   Kinlein, M.L. *Independent Nursing Practice with Clients*, Philadelphia: Lippincott, 1977.

45.   Knust, S.J. & Quarn, J.M. Integration of Self-Care Theory with Rehabilitation Nursing, *Rehabilitation Nursing*, 1983, 26–28.

46.   Orem, *Nursing*, 3rd ed., p. 76.

47.   Ibid, 74–75.

48.   Ibid, 80.

49.   Ibid, 153–154.

50.   Ibid, 157.

51.   Knust and Quarn, Integration of Self-Care, p. 27.

52.   Orem, *Nursing*, 3rd ed., pp. 49–50.

53.   Ibid, 148.

54.   Bromley, B. Applying Orem's Self-Care Theory in Enterostomal Therapy, *American Journal of Nursing*, 1980, *80*, 245–249.

55.   Fitzgerald, S. Utilizing Orem's Self-Care Model in Designing an Educational Program for the Diabetic, *Topics in Clinical Nursing*, 1980, *2*, 57–65.

56.   Scrak, B.M., Zimmerman, J., Wilson, M., & Greenstein, R. Moving from the Gas Station to a Nurse-Managed Psych Clinic, *American Journal of Nursing*, 1987, *87*, 188–190.

57.   Wyatt, G.K. & Omar, M.A. Interventions Useful to the Public Health Nurse: Improving Health Behaviors, *Journal of Nursing Education*, 1985, *24*, 168–170.

58.(a) Chang, B.L., Cuman, G., Linn, L.S., Ware, J.E., & Kane, R.L. Adherence to Health Care Regimens among Elderly Women, *Nursing Research*, 1985, *34*, 27–31.

58.(b) Reed, P.G. Developmental Resources and Depression in the Elderly, *Nursing Research*, 1986, *35*, 368–374.

59.   Murphy, P. A Hospice Model and Self-Care Theory, *Oncology Nursing Forum*, 1981, *8*, 19–21.

CHAPTER 8

Dorothy E. Johnson

Marie L. Lobo

Dorothy Johnson was born in Savannah, Georgia, in 1919. Her Bachelor of Science in Nursing was from Vanderbilt University, Nashville, Tennessee, and her Masters in Public Health from Harvard. She began publishing her ideas about nursing soon after graduation from Vanderbilt. Most of her teaching career was at the University of California, Los Angeles. She retired as Professor Emeritus, January 1, 1978, and is currently residing in Florida.

Dorothy Johnson has been influencing nursing through her publications since the 1950s.[1a-1f] Throughout her career, Johnson has stressed the importance of research-based knowledge about the effect of nursing care on clients. Johnson was an early proponent of nursing as a science as well as an art. She also believed nursing had a body of knowledge reflecting both the science and the art. From the beginning, Johnson proposed that the knowledge of the science of nursing necessary for effective nursing care included a synthesis of key concepts drawn from basic and applied sciences.[2]

In 1961, Johnson proposed that nursing care facilitated the client's maintenance of a state of equilibrium.[3] Johnson proposed that clients were "stressed" by a stimulus of either an internal or external nature. These stressful stimuli created such disturbances, or "tensions," in the patient that a state of disequilibrium occurred. Johnson identified two areas of foci for nursing care based on returning the client to a state of equilibrium. First, nursing care should reduce stimuli that are stressors, and second, "nursing care should provide support of the client's 'natural' defenses and adaptive processes."[4]

In 1968, Johnson first proposed her model of nursing care as the fostering of "the efficient and effective behavioral functioning in the patient to prevent illness."[5] The patient is identified as a behavioral system with multiple subsystems. At this point Johnson began to integrate concepts related to systems models into her work. Johnson's integration of systems concepts into her work was further illustrated by her statement of belief that nursing was "concerned with man as an integrated whole and this is the specific knowledge of order we require."[6] Not only did nurses need to care for the "whole" client but the generation of nursing knowledge needed to take a course in the direction of concern with the entire needs of the client.

In the mid to late 1970s, several nurses published conceptualizations of nursing based on Johnson's behavioral systems model. Grubbs, Holaday, Skolny and Riehl, Damus, and Auger are some of the authors who have interpreted Johnson.[7a-7e] Roy and Wu and others were sharing their beliefs about nursing at the same time, and Johnson's influence, as their professor, is clearly reflected in their works.[8a,8b] In 1980, Johnson published her conceptualization of the "Behavioral System Model for Nursing." This is the first work published by Johnson that explicates her definitions of the behavioral system model.[9] Her evolution in the development of this complex model is clearly demonstrated in the progression of her ideas from works published in the 1950s to her latest available work published in 1980.[1a-1f]

DEFINITION OF NURSING

Johnson developed her behavioral system model for nursing from a philosophical perspective "supported by a rich, sound and rapidly expanding body of empirical and theoretical knowledge."[10] From her early beliefs, which focused on the impaired individual, Johnson evolved a much broader definition of nursing. By 1980, she defined nursing as "an external regulatory force which acts to preserve the organization and integration of the patient's behavior at an optimal level under those conditions in which the behavior constitutes a threat to physical or social health, or in which illness is found."[11] Based on this definition, the four goals of nursing are to assist the patient to become a person[12]:

1. Whose behavior is commensurate with social demands.
2. Who is able to modify his behavior in ways that support biologic imperatives.
3. Who is able to benefit to the fullest extent during illness from the physician's knowledge and skill.
4. Whose behavior does not give evidence of unnecessary trauma as a consequence of illness.

ASSUMPTIONS OF THE BEHAVIORAL SYSTEM MODEL

There are several layers of assumptions that Johnson makes in the development of her conceptualization of the behavioral system model. Assumptions are made about the system as a whole as well as about the subsystems. Another set of assumptions deals with the knowledge base necessary to practice nursing.

As with Rogers and Roy, Johnson believes that nurses need to be well grounded in the physical and social sciences.[13a,13b] Particular emphasis should be placed on the knowledges in areas from both the physical and social sciences that are found to influence behavior. Thus Johnson believes it would be equally important to have information available on endocrine influences on behavior as well as on psychological influences on behavior.

In developing assumptions about behavioral systems, Johnson was influenced by Buckley, Chin, and Rapport, early leaders in the development of systems concepts. Johnson cites Chin as the source for her first assumption about systems. In constructing a behavioral system, the assumption is made that there is "organization, interaction, interdependency and integration of the parts and elements [14a] of behavior that go to make up the system."[14] It is the interrelated parts that contribute to the development of the whole.

The second assumption about systems also evolves from the work of Chin. A system " 'tends to achieve a balance among the various forces operating within and upon it'[14a], and that man strives continually to maintain a behavioral system balance and steady state by more or less automatic adjustments and adaptations to the 'natural' forces impinging upon him."[14] The individual is continually presented with situations in everyday life that require the individual to adapt and adjust. These adjustments are so natural that they occur without conscious effort by the individual.

The third assumption about a behavioral system is that a

> behavioral system, which both requires and results in some degree of regularity and constancy in behavior, is essential to man; that is to say, it is functionally significant in that it serves a useful purpose, both in social life and for the individual.[14]

The patterns of behavior characteristic of the individual have a purpose in the maintenance of homeostasis by the individual. The development of behavioral patterns that are acceptable to both society and the individual foster the individual's ability to adapt to minor changes in the environment.

The final assumption about the behavioral system is that the "system balance reflects adjustments and adaptations that are successful in some way and to some degree."[14] Johnson acknowledges that the achievement of this balance may and will vary from individual to individual. At times this balance may *not* be exhibited as behaviors that are acceptable or meet society's norms. What may be adaptive for the individual in coping with impinging forces may be disruptive to society as a whole. Most individuals are flexible enough, however, to be in some state of balance that is "functionally efficient and effective" for them.[15]

The integration of these assumptions by the individual provides the behavioral system with the patterns of action to form "an organized and integrated functional unit that determines and limits the interaction between the person and his environment and establishes the relationship of the person to the objects, events and situations in his environment."[15] The function of the behavioral system then is to regulate the individual's response to input from the environment so that the balance of the system can be maintained.

There are four assumptions made about the structure and function of each subsystem. These four assumptions are the "structural elements" common to each of the seven subsystems. The first assumption is "from the form the behavior takes and the consequences it achieves can be inferred what *drive* has been stimulated or what *goal* is being sought."[16] The ultimate goal for each subsystem is expected to be the same for all individuals. However, the methods of achieving the goal may vary depending on culture or other individual variations.

The second assumption is that each individual has a "predisposition to act, with reference to the goal, in certain ways rather than in other ways."[17] This predisposition to act is labeled "set" by Johnson. The concept of "set" implies that despite having only a few alternatives from which to select a behavioral response, the individual will rank those options and choose the option considered most desirable.

The third assumption is that each subsystem has a repertoire of choices or "scope of action" alternatives available from which choices can be made.[18] Johnson subsumes under this assumption that larger behavioral repertoires are available to more adaptable individuals.[18] As life experiences occur, individuals add to the number of alternative actions available to them. At some point, however, the acquisition of new alternatives of behavior decreases as the individual is comfortable with the available repertoire. The point at which the individual loses the desire or ability to acquire new options is not identified by Johnson.

The fourth assumption about the behavioral subsystems is that they produce observable outcomes; that is, the individual's behavior.[18] The observable behaviors allow an outsider—in this case the nurse—to note the actions the individual is taking to reach a goal related to a specified subsystem. The nurse can then evaluate the effectiveness and efficiency of these behaviors in assisting the individual in reaching one of these goals.

In addition, each of the subsystems has three functional requirements. First, each subsystem must be "*protected* from noxious influences with which the system cannot cope."[19] Second, each subsystem must be "*nurtured* through the input of appropriate supplies from the environment."[19] Finally, each subsystem must be "*stimulated* for use to enhance growth and prevent stagnation."[19] As long as the subsystems are meeting these functional requirements, the system and the subsystems are viewed as self-maintaining and self-perpetuating. The internal and external environments of the system need to remain orderly and predictable for the system to maintain homeostasis or remain in balance. The interrelationships of the structural elements of the subsystem are critical for each subsystem to function at a maximum state. The interaction of the structural elements allows the subsystem to maintain a balance that is adaptive to that individual's needs.

An imbalance in a behavioral subsystem produces "tension," which results in disequilibrium. The presence of tension resulting in an unbalanced behavioral system requires the system to increase energy usage to return the system to a state of balance.[20] Nursing is viewed as a part of the external environment that can assist the client to return to a state of equilibrium or balance.

JOHNSON'S BEHAVIORAL SYSTEM MODEL

Johnson believes each individual has patterned, purposeful, repetitive ways of acting that comprise a behavioral system specific to that individual. These actions or behaviors form an "organized and integrated functional unit that determines and limits the interaction between the person and his environment and establishes the relationship of the person to the objects, events and situations in his environment."[21] These behaviors are "orderly, purposeful and predictable . . . [and] sufficiently stable and recurrent to be amenable to description and explanation."[21] Johnson identifies seven subsystems within the behavioral system model. This identification of seven subsystems is at variance with others who have published interpretations of Johnson's model. Johnson states that the seven subsystems identified in her 1980 publication are the only ones to which she subscribes and recognizes they are at variance with Grubb.[22] These seven subsystems were originally identified in Johnson's 1968 paper presented at Vanderbilt University.[23] The seven subsystems are considered to be interrelated, and changes in one subsystem affect all of the subsystems.

Johnson has never produced a schematic representation of her system. Marriner, Loveland-Cherry and Wilkerson, and Torres[24a–24c] have produced similar schematic representations of Johnson's model (see Fig. 8–1).

Johnson's Seven Behavioral Subsystems

The *attachment* or *affiliative* subsystem is identified as the first response system to develop in the individual. The optimal functioning of the affiliative subsystem allows "social inclusion, intimacy and the formation and attachment of a strong social bond."[25] Attachment to a significant care giver has been found to be critical for the survival of an infant. As the individual matures, the attachment to the caretaker continues and there are additional attachments to other significant individuals as they enter both the child's and the adult's network. These "significant others" provide the individual with a sense of security.

The second subsystem identified by Johnson is the *dependency* subsystem. Johnson distinguishes the dependency subsystem from the attachment or affiliative subsystem. Dependency behaviors are "succoring" behaviors

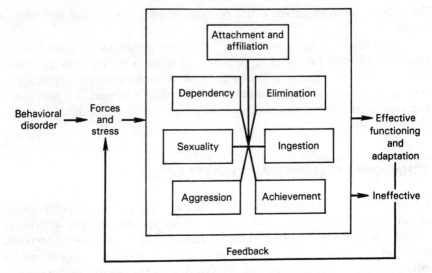

Figure 8–1. Johnson's model. *From Torres, G.* Theoretical Foundations of Nursing, *Norwalk, CT: Appleton-Century-Crofts, 1986, p. 121. Used with permission.*

that precipitate nurturing behaviors from other individuals in the environment. The result of dependency behavior is "approval, attention or recognition and physical assistance."[26] It is difficult to separate the dependency subsystem from the affiliative or attachment subsystem because without someone invested in or attached to the individual to respond to that individual's dependency behaviors, the dependency subsystem has no animate environment in which to function.

The *ingestive* subsystem relates to the behaviors surrounding the intake of food.[26] It is related to the biological system. However, the emphasis for nursing, from Johnson's perspective, is the meanings and structures of the social events surrounding the occasions when food is eaten. Behaviors related to the ingestion of food may relate more to what is socially acceptable in a given culture than to the biological needs of the individual.

The *eliminative* subsystem relates to behaviors surrounding the excretion of waste products from the body.[26] Johnson admits this may be difficult to separate from a biological systems perspective. However, as with behaviors surrounding the ingestion of food, there are socially acceptable behaviors for the time and place for humans to excrete waste. Human cultures have defined different socially acceptable behaviors for excretion of waste, but the existence of such a pattern remains from culture to culture. Individuals who have gained physical control over the eliminative subsystem will control those subsystems rather than behave in a socially unacceptable manner. For example, biological cues are often ignored if the social situation dictates it is objectionable to eliminate wastes at a given time.

The *sexual* subsystem reflects behaviors related to procreation.[26] Both biological and social factors affect behaviors in the sexual subsystem. Again, the behaviors are related to culture and will vary from culture to culture. Behaviors will also vary according to the gender of the individual. The key is that the goal in all societies has the same outcome—behaviors acceptable to society at large.

The *aggressive* subsystem relates to behaviors concerned with protection and self-preservation. Johnson views the aggressive subsystem as one that generates defensive responses from the individual when life or territory is being threatened.[26] The aggressive subsystem does not include those behaviors with a primary purpose of injuring other individuals.

Finally, the *achievement* subsystem provokes behaviors that attempt to control the environment. Intellectual, physical, creative, mechanical, and social skills achievement are some of the areas that Johnson recognizes.[26] Other areas of personal accomplishment or success may also be included in this subsystem.

JOHNSON'S BEHAVIORAL SYSTEM MODEL AND THE FOUR MAJOR CONCEPTS

Johnson views *human beings* as having two major systems, the biological system and the behavioral system. It is the role of medicine to focus on the biological system, whereas nursing's focus is the behavioral system. There is recognition of the reciprocal actions that occur between the biological and behavioral systems when some type of dysfunction occurs in one or the other of the systems.

Society relates to the environment in which an individual exists. According to Johnson, an individual's behavior is influenced by all the events in the environment. Cultural influences on the individual's behavior are viewed as profound. However, it is felt that there are many paths, varying from culture to culture, that influence specific behaviors in a group of people, although the outcome for all of the groups or individuals is the same.

Health is a "purposeful, adaptive response, physically, mentally, emotionally, and socially, to internal and external stimuli in order to maintain stability and comfort."[27] Johnson's behavioral model supports that the individual is attempting to maintain some balance or equilibrium. The individual's goal is to maintain the entire behavioral system efficiently and effectively, but with enough flexibility to return to an acceptable balance if a malfunction disrupts the original balance.

Nursing has a primary goal that is to foster equilibrium within the individual. This allows for the practice of nursing with individuals at any point in the health–illness continuum. Nursing implementations may focus on alterations of a behavior that is not supportive to maintaining equilibrium for the individual. In earlier works, Johnson focused nursing on impaired individuals. By 1980, she stated that nursing is concerned with the organized and integrated whole, but that the major focus is on maintaining a balance in the behavioral system when illness occurs in the individual.[28]

JOHNSON'S BEHAVIORAL SYSTEM AND THE NURSING PROCESS

Johnson's behavioral system model easily fits the nursing process model. Grubbs developed an assessment tool based on Johnson's seven subsystems, plus a subsystem she labeled "restorative," which focused on activities of daily living.[29] Activities of daily living are considered to include such areas as patterns of rest, hygiene, and recreation. A diagnosis can be made related to insufficiencies or discrepancies within a subsystem or between subsystems. Planning for the implementation of nursing care should start at the subsystem level with the ultimate goal of effective behavioral functioning of the entire system. Implementations by the nurse present to the client an external force for the manipulation of the subsystem back to the state of equilibrium. Evaluation of the result of this implementation is readily possible if the state of "balance" that is the goal has been defined during the planning phase that occurs before the implementation.

Assessment

In the assessment phase of the nursing process, questions related to specific subsystems are developed. Holaday, Small, and Damus propose that the assessment focus on the subsystem related to the presenting health problem.[30a–30c] An assessment based on the behavioral subsystems does not easily permit the nurse to gather detailed information about the biological systems. Assessment questions related to the affiliative subsystem might focus on the presence of a significant other or on the social system of which the individual is a member. In the assessment of the dependency subsystem, attention is placed on understanding how the individual makes needs known to significant others, so the significant others in the environment can assist the individual in meeting those needs. Assessment of the ingestive subsystem would examine patterns of food and fluid intake, including the social environment in which the food and fluid are ingested. The eliminative subsystem generates questions related to patterns of defecation and urination and the social context in which the patterns occur. The sexual subsystem assessment would include information about sexual patterns and behaviors. The aggressive subsystem generates questions about how individuals protect themselves from perceived threats to safety. Finally, the achievement subsystem allows for assessment of how the individual changes the environment to facilitate the accomplishment of goals.

There are many gaps in information about the whole individual if only Johnson's behavioral system model is used to guide the assessment. There is little physiological data on the individual's present or past health status. The exception might be when an impaired health state is demonstrated in the ingestive or eliminative subsystems. Family interaction and patterns are only touched on in the affiliative and dependency subsystems. Basic information relating to education, socioeconomic status, and type of dwelling is tangentially related to most of the subsystems. However, these factors are not clearly identified as an important aspect of any of the subsystems.

Diagnosis

Diagnosis using Johnson's behavioral system model becomes cumbersome. Diagnosis tends to be general to a subsystem rather than specific to a problem. Grubbs has proposed four categories of nursing diagnoses derived from Johnson's behavioral system model.[31]

1. Insufficiency—a state which exists when a particular subsystem is not functioning or developed to its fullest capacity due to inadequacy of functional requirements.
2. Discrepancy—a behavior that does not meet the intended goal. The incongruency usually lies between the action and the goal of the subsystem, although the set and choice may be strongly influencing the ineffective action.
3. Incompatibility—the goals or behaviors of two subsystems in the same situation conflict with each other to the detriment of the individual.
4. Dominance—the behavior in one subsystem is used more than any other subsystem regardless of the situation or to the detriment of the other subsystems.

Since Johnson has never written about the use of nursing diagnosis with her model, it is difficult to evaluate whether these diagnostic classifications are Johnson's or if they are an extension of Johnson's work by Grubbs.

Planning and Implementation

Planning for implementation of the nursing care related to the diagnosis may be difficult because of the lack of client input into the plan. The plan will focus on the nurse's action to modify client behavior. These plans then have a goal, to bring about homeostasis in a subsystem, based on the nurse's assessment of the individual's drive, set, behavioral repertoire, and observable behavior. The plan may include protection, nurturance, or stimulation of the identified subsystem.

Planning and implementation for clients based on Johnson's behavioral system model would focus on maintaining or returning an individual's subsystem to a state of equilibrium. Implementation would focus on achieving the goals of nursing.* Although Johnson refers to biological systems in

---

* See page 114.

her goals of nursing, they are not included in her behavioral system model and can and do produce incongruities for the planning and implementation of nursing care in relation to a specific diagnosis.

Evaluation

Evaluation is based on the attainment of a goal of balance in the identified subsystems. If base-line data are available for the individual, the nurse may have a goal for the individual to return to the base-line behavior. If the alterations in behavior that are planned do occur, the nurse should be able to observe the return to previous behavior patterns.

There is little or no recognition by either Johnson or Grubbs of the client's input into plans for nursing implementation. They use the term of *nursing intervention.* Holaday's example of implementation also does not contain strong client input.[32] Using Johnson's behavioral system model with the nursing process is a nurse-centered activity, with the nurse determining the client's needs and the state of behavior appropriate to those needs.

Holaday demonstrates the flexibility available in the use of the Johnson behavioral system model with the nursing process by using a very specific assessment tool to determine appropriate "interventions."[32] Holaday used tests of cognitive development developed by Piaget to determine the level of information to present to a child during a preoperative teaching session.

Situation. An example of the use of the nursing process with Johnson's behavioral system model is demonstrated with Johnny Smith, age 6 weeks, brought into the clinic for a routine checkup. He presents with no weight gain since his checkup at age 2 weeks. His mother states she feeds him but he does not seem to eat much. He sleeps 4 to 5 hours between feedings. His mother holds him in her arms without making trunk-to-trunk contact. As the assessment is made the nurse notes that Mrs. Smith never looks at Johnny and never speaks to him. She states he was a planned baby but that she never "realized how much work an infant could be." She says her mother told her she was not a good mother because Johnny is not gaining weight like he should. She states she had not called the nurse when she knew Johnny was not gaining weight because she thought the nurse would think she was a "bad mother" just like her own mother thought she was a "bad mother."

Based on the information available and using the Johnson behavioral system model, assessment would focus on the affiliative and dependency subsystems between mother and Johnny. Further assessment of Mrs. Smith's relationship with her own mother needs to be done. The critical need is for Johnny to begin gaining weight. The secondary need is for Mrs. Smith to resolve her own conflict with her mother. The assessment of the affiliative subsystem would focus on the specific behaviors manifested by Johnny to indicate attachment to his mother. The assessment of the dependency subsystem would focus on the specific behaviors manifested by Johnny to cue his mother to his needs. Because of the nature of his problem, a decision is made to use a tool that specifically focuses on parent–infant interaction during a feeding situation. Thus the Nursing Child Assessment Feeding Scale is used during a feeding that takes place at a normal feeding time for Johnny.[33] Johnny cries at the beginning of the feeding and turns toward his mother's hand when she touches his cheek. Mrs. Smith does not speak to Johnny, or in any verbal way acknowledge his hunger. When Johnny slightly chokes on some formula, she does not remove the bottle from his mouth. Mrs. Smith does not describe any of the environment to Johnny, nor does she stroke his body or make eye contact with him. Johnny does not reach out to touch his mother nor does he make any vocalizations. The assessment scale indicates that both mother and baby are not cueing each other at a level where they can respond appropriately.

The diagnoses based on this assessment, using Johnson's behavioral system model, are, "insufficient development of the affiliative subsystem" and "insufficient development of the dependency subsystem." Based on these diagnoses, nursing implementations would focus on increasing Mrs. Smith's awareness of the meaning of Johnny's infrequent cues. By increasing her awareness of the meaning of his cues, she can begin to reinforce them so that he begins to know there is someone in the environment who cares about him, thus fostering his attachment to her. Further assistance needs to be given in assisting Mrs. Smith in communicating with her infant. If further assessment indicates Mrs. Smith is uncomfortable talking with an infant who does not respond with words, it may be suggested that she read to Johnny from a book, thus providing him with needed verbal stimulation. Another implementation may include the nurse placing herself in Johnny's role and "talking" for him to his mother. The nurse may sit, watching Mrs. Smith hold Johnny, and say such things as "I like it when you pat me," "It feels good when you cuddle me," "When I turn my head like this, I'm hungry."

Evaluation of these implementations would be based on two criteria. First, Johnny's weight gains or losses would be carefully assessed. Not gaining weight would place him in a life-threatening situation; therefore it is critical that a pattern of weight gain be initiated. Second, the mother–infant interaction could be reassessed, again using the Nursing Child Assessment Feeding Scale, which would allow for comparison of the first observation with a series of subsequent observations.

JOHNSON'S WORK AND THE CHARACTERISTICS OF A THEORY

Johnson states that she is presenting a model related to subsystems of the human being that have observable behaviors leading to specific outcomes, although the method of attaining the specific outcomes may vary according to the culture of the individual. The characteristics of a theory discussed in Chapter 1 are that theories must (1) interrelate concepts to create a different way of viewing a particular phenomenon, (2) be logical in nature, (3) be relatively simple yet generalizable, (4) be the bases for testable hypotheses, (5) contribute to the general body of knowledge of the discipline, (6) be utilized to guide and improve practice, and (7) be consistent with other validated theories, laws, and principles while allowing the investigation of unanswered questions. Using these as a guide, it is clear that Johnson has indeed developed a model. Johnson's behavioral system model is based on general system concepts. However, the definitions related to the terms used to label her concepts have not been made explicit by Johnson. Grubbs has presented her definitions of Johnson's terms and those are the definitions most often reflected in the literature of other investigators claiming to use Johnson's model.[34]

Johnson does not clearly interrelate her concepts of subsystems comprising the behavioral system model. Thus the logic of her work is difficult to follow. The definitions of the concepts are so abstract that they are difficult to use. For example, intimacy is identified as an aspect of the affilitative subsystem, but the concept is not defined or described. An advantage of the abstract definition is that individuals using the model may identify an assessment tool that most specifically fits a problem and use it in their work. There are two major disadvantages. First, the abstract level and multiplicity of definitions make it difficult to compare the same subsystem across studies. Second, the lack of clear definitions for the interrelationships among and between the subsystems makes it difficult to view the entire behavioral system as an entity.

It is difficult to test Johnson's model by the development of hypotheses. Subsystems of the model can be examined, but the lack of definitions and connections of the subsystems makes hypothesis testing difficult.

Johnson's behavioral model can be generalized across the life span and across cultures. However, the focus on the behavioral system may make it difficult for nurses working with physically impaired individuals to use the model. Johnson's model is also very individual oriented, so that nurses working with groups of individuals with similar problems would have difficulty using the model. The subsystems in Johnson's behavioral system model are individual oriented to such an extent that the family can only be considered as the environment in which the individual presents behaviors and not as the focus of care.

Johnson's behavioral system model provides a framework for organizing human behavior. However, it is a different framework than that provided by other nursing theorists, such as Roy or Rogers.[35] Johnson believes that she is the first person to view "man as a behavioral system." Others have viewed the behavioral subsystem as just one piece of the biopsychosocial human being. Johnson's framework does contribute to the general body of nursing knowledge but needs further development.

Johnson does not clearly define the expected outcomes when one of the subsystems is being affected by nursing implementation. An implicit expectation is made that all humans in all cultures will attain the same outcome—homeostasis. Because of the lack of definitions, the model does not allow for control of the areas of interest, so it is difficult to use the model to guide practice. The authors reportedly using the model to guide practice have not integrated the subsystems to the degree necessary to label this model a theory. In general, the Johnson behavioral system model does not meet the criteria for a theory. However, it must be stressed that Johnson does not suggest that she has developed a theory, although other nurse scholars have identified and used Johnson as a theorist.

Johnson's behavioral system model is based on principles of general system theory. Her statements on the multiple modes of attaining the same subsystem goal, regardless of culture, are an example of the principle of "equifinality." As with Rogers, this allows individuals to develop and change through time at unique rates but with the same outcomes at the end of the process: mature, adult behaviors that are culturally acceptable.[36]

Johnson's behavioral system model is not as flexible as Rogers' concept of homeodynamics or Roy's adaptation model. Rogers' concepts are so broadly applicable that nursing care can take place at any level, individual, family, or community. All systems within the human being can be considered for the focus of nursing implementations.[36] With Roy's model, the focus is still at the individual level, but the total human being can be considered. Roy's assumptions include that the human being is a biopsychosocial being.[37] This allows for all of the subsystems of a human being to be included for nursing assessment and implementation.

Johnson's behavioral system model is congruent with many of the nursing models in the belief that the individual is influenced by the environment. Since Nightingale first presented her beliefs about nursing, nurses have been concerned with the individual's relationship with the environment.[38] In practice, nurses often have the necessary control over the environment to promote a healthier state for the individual.

SUMMARY

Although Johnson's behavioral system model has many limitations, she does provide a frame of reference for nurses concerned with specific client behaviors. It must also be noted that Johnson, through her work at the University of California, Los Angeles, has had a profound influence on the development of nursing models and nursing theories. Through her position as a faculty member she influenced Roy, Grubbs, Holaday, and others. As a peer she influenced Riehl, Neuman, Wu, and others, scholars who have generated many ideas about nursing concepts and theories.

Johnson's behavioral system model is a model of nursing care that advocates the fostering of efficient and effective behavioral functioning in the patient to prevent illness. The patient is identified as a behavioral system composed of seven behavioral subsystems. The seven behavioral subsystems are affiliative, dependency, ingestive, eliminative, sexual, aggressive, and achievement. Each subsystem is composed of four structural characteristics. These characteristics are drive, set, choices, and observable behaviors. The three functional requirements for each subsystem include: protection from noxious influences, provision for a nurturing environment, and stimulation for growth. An imbalance in any of the behavioral subsystems results in disequilibrium. It is nursing's role to assist the client to return to a state of equilibrium.

REFERENCES

1.(a) Johnson, D.E. The Nature of a Science of Nursing, *Nursing Outlook,* 1959, 7, 291–94.
1.(b) Johnson, D.E. The Significance of Nursing Care, *American Journal of Nursing,* 1961, *61,* 63–66.
1.(c) Johnson, D.E. One Conceptual Model of Nursing, paper presented April 25, 1968, Vanderbilt University, Nashville, Tennessee.
1.(d) Johnson, D.E. Theory in Nursing: Borrowed and Unique, *Nursing Research,* 1968*17,* 206–9.
1.(e) Johnson, D.E. Development of Theory: A Requisite for Nursing as a Profession, *Nursing Research,* 1974, *23,*372–77.
1.(f) Johnson, D.E. The Behavioral System Model for Nursing, in *Conceptual Models for Nursing Practice* (2nd ed.), Riehl, J.P., Roy, C., eds., New York: Appleton-Century-Crofts, 1980, 207–16.
2.   Johnson, The Nature of a Science of Nursing, p. 292.
3.   Johnson, The Significance of Nursing Care.
4.   Ibid, 66.
5.   Johnson, One Conceptual Model of Nursing, p. 2.
6.   Johnson, Theory in Nursing: Borrowed and Unique, p. 207.
7.(a) Grubbs, J. The Johnson Behavioral System Model, in *Conceptual Models for Nursing Practice,* Riehl, J.P., Roy, C. eds., New York: Appleton-Century-Crofts, 1974.
7.(b) Holaday, B. Implementing the Johnson Model for Nursing Practice, in *Conceptual Models for Nursing Practice.*
7.(c) Skolny, M.A., Riehl, J.P. Hope: Solving Patient and Family Problems by Using a Theoretical Framework, in *Conceptual Models for Nursing Practice.*
7.(d) Damus, K. An Application of the Johnson Behavioral System Model for Nursing Practice, in *Conceptual Models for Nursing Practice.*
7.(e) Auger, J.R. *Behavioral Systems and Nursing,* Englewood Cliffs, N. J.: Prentice-Hall, 1976.
8.(a) Roy, C. The Roy Adaptation Model, in *Conceptual Models for Nursing Practice.*
8.(b) Wu, R. *Behavior and Illness,* Englewood Cliffs, N.J.: Prentice-Hall, 1973.

9.   Johnson, The Behavioral System Model for Nursing.
10.   Ibid, 207.
11.   Ibid, 214.
12.   Ibid, 207.
13.(a) Rogers, M. *The Theoretical Basis for Nursing*, Philadelphia: F. A. Davis Co., 1970,
13.(b) Roy, C. The Roy Adaptation Model, in *Conceptual Models for Nursing Practice*.
14.   Johnson, The Behavioral System Model. p. 208.
14(a) Chin, R. The utility of system models and developmental models for practitioners. In Benne, K., Bennis, W., and Chin, R. (eds): *The Planning of Change*. New York: Holt, 1961.
15.   Ibid, 209.
16.   Ibid, 210. [Italics in original]
17.   Ibid, 210–11.
18.   Ibid, 211.
19.   Ibid, 212. [Italics in original]
20.   Johnson, One Conceptual Model of Nursing, p. 4.
21.   Johnson, The Behavioral System Model for Nursing, p. 209.
22.   Ibid, 214.
23.   Johnson, One Conceptual Model of Nursing.
24.(a) Conner, S.S., Watt, J.K. Dorothy E. Johnson: Behavioral System Model in *Nursing Theorists and Their Work*, Marriner, A. ed., St Louis: C.V. Mosby; p. 121.
24.(b) Loveland-Cherry, C. & Wilkerson, S.A. Dorothy Johnson's Behavioral System Model in *Conceptual Models of Nursing: Analysis and Application*, Fitzpatrick, J. & Whall, A. eds., Bowie, MD: Robert J. Brady, p. 123.
24.(c) Torres, G. *Theoretical Foundations of Nursing*, Norwalk, CT: Appleton-Century-Crofts, 1986, p. 121.
25.   Johnson, The Behavioral System Model for Nursing, p. 212.
26.   Ibid, 213.
27.   Murray, R.B., Zentner, J.P. *Nursing Concepts for Health Promotion*, Englewood Cliffs, N.J.: Prentice-Hall, 1979, pp. 5–6.
28.   Johnson, One Conceptual Model of Nursing and The Behavioral System Model for Nursing.
29.   Grubbs, The Johnson Behavioral System Model.
30.(a) Holaday, B. Implementing the Johnson Model for Nursing Practice.
30.(b) Small, B. Nursing Visually Impaired Children with Johnson's Model as a Conceptual Framework, in *Conceptual Models for Nursing Practice*.
30.(c) Damus, K. An Application of the Johnson Behavioral System Model for Nursing Practice.
31.   Grubbs, The Johnson Behavioral System Model, pp. 240–41.
32.   Holaday, Implementing the Johnson Model, 1980.
33.   Barnard, K.E. Nursing Child Assessment Feeding Scale, University of Washington, Seattle, 1978.
34.   Grubbs, The Johnson Behavioral System Model.
35.   Roy, The Roy Adaptation Model and Rogers, *The Theoretical Basis of Nursing*.
36.   Rogers, *The Theoretical Basis of Nursing*.
37.   Roy, The Roy Adaptation Model.
38.   Nightingale, F. *Notes on Nursing*, Philadelphia: Lippincott, 1859.

BIBLIOGRAPHY

Hardy, Margaret E., Theories: Components, Development, Evaluation, *Nursing Research*, 1974, *23*, 100–107.

Johnson, Dorothy E., Behavioral System Model for Nursing. Supplemental materials for Nursing Theorists General Session, the Second Annual Nurse Education Conference, December 4–6, 1978.

Kaplan, Abraham, *The Conduct of Inquiry*, New York: Thomas Y. Crowell, 1964.

Meleis, Afaf I. *Theoretical Nursing: Development & Progress*, Philadelphia: Lippincott, 1985.

Neuman, Betty, The Betty Neuman Health-Care Systems Model: A Total Person Approach to Patient Problems, in *Conceptual Models for Nursing Practice* (2nd ed.), Riehl, J.P. & Roy, C., eds., New York: Appleton-Century-Crofts, 1980.

Newman, Margaret, *Theory Development in Nursing*. Philadelphia: F. A. Davis Co., 1979.

Rogers, Martha E., Nursing, A Science of Unitary Man in *Conceptual Models for Nursing Practice* (2nd ed), Riehl, J.P. & Roy, C., eds. New York: Appleton-Century-Crofts, 1980.

Stevens, Barbara J., *Nursing Theory: Analysis, Application, Evaluation*. Boston: Little, Brown, 1979.

Yura, Helen, and Walsh, Mary, *The Nursing Process* (3rd ed.) New York: Appleton-Century-Crofts, 1978.

CHAPTER 9

Faye Glenn Abdellah

Suzanne M. Falco

Faye Glenn Abdellah was born in New York City and graduated magna cum laude from Fitkin Memorial Hospital School of Nursing in Neptune, New Jersey in 1942. She received her BS (1945), MA (1947), and EdD (1955) from Teachers College, Columbia University. She has been granted honorary doctorates by a number of institutions, including Case Western Reserve, Rutgers, University of Akron, Catholic University of America, Eastern University, and Monmouth College.

Dr. Abdellah is Deputy Surgeon General and former Chief Nurse Officer for the U.S. Public Health Service, Department of Health and Human Services, Washington, D.C. She is the recipient of both national and international awards and is a Fellow in the American Academy of Nursing. She has been a leader in nursing research and has over one hundred publications related to nursing care, education for advanced practice in nursing, and nursing research.

In 1960, influenced by the desire to promote client-centered comprehensive nursing care, Abdellah described nursing as a service to individuals, to families, and, therefore, to society. According to Abdellah, nursing is based on an art and science that mold the attitudes, intellectual competencies, and technical skills of the individual nurse into the desire and ability to help people, sick or well, cope with their health needs. Nursing may be carried out under general or specific medical direction. As a comprehensive service, nursing includes[1]:

1. Recognizing the nursing problems of the patient
2. Deciding the appropriate courses of action to take in terms of relevant nursing principles
3. Providing continuous care of the individual's total health needs
4. Providing continuous care to relieve pain and discomfort and provide immediate security for the individual
5. Adjusting the total nursing care plan to meet the patient's individual needs
6. Helping the individual to become more self-directing in attaining or maintaining a healthy state of mind and body
7. Instructing nursing personnel and family to help the individual do for himself that which he can within his limitations

8. Helping the individual to adjust to his limitations and emotional problems
9. Working with allied health professions in planning for optimum health on local, state, national, and international levels
10. Carrying out continuous evaluation and research to improve nursing techniques and to develop new techniques to meet the health needs of people

These original premises have undergone an evolutionary process. As a result, in 1973, item 3—"providing continuous care of the individual's total health needs"—was eliminated.[2] Although no reason was given, it can be hypothesized that the words *continuous* and *total* render that service virtually impossible to provide. From these premises, Abdellah's theory was derived.

ABDELLAH'S THEORY

Although Abdellah's writings are not specific as to a theoretical statement, such a statement can be derived by using her three major concepts of health, nursing problems, and problem solving. Abdellah's theory would state that nursing is the use of the problem-solving approach with key nursing problems related to the health needs of people. Such a theoretical statement maintains problem solving as the vehicle for the nursing problems as the client is moved toward health—the outcome. It is also a relatively simple statement and can be used as a basis for nursing practice, education, and research.

Health
Although Abdellah never defined it per se, her concept of health may be defined as the dynamic pattern of functioning whereby there is a continued interaction with internal and external forces that results in the optimal use of necessary resources that serve to minimize vulnerabilities.[3a,3b] Emphasis should be placed upon prevention and rehabilitation with wellness as a lifetime goal. By performing nursing services through a holistic approach to the client, the nurse helps the client achieve a state of health. However, in order to effectively perform these services, the nurse must accurately identify the lacks or deficits regarding health that the client is experiencing. These lacks or deficits are the client's health needs.

Nursing Problems
The client's health needs can be viewed as problems. These problems may be *overt* as an apparent condition, or *covert* as a hidden or concealed one. Because covert problems can be emotional, sociological, and interpersonal in nature, they are often missed or perceived incorrectly. Yet, in many instances, solving the covert problems may solve the overt problems as well.[4]

Such a view of problems implies a client-centered orientation. Abdellah, however, seems to imply a different viewpoint. She says a nursing problem presented by a client is a condition faced by the client or client's family that the nurse through the performance of professional functions can assist them to meet.[4] Abdellah's use of the term *nursing problems* is more consistent with "nursing functions" or "nursing goals" than with client-centered problems. This view-point leads to an orientation that is more nursing-centered than client-centered.[5]

This nursing-centered orientation to client care seems contrary to the client-centered approach that Abdellah professes to uphold. The apparent contradiction can be explained by her desire to move away from a disease-centered orientation. In her attempt to bring nursing practice into its proper relationship with restorative and preventative measures for meeting total client needs,[6] she seems to swing the pendulum to the opposite pole, from the disease orientation to nursing orientation, while leaving the client somewhere in the middle (see Fig. 9–1).

It is noted that Abdellah recognized the need to shift from nursing problems to patient problems.[7] However, there has been no further development of the framework to accomplish this.

Problem Solving

Quality professional nursing care requires that nurses be able to identify and solve overt and covert nursing problems. This can be accomplished by the problem-solving approach. The problem-solving process involves identifying the problem, selecting pertinent data, formulating hypotheses, testing hypotheses through the collection of data, and revising hypotheses where necessary on the basis of conclusions obtained from the data.[8]

Many of these steps parallel the steps of the nursing process of assessment, diagnosis, planning, implementation, and evaluation. The problem-

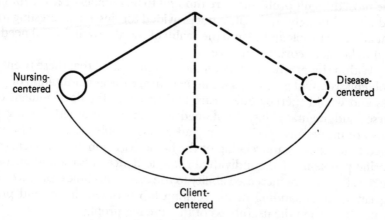

Figure 9–1. The focus of care pendulum.

solving approach was selected because of the assumption that the correct identification of nursing problems influences the nurse's judgment in selecting the next steps in solving the client's nursing problems.[9] The problem-solving approach is also consistent with such basic elements of nursing practice espoused by Abdellah as observing, reporting, and interpreting the signs and symptoms that comprise the deviations from health and constitute nursing problems; and with analyzing the nursing problems and selecting the necessary course of action.[10]

THE TWENTY-ONE NURSING PROBLEMS

The crucial element within Abdellah's theory is the identification of correct nursing problems. To assist in this identification, the need was defined for a systematic classification of nursing problems presented by the client. It was felt that such problems could be classified into three major categories.[11]

1. Physical, sociological, and emotional needs of clients
2. Types of interpersonal relationships between the nurse and client
3. Common elements of client care

Over a five-year period, several studies were carried out to establish the classification. As the result of this research, twenty-one groups of common nursing problems were identified (see Table 9–1). It is these twenty-one common nursing problems of Abdellah's that are most widely known, and they will be the focus of the rest of the chapter.

These twenty-one nursing problems focus on the physical, biological, and social–psychological needs of the client and attempt to provide a more meaningful basis for organization than the categories of systems of the body. The most difficult problems were thought to be numbers 12, 14, 15, 17, 18, and 19.[12] Although a rationale is not provided for this, it is interesting to note that all these problems fall into the realm of social–psychological needs and tend to be more covert in nature.

Within the practice of nursing, it was anticipated that these twenty-one problems as broad groupings would encourage the generalization of principles and would thereby guide care and promote the development of the nurse's judgmental ability. Contained in each of the broad nursing problems are numerous specific overt and covert problems. It was also anticipated that the constant relating of the broad basic nursing problems to the specific problems of the individual client and vice versa would encourage the development of increased ability to use theory in clinical practice. Thus, a greater understanding of the relationship between theory and practice would strengthen the usefulness of the nursing problems.[13]

TABLE 9–1. ABDELLAH'S TWENTY-ONE NURSING PROBLEMS

1. To maintain good hygiene and physical comfort.
2. To promote optimal activity: exercise, rest, and sleep.
3. To promote safety through the prevention of accidents, injury, or other trauma and through the prevention of the spread of infection.
4. To maintain good body mechanics and prevent and correct deformities.
5. To facilitate the maintenance of a supply of oxygen to all body cells.
6. To facilitate the maintenance of nutrition of all body cells.
7. To facilitate the maintenance of elimination.
8. To facilitate the maintenance of fluid and electrolyte balance.
9. To recognize the physiological responses of the body to disease conditions— pathological, physiological, and compensatory.
10. To facilitate the maintenance of regulatory mechanisms and functions.
11. To facilitate the maintenance of sensory function.
12. To identify and accept positive and negative expressions, feelings, and reactions.
13. To identify and accept the interrelatedness of emotions and organic illness.
14. To facilitate the maintenance of effective verbal and nonverbal communication.
15. To promote the development of productive interpersonal relationships.
16. To facilitate progress toward achievement of personal spiritual goals.
17. To create and/or maintain a therapeutic environment.
18. To facilitate awareness of self as an individual with varying physical, emotional, and developmental needs.
19. To accept the optimum possible goals in the light of limitations, physical and emotional.
20. To use community resources as an aid in resolving problems arising from illness.
21. To understand the role of social problems as influencing factors in the case of illness.

From Abdellah, F.G., and others, Patient-Centered Approaches to Nursing, *New York: Macmillan Publishing Co., Inc., 1960, pp. 16–17. Used with permission.*

COMPARISON WITH OTHER THEORIES

An examination of these twenty-one problems yields similarities with other theories. Most notable is their similarity to Henderson's fourteen components of basic nursing care.[14] (See Table 9–2.) As can be seen in this table, Abdellah has consolidated some components, such as number 7—Select suitable clothing, and number 8—Keep body clean and well groomed; and has expanded others, most notably number 14—Learn, discover, and satisfy curiosity. The strong similarity may be the result of both Henderson's and Abdellah's exposure to the same environment—Teachers College, Columbia University, New York. It might be hypothesized that Abdellah moved from the rather simplistic form of Henderson's theory to a more complex structure.

TABLE 9–2. COMPARISON OF MASLOW'S, HENDERSON'S, AND ABDELLAH'S FRAMEWORKS

Maslow	Henderson	Abdellah[a]
1. Physiological needs	1. Breathe normally	5. To facilitate the maintenance of a supply of oxygen to all body cells
	2. Eat and drink adequately	6. To facilitate the maintenance of nutrition of all body cells
		8. To facilitate the maintenance of fluid and electrolyte balance
	3. Eliminate by all avenues of elimination	7. To facilitate the maintenance of elimination
	4. Move and maintain desirable posture	4. To maintain good body mechanics and prevent and correct deformities
	5. Sleep and rest	2. To promote optimal activity: exercise, rest, and sleep
	6. Select suitable clothing	10. To facilitate the maintenance of regulatory mechanisms and functions
	7. Maintain body temperature	1. To maintain good hygiene and physical comfort
	8. Keep body clean and well groomed & protect the integument	
2. Safety needs	9. Avoid environmental dangers and avoid injuring others	3. To promote safety through the prevention of accident, injury, or other trauma and through the prevention of the spread of infection
		11. To facilitate the maintenance of sensory function

3. Belonging and love
   needs

   10. Communicate with others

   11. Worship according to faith

   14. To facilitate the maintenance of effective verbal and non-verbal communication

   15. To promote the development of productive interpersonal relationships

   16. To facilitate progress toward achievement of personal spiritual goals

4. Esteem needs

   12. Work at something providing a sense of accomplishment

   13. Play or participate in various forms of recreation

   19. To accept the optimum possible goals in the light of limitations, physical and emotional

   14. Learn, discover, or satisfy curiosity

   9. To recognize the physiological responses of the body to disease conditions—pathological, physiological, and compensatory

   12. To identify and accept positive and negative expressions, feelings, and reactions

   13. To identify and accept the interrelatedness of emotions and organic illness

   17. To create and/or maintain a therapeutic environment

   18. To facilitate awareness of self as an individual with varying physical, emotional, and developmental needs

   20. To use community resources as an aid in resolving problems arising from illness

   21. To understand the role of social problems as influencing factors in the cause of illness

5. Self-actualization
   needs

[a] Numbers in column 3 refer to the twenty-one problems as listed in Table 9-1.

Despite the noted similarity, a major difference is evident. Henderson's components are written in terms of client behaviors, whereas Abdellah's problems are formulated in terms of the nursing services that should be incorporated into the determination of the client's needs.[15] This emphasis on nursing services is consistent with Abdellah's apparent nurse-centered orientation mentioned earlier. Henderson seems to have maintained the client orientation, whereas Abdellah seems to have moved beyond it (see Table 9–2).

Abdellah's nursing problems are also comparable to Maslow's hierarchy of needs.[16] In contrast to Henderson's components, which have a strong physiological orientation, Abdellah's expansion in the *esteem needs area* provides a more balanced set of nursing problems between the physical and nonphysical areas (Table 9–2). As with Henderson's components, Abdellah's problems do not meet the self-actualization needs of Maslow. This is not surprising as self-actualization is not a goal to be accomplished but a process that is ongoing—the dynamic process of beginning. To place elements in this area would negate the dynamism of self-actualization. From a different viewpoint, if Henderson's components and Abdellah's problems are fulfilled, then the client will move toward becoming and self-actualization.

ABDELLAH'S THEORY AND THE FOUR MAJOR CONCEPTS

Abdellah does not clearly specify each of the four major concepts—the individual or human, health, environment/society, and nursing. She does describe the recipients of nursing as *individuals* (and families), although she does not delineate her beliefs or assumptions about the nature of human beings. Her twenty-one nursing problems deal with biological, psychological, and social areas of individuals and can be considered to represent areas of importance to them.

Health, or the achieving of it, is the purpose of nursing services. Although Abdellah does not give a definition of health, she speaks to "total health needs" and "a healthy state of mind and body" in her description of nursing as a comprehensive service.[17]

Society is included in "planning for optimum health on local, state, national, and international levels."[18] However, as Abdellah further delineated her ideas, the focus of nursing service is clearly the individual. Society is negated when she discusses implementation.

Nursing is broadly grouped into the twenty-one problem areas to guide care and promote the use of nursing judgment. Abdellah considers nursing to be a comprehensive service that is based on an art and science and aims to help people, sick or well, cope with their health needs.

USE OF THE TWENTY-ONE PROBLEMS IN THE NURSING PROCESS

Because of the strong nurse-centered orientation in the twenty-one nursing problems, their use in the nursing process is primarily to direct the nurse. Indirectly, the client benefits. If the nurse helps the client reach all the goals stated in the nursing problems, then the client will be moved toward health.

Within the *assessment* phase, the nursing problems provide guidelines for the collection of data. A principle underlying the problem-solving approach is that for each identified problem, pertinent data are collected. Thus, for each of the identified twenty-one nursing problems, relevant data are collected. The overt or covert nature of the problems necessitates a direct or indirect approach, respectively. For example, the overt problem of nutritional status can be assessed by direct measures of weight, food intake, and body size; whereas the covert problem of maintaining a therapeutic environment requires more indirect approaches to data collection.

The nursing problems can be divided into those that are basic to all clients and those that reflect sustenal, remedial, or restorative care needs, as seen in Table 9–3. By facilitating data collection, such a classification promotes investigating those problems consistent with the client's stage of illness. However, such a classification promotes the thinking that the client's stage of illness determines appropriate or acceptable problems. Such thinking is contrary to the philosophy of holism. If clients are holistic, then they can have needs in any and all areas regardless of the stage of illness. A varied multitude of nursing problems could then exist.

The results of the data collection would determine the client's specific overt or covert problems. These specific problems would be grouped under one or more of the broader nursing problems. This step is consistent with that involved in *nursing diagnosis*. Within this framework, the nursing diagnoses are derived from the exhibited nursing problems.

The twenty-one nursing problems can have a great impact on the *planning* phase of the nursing process. The statements of the nursing problems most closely resemble goal statements. Therefore, once the problem has been diagnosed, the goals have been established. Many of the nursing problem statements can be considered goals for either the nurse or the client. Given that these problems are called *nursing problems*, then it becomes reasonable to conclude that these goals are basically nursing goals.

Using the goals as the framework, a plan is developed and appropriate nursing interventions are determined. Table 9–3 summarizes the kinds of interventions that would be appropriate for the categories of nursing problems. Again, holism tends to be negated in *implementation* because of the isolated, particulate nature of the nursing problems.

Following implementation of the plan, *evaluation* takes place. According to the American Nurses' Association *Standards of Nursing Practice*,[19] the

TABLE 9–3. THE RELATIONSHIPS AMONG THE CLASSIFICATION AND APPROACH OF THE TWENTY-ONE NURSING PROBLEMS AND STAGES OF ILLNESS, NURSING INTERVENTIONS, AND CRITERION MEASURES

Stages of Illness[a]	Nursing Problems	Classification and Approach[b]	Nursing Interventions[c]	Criterion Measures[a]
Basic to all patients	1. To maintain good hygiene and physical comfort	Overt problems, covert problems, or both	Measures necessary to maintain hygiene, physical comfort, activity, rest and sleep, safety, and body mechanics	Related to preventive care needs
	2. To promote optimal activity: exercise, rest, and sleep	Direct methods, indirect methods, or both		
	3. To promote safety through prevention of accident, injury, or other trauma and through the prevention of the spread of infection			
	4. To maintain good body mechanics and prevent and correct deformities			
Sustenal care needs	5. To facilitate the maintenance of a supply of oxygen to all body cells	Usually overt problems	Measures necessary to maintain oxygen supply, nutrition, elimination, fluid and electrolyte balance, regulatory mechanisms, and sensory functions. Interventions imply recognition of body's response to disease	Related to sustenal and restorative care needs—the normal and disturbed physiological body processes that are vital to sustaining life
	6. To facilitate the maintenance of nutrition of all body cells	Direct methods		
	7. To facilitate the maintenance of elimination			
	8. To facilitate the maintenance of fluid and electrolyte balance			
	9. To recognize the physiological responses of the body to disease conditions—pathological, physiological, and compensatory			
	10. To facilitate the maintenance of regulatory mechanisms and functions			
	11. To facilitate the maintenance of sensory function			

Remedial care needs	12. To identify and accept positive and negative expressions, feelings, and reactions	Usually overt problems Indirect methods	Measures that are helpful to the client and his or her family during their emotional reactions to client's illness	Related to rehabilitation needs, particularly those involving emotional and interpersonal difficulties
	13. To identify and accept the interrelatedness of emotions and organic illness			
	14. To facilitate the maintenance of effective verbal and nonverbal communication			
	15. To promote the development of productive interpersonal relationships			
	16. To facilitate progress toward achievement of personal and spiritual goals			
	17. To create and maintain a therapeutic environment			
	18. To facilitate awareness of self as an individual with varying physical, emotional, and developmental needs			
Restorative care needs	19. To accept the optimum possible goals in in the light of limitations, physical and emotional	Overt problems, covert problems, or both Direct methods, indirect methods, or both	Measures that will assist the client and his or her family to cope with the illness and necessary life adjustment	Related to sociological and community problems affecting client care
	20. To use community resources as an aid in resolving problems arising from illness			
	21. To understand the role of social problems as influencing factors in the cause of illness			

[a] From Abdellah, F.G. and Levine, E. Better Patient Care Through Nursing Research, New York: Macmillan Publishing Co., Inc., 1965, pp. 78–79, 280–81.
[b] From Abdellah, F.G. and others, Patient-Centered Approaches to Nursing, New York: Macmillan Publishing Co., Inc., 1973, pp. 81–82.
[c] From Carter, J.H. and others, Standards of Nursing Care, New York: Springer Publishing Co., Inc., 1976, pp. 8–9.

plan is evaluated in terms of the client's progress or lack of progress toward the achievement of the stated goals. This would be extremely difficult if not impossible to do for Abdellah's nursing problem approach since it has been determined that the goals are *nursing* goals, not *client* goals. Thus, the most appropriate evaluation would be the *nurse's* progress or lack of progress toward the achievement of the stated goals.

Abdellah postulates that criterion measures can be determined from the groupings of the nursing problems, as shown in Table 9–3. A criterion is a value-free name of a measurable variable believed or known to be a relevant indicator of the quality of client care.[20] These criteria can be used to measure client care. Although it is not clear in her writings, the measurement of criteria seems to have been substituted for evaluating a client's progress toward goal achievement.

The use of Abdellah's twenty-one nursing problems in an example might be beneficial. Consider the case of Ron who experienced severe crushing chest pain following a board meeting at his place of business. In addition to the pain, he experienced shortness of breath, tachycardia, and profuse diaphoresis. Upon admission to the hospital, assessment indicated that Ron might have sustained some cardiac damage. Investigation into his history revealed that he has been having episodes of chest pain for the past two months. With this as the data base, the specific problems of pain, impaired cardiac functioning, work-related stress, and failure to seek medical assistance can be identified. These specific problems can be related to selected nursing problems defined by Abdellah, and the nursing problems can be related to the stage of Ron's illness. Nursing strategies and criterion measures can then be determined. Table 9–4 illustrates the implementation of Abdellah's framework. The results of fractionalizing care can be readily seen by the repetition of intervention strategies for the two problems of pain and impaired cardiac functioning. (This table is in no way designed to be inclusive. Rather, it is offered as an attempt to make the theory operational.)

ABDELLAH'S WORK AND THE CHARACTERISTICS OF A THEORY

In comparing Abdellah's work with the characteristics of a theory presented in Chapter 1, it may be seen that Abdellah's theory has interrelated the concepts of health, nursing problems, and problem solving as she attempts to create a different way of viewing nursing phenomena (characteristic 1). The result was the statement that nursing is the use of the problem-solving approach with key nursing problems related to the health needs of people. Problem solving is an activity that is inherently logical in nature (characteristic 2).

Because of the failure of the framework to provide a perspective on humans and society in general, the theory appears to be limited to use with

TABLE 9—4. AN ILLUSTRATION OF THE IMPLEMENTATION OF ABDELLAH'S FRAMEWORK IN RON'S CARE

Stages of Illness	Selected Abdellah Nursing Problems	Classification and Approach	Selected Nursing Interventions	Criterion Measures
Basic to care	1. To maintain good hygiene and physical comfort	Overt problem of pain Direct and indirect methods	1. Administer oxygen 2. Elevate headrest 3. Reposition client 4. Administer prescribed analgesic 5. Remain with client	Amount of pain
Sustenal care needs	5. To facilitate the maintenance of a supply of oxygen to all body cells	Overt problem of impaired cardiac functioning Direct methods	1. Promote rest 2. Place in sitting position 3. Promote deep breathing and coughing 4. Implement exercise program as tolerated	Vital signs
Remedial care needs	13. To identify and accept the interrelatedness of emotional and organic illness	Covert problem of effects of work-related stress on cardiac functioning Indirect methods	1. Investigate the nature of his job and activities involved 2. Explore his work-related goals 3. Explore the kinds of stress associated with his job	Knowledge of relationship between stress and his illness
Restorative care needs	20. To use community resources as an aid in resolving problems arising from illness	Overt problem of failure to seek medical assistance when needed Direct methods	1. Teach early warning signs and symptoms of cardiac distress 2. Teach course of action should specific symptoms occur	Knowledge of appropriate use of certain community resources

those who have health needs or nursing problems. This may well be intentional as the framework seems to focus quite heavily on nursing practice with individuals. This somewhat limits the ability to generalize, although the problem-solving approach is readily generalizable to clients with specific health needs and specific nursing problems (characteristic 3).

One of the most important questions that arises when considering Abdellah's work is the role of the client within the framework. This question could generate hypotheses for testing and thus demonstrates the ability of Abdellah's work to generate hypotheses for testing (characteristic 4). The results of testing such hypotheses would contribute to the general body of nursing knowledge (characteristic 5).

As a logical and simple statement, Abdellah's problem-solving approach can easily be used by practitioners to guide various activities within their nursing practice. This is especially true when considering nursing practice that deals with clients who have specific needs and specific nursing problems (characteristic 6).

Abdellah's theory is consistent with other theories such as those of Maslow and Henderson. Although this consistency exists, many questions remained unanswered (characteristic 7).

LIMITATIONS

The major limitation to Abdellah's theory and the twenty-one nursing problems is their very strong nursing-centered orientation. With this orientation, appropriate uses might be the organization of teaching content for nursing students, the evaluation of a student's performance in the clinical area or both. But in terms of client care, there is little emphasis on what the client is to achieve.

Abdellah's framework is inconsistent with the concept of holism. The classification of the twenty-one nursing problems according to stages of illness and the particulate nature of the problems attests to this. As a result, the client may be diagnosed as having numerous problems that would lead to fractionalized care efforts, and potential problems might be overlooked because the client is not deemed to be in a particular stage of illness.

CONCLUSIONS

Abdellah's theory and framework provide a basis for determining and organizing nursing care. If all of the problems are investigated, the client would be likely to be thoroughly assessed. The problems also provide a basis for organizing appropriate nursing strategies. It is anticipated that by solving the nursing problems, the client would be moved toward health. The nurse's philosophical frame of reference would determine whether this theory and the twenty-one nursing problems could be implemented in practice.

SUMMARY

Using Abdellah's concepts of health, nursing problems, and problem solving, the theoretical statement of nursing that can be derived is the use of the problem-solving approach with key nursing problems related to the health needs of people. From this framework, twenty-one nursing problems were developed. These problems are compared to Henderson's fourteen components of nursing and Maslow's hierarchy of needs. Ways to use the nursing problems in the nursing process are explored. The major limitation of Abdellah's theory is its strong nursing-centered orientation. Some modification of the nursing problems to promote a more client-centered orientation would encourage effective utilization of the theory in professional nursing practice.

REFERENCES

1. Abdellah, F.G., and others, *Patient-Centered Approaches to Nursing*, New York: Macmillan Publishing Co., Inc., 1960, pp. 24–25.
2. Abdellah, F.G., and others, *New Directions in Patient-Centered Nursing*, New York: Macmillan Publishing Co., Inc., 1973, p. 19.
3.(a) Torres, G. & Stanton, M. *Curriculum Process in Nursing: A Guide to Curriculum Development*, Englewood Cliffs, N.J.: Prentice-Hall, 1982, p. 126.
3.(b) Abdellah, F.G. & Levine, E. *Better Patient Care Through Nursing Research* (3rd ed.), New York: Macmillan, 1986, p. 54.
4. Abdellah and others, *Patient-Centered Approaches*, pp. 6–7.
5. Nicholls, M.E. & Wessells, V.G., eds. *Nursing Standards and Nursing Process*, Wakefield, Mass.: Contemporary Publishing, Inc., 1977, p. 6.
6. Abdellah and others, *Patient-Centered Approaches*, pp. 30–31.
7. Abdellah & Levine, *Better Patient Care Through Nursing Research*, p. 54.
8. Abdellah and others, p. 27.
9. Abdellah, F.G. & Levine, E. *Better Patient Care Through Nursing Research*, p. 492.
10. Abdellah and others, *Patient-Centered Approaches*, p. 26.
11. Ibid, 11.
12. Abdellah and others, *New Directions*, p. 79.
13. Abdellah and others, *Patient-Centered Approaches*, p. 27.
14. Henderson, V. & Nite, G. *Principles and Practice of Nursing* (6th ed.) New York: Macmillan, 1978, p. 94.
15. DeYoung, L. *The Foundations of Nursing*, St. Louis, Mo.: C. V. Mosby, 1976, p. 112.
16. Maslow, A. *Motivation and Personality*, New York: Harper & Row, 1954.
17. Abdellah and others, *Patient-Centered Approaches*, pp. 24–25.

18.   Ibid, 25.
19.   Congress for Nursing Practice, *Standards of Nursing Practice*, Kansas City, Mo.: American Nurses' Association, 1973.
20.   Bloch, D. Criteria, Standards, Norms—Crucial Terms in Quality Assurance, *Journal of Nursing Administration*, 1977, 7, 22.

CHAPTER 10

Ida Jean Orlando

Mary Kathryn Leonard
Mary Disbrow Crane

Ida Jean Orlando Pelletier (b. 1926) has had a varied career as a practitioner, educator, researcher, and consultant in nursing. During the early part of her career she worked as a staff nurse in such areas as obstetrics, medicine and surgery, and the emergency room. She has also held supervisory positions and the title of Second Assistant Director of Nurses. She received a diploma in nursing from New York Medical College, Flower Fifth Avenue Hospital School of Nursing in 1947 and a BS in Public Health Nursing from St. John's University in Brooklyn, New York in 1951. In 1954, she received her MA in mental health consultation from Columbia University, New York. She then went to Yale University where she became a research associate and principal investigator on a project studying the integration of mental health concepts into the basic curriculum. This led to the publication of her first book, The Dynamic Nurse–Patient Relationship: Function, Process, and Principles, *in 1961.[1] She has also served as director of the graduate program in mental health and psychiatric nursing at Yale.*

In 1962, Orlando moved to Massachusetts. She became a clinical nursing consultant to a psychiatric hospital, McLean Hospital, and at a veterans' hospital. At McLean Hospital, she carried out the research that led to the publication in 1972 of her second book, The Discipline and Teaching of Nursing Process.[2]

Since 1972, Orlando has been associated intermittently with Boston University School of Nursing, teaching nursing theory and supervising graudate students in the clinical area. The New England Board of Higher Education has employed her as a project consultant in their Mental Health Project for Associate Degree Faculties. Her most recent position is as a nurse educator at Metropolitan State Hospital in Waltham, Massachusetts.

Throughout her career, Orlando has been active in a variety of organizations including the Massachusetts Nurses' Association and the Harvard Community Health Plan. She has also lectured and offered workshops and consultation to a wide variety of agencies.

Ida Jean Orlando Pelletier is a significant contributor to the developing body of nursing knowledge. She describes a nursing process based on the interaction at a specific time between a patient and a nurse. Two books present her ideas. Her initial work, *The Dynamic Nurse–Patient Relationship: Function, Process and Principles* was published in 1961.[3] *The Discipline and*

Teaching of Nursing Process, showing further refinement of her theory, appeared in 1972.[4]

Orlando's educational background and the work that led her to publish provide insight into the content of her theory. Her advanced nursing preparation and area of teaching responsibility and practice were in mental health and psychiatric nursing. Although she applied her ideas to many nursing speciality areas, her interactive focus is dominant. Her position as an educator also influenced her work. Both of her books were the result of studies designed to improve the teaching of nurses.

The Dynamic Nurse–Patient Relationship was written after the completion of a five-year project at Yale University in the mid-1950s. The purpose of this project, supported by a grant from the National Institute of Mental Health, was "to identify the factors which enhanced or impeded the integration of mental health principles in the basic nursing curriculum."[5] The book describes the curriculum content developed from the study. Its stated purpose is "to offer the professional nursing student a theory of effective nursing practice."[6]

After completing her first book, Orlando refined her ideas and put them into practice at a private psychiatric facility, McLean Hospital in Belmont, Massachusetts. Again with a National Institute of Mental Health grant, she studied an objective means to evaluate her process and training in its discipline. This work, done during the 1960s, led to *The Discipline and Teaching of Nursing Process.*[7] In this book, she is concerned with the specific definition of nursing function and with incorporating nursing activities beyond the nurse–patient relationship into a total nursing system. She also developed more readily measured criteria to guide the nurse in her reaction to patient behavior.*

Orlando's work spans a fertile period of nursing thinking. She was probably influenced by, as well as an influence upon, other nursing theorists. For example, Orlando sounds similar to Nightingale when she states, "It is important for the nurse to concern herself with the patient's distress because the treatment and prevention of disease proceeds best when conditions extraneous to the disease itself and its management do not cause the patient additional suffering."[8] Another nursing theorist, Peplau, published her highly interpersonal theory two years before Orlando began her first study.[9] Henderson also was redefining her definition of nursing during Orlando's first study. Henderson's 1955 definition is consistent with Orlando when she states, "Nursing is primarily assisting the individual . . . in the performance of those activities . . . that he would perform unaided if he had the necessary strength, will, or knowledge."[10] Thus the majority of the

---

* In this chapter, the feminine pronoun is used when referrring to the nurse and the masculine pronoun when referring to the patient. This is consistent with Orlando's use of these pronouns and terms.

nursing theorists described in this book published during the time that Orlando was actively working on her theory.

ORLANDO'S KEY CONCEPTS

Certain major concepts are evident in Orlando's theory of nursing. She believes that nursing is *unique* and *independent* because it concerns itself with an *individual's need for help,* real or potential, in an *immediate* situation. The process by which nursing resolves this helplessness is *interactive* and is pursued in a *disciplined* manner that requires *training.*

Throughout her career, Orlando has been concerned with identifying that which is *uniquely* nursing. In her first book she presents principles to guide nursing practice.[11] She believes that the use of general principles from other fields is not sufficient to help the nurse in her interaction with patients. In this book, she identifies nursing's role as follows, "It is the nurse's direct responsibility to see to it that the patient's needs for help are met either by her own activity or by calling in the help of others."[12]

By the time of her second book, Orlando suggests that nursing's failure to establish its uniqueness results from the lack of a clearly identifiable function.[13] This leads to inadequate care and insufficient attention to the patient's reactions to his immediate experiences. Thus, nursing "is concerned with providing direct assistance to individuals in whatever setting they are found for the purpose of avoiding, relieving, diminishing, or curing the individual's sense of helplessness."[14]

It is this unique function that gives nurses the authority to work *independently.* Orlando recommends that "nurses . . . must radically shift their focus from assistance to physicians and institutions to assisting patients with what they cannot do alone."[15] Physicians' orders are directed to patients, not to nurses. Moreover, at times nurses may even assist patients *not* to comply with a medical order. Nurses must also resolve conflicts between the patient's need for help and institutional policies. Nursing's unique function allows nurses to work in any setting where persons experience a need for help that they cannot resolve themselves. Thus, nurses may practice with well or ill persons in an independent practice or in an institutional setting.

Orlando's theory focuses on the patient as an *individual.* Each person is different. Thus, appropriate nursing actions for two patients with the same presenting behavior are to be individualized. Nurses cannot automatically act based only on principles, past experience, or physicians' orders. They must first ascertain that their actions will meet the specific patient's need for help.

Nursing is concerned with "individuals who suffer or anticipate a sense of helplessness."[16] Orlando defines need as "a requirement of the patient which, if supplied, relieves or diminishes his immediate distress or improves his immediate sense of adequacy or well-being."[17] In many instances, people can meet their own needs, do so, and do not require the help of professional nurses. When they cannot do so, or do not clearly understand these needs, a *need for help* is present. The nurse's function is to correctly identify and relieve this need for help.

The *immediacy* of the nursing situation is a vital concept in Orlando's theory. Each patient's behavior must be assessed to determine whether it expresses a need for help. Furthermore, identical behaviors by the same patient may indicate different needs. The nursing action must also be specifically designed for the immediate encounter. Long-term planning has no part in Orlando's theory except as it pertains to providing adequate staff coverage for a job setting. Thus, Orlando's process is dynamic. In this area, her theory is consistent with Martha Roger's principles of homeodynamics.[18]

Orlando's nursing process is totally *interactive*. It describes, step by step, what goes on between a nurse and a patient in a specific encounter. A patient behavior causes the process to begin. The process involves the nurse's reaction to this behavior and the nurse's consequent action. The nurse shares her reaction with the patient to identify the need for help and the appropriate action. Orlando's principles are meant to guide the nurse at various stages of the interaction. She emphasizes the importance of interaction when she writes, "Learning how to understand what is happening between herself and the patient is the central core of the nurse's practice and comprises the basic framework for the help she gives to patients."[19]

The actual *process* of a nurse–patient interaction is the same as that of any interaction between two persons. When nurses use this process in caring for patients, Orlando calls it the "nursing process." It is the tool that nurses use to fulfill their function to patients. In an attempt to extend her theory to encompass all nursing activities, Orlando broadens the use of the process beyond the individual nurse–patient relationship in her book *The Discipline and Teaching of Nursing Process*. She applies the process to contacts between a nurse leader and those she supervises or directs. When used in this manner, she refers to the process as the "directive or supervisory job process in nursing."[20]

If the nursing process is the same as the interactive process between any two individuals, how can nursing call itself a profession? The key is *discipline* in use of the process. Orlando provides three criteria to evaluate this discipline. These criteria differentiate an "automatic personal response" from a "disciplined professional response."[21] Only the latter leads to effective nursing care, that is, relief of the patient's sense of helplessness. Learning to employ the process discipline requires *training*. This justifies the need for specific education in nursing. Orlando's nursing process and the criteria for its disciplined use provide the content for the following section.

ORLANDO'S NURSING PROCESS

Orlando's nursing process is based on the "process by which any individual acts."[22] The purpose of the process when used between a nurse and a patient is meeting the patient's need for help. Improvement in the patient's behavior that indicates resolution of the need is the result. The process is also used with other persons working in a job setting. The purpose here is to understand how the professional and job responsibilities of each affect the other. This allows each nurse to effectively fulfill her professional function for the patient within the organizational setting.

Patient Behavior

The nursing process is set in motion by *patient behavior*. All patient behavior, no matter how insignificant, must be considered as expression of need for help until its meaning to a particular patient in an immediate situation is understood. Orlando stresses this in her first principle: "The presenting behavior of the patient, regardless of the form in which it appears, may represent a plea for help."[23]

When the patient experiences a need that he cannot resolve, a sense of helplessness occurs. The patient's behavior reflects this distress. In *The Dynamic Nurse–Patient Relationship,* Orlando describes some categories of patient distress. These are "physical limitations, . . . adverse reactions to the setting and . . . experiences which prevent the patient from communicating his needs."[24] Feelings of helplessness due to physical limitations may result from incomplete development, temporary or permanent disability, or restrictions of the environment, real or imagined. Adverse reactions to the setting, on the other hand, usually result from incorrect or inadequate understanding of an experience there. Patients may become distressed from a negative reaction to any aspect of the setting despite its helpful or therapeutic intent. Frequently a need for help may also arise from the patient's inability to communicate effectively. This may be due to such factors as ambivalence concerning dependency brought on by illness, embarrassment related to the need, lack of trust in the nurse, and inability to state the need precisely.

Patient behavior may be verbal or nonverbal. Inconsistency between these two types of behavior may be the factor that alerts the nurse that the patient needs help. Verbal behavior encompasses all the patient's use of language. It may take the form of "complaints . . . , requests . . . , questions . . . , refusals . . . , demands . . . , and . . . comments or statements."[25] Nonverbal behavior includes physiological manifestations such as heart rate, perspiration, edema, and urination; and motor activity such as smiling, walking, and avoiding eye contact. Nonverbal patient behavior may also be vocal. This includes such actions as sobbing, laughing, shouting, and sighing.

Although all patient behavior may indicate a need for help, the behavior may not effectively communicate that need. When the behavior does not communicate the need, problems in the nurse–patient relationship can arise. Ineffective patient behavior "prevents the nurse from carrying out her concerns for the patient's care or from maintaining a satisfactory relationship to the patient."[26] Ineffective patient behavior may also indicate difficulties in the initial establishment of the nurse–patient relationship, inaccurate identification of the patient's need by the nurse, or negative patient reaction to automatic nursing action. Resolution of ineffective patient behavior deserves high priority as the behavior usually becomes worse over time if the need for help that it expresses remains unresolved.

Nurse Reaction.

The patient behavior stimulates a *nurse reaction*, which marks the beginning of the nursing process. This reaction is comprised of three sequential parts. First, the nurse perceives the behavior through any of her senses. Second, the perception leads to thought. Finally, the thought produces an automatic feeling.[27] For example, the nurse sees a patient smile, thinks he is happy, and feels good. This reaction forms the basis for determining the nursing action. However, the nurse must first share her reaction with the patient to ascertain that she has correctly identified the need for help and the nursing action appropriate to resolve it. Orlando offers a principle to guide the nurse in her reaction to patient behavior. "The nurse does not assume that any aspect of her reaction to the patient is correct, helpful, or appropriate until she checks the validity of it in exploration with the patient."[28]

Perception, thought, and feeling occur automatically and almost simultaneously. Therefore the nurse must learn to identify each part of her reaction. This helps her to analyze the reaction to determine why she reacted as she did. The process becomes logical rather than intuitive. The nurse is able to use her reaction for the purpose of helping the patient.

The discipline in the nursing process prescribes how the nurse shares her reaction with the patient. Orlando offers a principle to explain the usefulness of this sharing:

> Any observation shared and explored with the patient is immediately useful in ascertaining and meeting his need or finding out that he is not in need at that time.[29]

She provides the following three criteria to ensure that the nurse's exploration of her reaction with the patient is successful[30]:

> 1. What the nurse says to the individual in the contact must match (*be consistent with*) any or all of the items contained in the immediate reaction, and what the nurse does nonverbally must be verbally expressed and the expression must match one or all of the items contained in the immediate

reaction; 2. The nurse must clearly communicate to the individual that the item being expressed belongs to herself; 3. The nurse must ask the individual about the item expressed in order to obtain correction or verification from that same individual.

Which aspect of her reaction the nurse shares with the patient is not as important as that it be shared in the manner described in the criteria. From a practical standpoint, it may be more expeditious to share a perception than a thought or feeling. "You are grimacing" contains less assumption than "Are you in pain?" In this way the patient can more easily express his need for help without having to correct the nurse's misconception.

Feelings can and should be shared even when they are negative. The nonverbal action of the nurse will usually show her feelings if they are not verbally expressed. Thus, the nurse's verbal and nonverbal behavior will be inconsistent. Proper sharing of feelings can effectively help the patient to express his need for help. For example, a nurse may react to a patient's refusal of a medication with anger. If she says, "I am angry with your refusal of your medication. Could you explain to me why you have refused?" she invites the patient to explain the need for help that his refusal expressed. Her expression meets the three criteria, and the patient's need for help can be identified and resolved.

This example shows the importance of the nurse sharing her reaction as a fact about herself. She states, "I am angry," rather than, "You make me angry." This clear identification of the reaction as her own reduces the chance of patient misinterpretation. It also encourages the patient to share his reaction in a similar manner.

Adequate identification of the three aspects of the nurse's reaction helps to resolve extraneous feelings that may interfere with the patient's care. The nurse may find that her feelings come from her personal belief of how people should act or from stresses in the organizational setting. These feelings or stresses are unrelated to meeting the patient's need. If they are not resolved, the nurse's verbal and nonverbal behavior will again be inconsistent. This same process should be employed with nurses or other professionals in the job setting to resolve any conflicts that interfere with the nurse fulfilling her professional function for the patient.

Orlando used her three criteria in the study described in *The Discipline and Teaching of Nursing Process* and found that use of the process discipline is positively related to improvement in patient behavior.[31] The study also showed a positive relationship between the nurse's use of the process and its use by the patient.[31] Thus, use of the process alone can help the patient communicate his need more effectively.

Orlando offers a diagram depicting open sharing of the nurse's reaction versus keeping the reaction secret (see Figs. 10–1 and 10–2). The nurse action that results from the reaction becomes a behavior stimulating a reaction to the patient. Only openness in sharing of the reaction assures

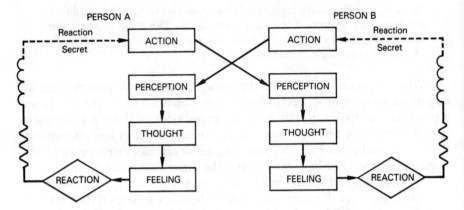

Figure 10–1. The action process in a person-to-person contact functioning in secret. The perceptions, thoughts, and feelings of each individual are not directly available to the perception of the other individual through the observable action. *(From Orlando, I.J., The Discipline and Teaching of Nursing Process, New York: G. P. Putnam's Sons, 1972, p. 26. Used with permission.)*

that the patient's need will be effectively resolved. This sharing, in the manner prescribed, differentiates professional nursing practice from automatic personal response.

Nurse's Action

Once the nurse has validated or corrected her reaction to the patient's behavior through exploration with him, she can complete the nursing process with the *nurse's action*. Orlando includes "only what she [the nurse] says

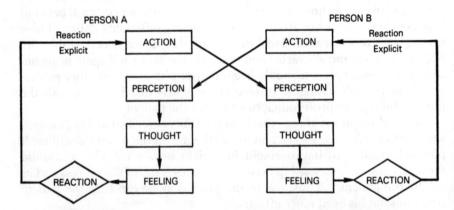

Figure 10–2. The action process in a person-to-person contact functioning by open disclosure. The perceptions, thoughts, and feelings of each individual are directly available to the perception of the other individual through the observable action. *(From Orlando, I.J., The Discipline and Teaching of Nursing Process, New York: G. P. Putnam's Sons, 1972, p. 26. Used with permission.)*

or does with or for the benefit of the patient" as professional nursing action.[32] The nurse must be certain that her action is appropriate to meet the patient's need for help. Orlando's principle guiding nursing action states, "The nurse initiates a process of exploration to ascertain how the patient is affected by what she says or does."[33]

The nurse can act in two ways: automatic or deliberative. Only the second manner fulfills her professional function. Automatic actions are "those decided upon for reasons other than the patient's immediate need," whereas deliberative actions ascertain and meet this need.[34] There is a distinction between the purpose an action actually serves and its intention to help the patient. For example, a nurse administers a sleeping pill because the physician orders it. Carrying out the physician's order is the purpose of the action. However, the nurse has not determined that the patient is having trouble sleeping or that a pill is the most appropriate way to help him sleep. Thus the action is automatic, not deliberative, and the patient's need for help is unlikely to be met.

The following list identifies the criteria for deliberative actions:

1. Deliberative actions result from the correct identification of patient needs by validation of the nurse's reaction to patient behavior.
2. The nurse explores the meaning of the action to the patient and its relevance to meeting his need.
3. The nurse validates the action's effectiveness immediately after completing it.
4. The nurse is free of stimuli unrelated to the patient's need when she acts.

Automatic actions fail to meet one or more of these criteria. Automatic actions are most likely to be done by nurses primarily concerned with carrying out physicians' orders, routines of patient care, or general principles for protecting health or by nurses who do not validate their reactions to patient behaviors.

Professional Function

Nurses often work within organizations with other professionals, and are subject to the authority of the organization that employs them. It is inevitable, therefore, that at times conflicts will arise between the actions appropriate to the nurse's profession and those required by the job. Nonprofessional actions can prevent the nurse from carrying out her professional function, and this can lead to inadequate patient care. A well-defined function of the profession can help to prevent and resolve this conflict.

Nurses should not accept positions that do not allow them to meet their patient's need for help. If a conflict does arise, the nurse must present data to show that nursing is unable to fulfill its professional function. Orlando believes that an employer is unlikely to continue to require job activities that interfere with a well-defined function of a profession. For an agency to do so "would be to completely abandon the whole point of having enlisted the services of that profession in the agency or institution."[35]

Nurses must be constantly aware that their "activity is professional only when it deliberately achieves the purpose of helping the patient."[36] Some automatic activities may be necessary to the running of an institution. These should, however, be kept to a minimum and should be carried out, as much as possible, by support personnel. The nurse must attend to helping the patients resolve any conflict between these routines and their needs for help.

In most acute care institutions today, the potential demand for nursing skill and judgment exceeds the availability of such. As a result, nursing care delivery systems are being evaluated and revised to enable the nurse to practice in those situations or areas where she is most needed. Some of these situations have been specifically identified by the Professional Nursing Accreditation Committee and, through their input, reflected in the accreditation standards of the Joint Commission on Accreditation for Health Care Organizations. These are: (1) when the patient is admitted, a professional nursing assessment is needed to identify the patient's need for help; (2) when the patient has a need for education commonly called patient education; and (3) when the patient is being prepared for discharge.[37] In each of these situations, the use of Orlando's theory would guide the nurse in expeditiously meeting the patient's need. At this time, nurses in acute care facilities are being looked to to use their professional skills and knowledge to recognize and resolve the patient's need for help. Some of this recognition of the nursing contribution may be related to the situational pressures arising out of the prospective payment reimbursement system affecting health care institutions today. Under this system, emphasis is placed on the patient being treated and discharged within a predetermined number of days. Nursing can capitalize on this situation and use it to the patient's and profession's best interests. Orlando's theory, while simple in nature, provides direction and focus for identifying and understanding the patient's need.

Thus, the nursing process is set in motion by a patient behavior that may indicate a need for help. The nurse reacts to this behavior with perceptions, thoughts, and feelings. She shares an aspect of her reaction with the patient, making sure that her verbal and nonverbal actions are consistent with her reaction, that she identifies the reaction as her own, and that she invites the patient to comment on the validity of her reaction. A properly shared reaction by the nurse helps the patient to use the same process to more effectively communicate his need. Next, an appropriate action to resolve the need is mutually decided upon by the patient and nurse. After the nurse acts, she immediately asks the patient if the action has been effective. Throughout the interaction, the nurse makes sure that she is free of any extraneous stimuli that interfere with her reaction to the patient.

ORLANDO'S THEORY AND THE FOUR MAJOR CONCEPTS

Orlando includes material specific to three of the four major concepts: the human, health, and nursing. The fourth concept, society, is not included in her theory.

She uses the concept of *human* as she emphasizes individuality and the dynamic nature of the nurse–patient relationship.

While *health* is not specified, it is implied. In her initial work, Orlando focused on illness. Later, she indicated that nursing deals with the individual whenever there is a need for help. Thus, a sense of helplessness replaces the concept of health as the initiator of a need for nursing.

Orlando largely ignores *society*. She deals only with the interaction between a nurse and a patient in an immediate situation and speaks to the importance of individuality. She does make some attempt to discuss the overall nursing system in an institutional setting. However, she does not discuss how the patient is affected by the society in which he lives nor does she use society as a focus of nursing action.

Nursing is, of course, the focus of Orlando's work. She speaks of nursing as unique and independent in its concerns for an individual's need for help in an immediate situation. The efforts to meet the individual's need for help are carried out in an interactive situation and in a disciplined manner that requires proper training.

COMPARISON OF ORLANDO'S PROCESS AND THE NURSING PROCESS

Orlando's nursing process may be compared with the nursing process described in Chapter 2. Figure 10–3 helps to guide this comparison.

Certain overall characteristics are similar in both processes. For example, both are interpersonal in nature and require interaction between patient and nurse. The patient is asked for input throughout the process. Both processes also view the patient as a total person. He is not merely a disease process or body part. Orlando does not use the term *holistic*, but she effectively describes a holistic approach. Both processes are also used as a method to provide nursing care and as a means to evaluate that care. Finally, both are deliberate intellectual processes.

The *assessment* phase of the nursing process corresponds to the sharing of the nurse reaction to the patient behavior in Orlando's process. The patient behavior initiates the assessment. The collection of data includes only information relevant to identifying the patient's need for help. An ongoing data base is not useful to the immediate situation of the patient. The nurse's reaction, however, is probably influenced somewhat by her past experiences with the patient.

Orlando discusses data collection in her first book, *The Dynamic Nurse–*

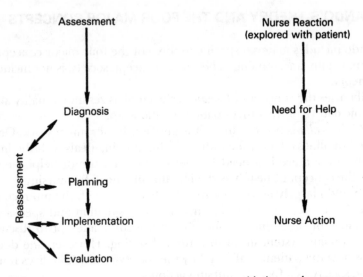

Figure 10–3. Comparison of Orlando's process with the nursing process.

Patient Relationship. She defines observation as "any information pertaining to a patient which the nurse acquires while she is on duty."[38] Direct data are comprised of "any perception, thought, or feeling the nurse has from her own experience of the patient's behavior at any or several moments in time."[39] Indirect data come from sources other than the patient, such as records, other health team members, or the patient's significant others. Both types of data require exploration with the patient to determine their relevance to the specific situation. Both verbal and nonverbal patient behaviors are important. Their consistency or inconsistency is a data piece in itself. This corresponds somewhat with subjective and objective data in the nursing process.

The sharing of the nurse's reaction in Orlando's process has components similar to the analysis in the nursing process. Although the nurse's reaction is automatic, her awareness of it and how she shares it is a deliberate intellectual activity. Orlando's sharing of the reaction, however, is a process of exploration with the patient. The nursing process, on the other hand, makes use of nursing's theoretical base and principles from the physical and behavioral sciences.

The product of the analysis in the nursing process is the *nursing diagnosis.* Exploration of the nurse's reaction with the patient in Orlando's process leads to identification of his need for help. The statement of the nursing diagnosis is a more formal process than that of need. Many nursing diagnoses may be made, given priority ratings, and resolved over time. Since Orlando deals with immediate nurse–patient interaction, only one need is dealt with at a time. Current efforts to develop a taxonomy of nursing diagnosis would be inappropriate in Orlando's theory since each patient encounter is different. Using Orlando's theory, nursing might develop categories of such areas as causes of patient's needs for help. These would, of course, have to be modified to fit the particular patient situation.

The *planning* phase of the nursing process involves writing goals and objectives and deciding upon appropriate nursing action. This corresponds to the nurse's action phase of Orlando's process. Any type of goal beyond the immediate situation is not possible in Orlando's process. Her goal is always relief of the patient's need for help; the objective relates to improvement in the patient's behavior. The nursing process mandates a more formal action of writing and giving priority to goals and objectives.

Both processes require patient participation in determining the appropriate action. In the nursing process this occurs mostly in goal setting. Orlando's process sees the patient as an active participant in determining the actual nurse action. The nursing process, on the other hand, relies more heavily on scientific principles and nursing theories in deciding how the nurse will act.

Implementation involves the final selection and carrying out of the planned action. This is also part of the nurse's action phase of Orlando's process. Both processes mandate that the action be appropriate for the patient as a unique individual. The nursing process expects the nurse to consider all possible effects of the action upon the patient. Orlando's process is concerned only with the effectiveness of the action in resolving the immediate need for help.

Evaluation is inherent in Orlando's action phase of her process. For an action to be deliberative, the nurse must evaluate its effectiveness when it is completed. Failure to do this can result in a series of ineffective actions with failure to meet the patient's need and an increase in the cost of nursing care and materials.

Evaluation in both processes is based on objective criteria. In the nursing process, evaluation asks whether the behaviorally stated objectives were met. In Orlando's process, the nurse observes patient behavior to see whether the patient has been helped. Thus, both processes evaluate in terms of outcomes of care.

Both the nursing process and Orlando's process are described as a series of sequential steps. The steps do not actually occur discretely and in order in either process. As new information becomes available, earlier steps may be repeated. Thus, new assessment data may alter the nursing diagnosis or the plan. Orlando's process is almost a continuous interchange— where patient behavior leads to nurse reaction, which leads to nurse behavior, which leads to patient reaction (see Figs. 10–2 and 10–3). Thus, both processes are dynamic and responsive to changes in the patient's situation.

The nursing process used today and Orlando's process have many similarities. They do, however, have important differences. The nursing process is far more formal and has more detailed phases than Orlando's. It requires the nurse to bring her knowledge of scientific principles and nursing theory to guide her behavior. Orlando demands only that the nurse follow the principles she lays down to guide nursing care. Long-term planning is part of the nursing process but is not relevant to Orlando's process. Although both processes call for patient involvement in the process of his care, Orlando's demands this participation more comprehensively.

ORLANDO'S WORK AND THE CHARACTERISTICS OF A THEORY

Can Orlando's work be called a theory of nursing as described in Chapter 1? In the sense of a "vision" of what nursing is, her work certainly qualifies. Does she combine concepts for the purpose of deriving hypotheses about practice? An exploration to see whether Orlando's work meets all of the basic characteristics of a theory helps to answer this question.

Before this is done, a comment on Orlando's use of the term *principle* is appropriate. Principles, as are laws, are truly predictable. They are most useful in the pure sciences. Human beings are too individualistic to be predictable, especially in relation to their behavior. Orlando's principles tell the nurse how to act. They predict only in the general sense that if the nurse uses the principles, the patient's behavior will improve. Thus, *guides for practice* would be a more appropriate term for them than principles.

1. Theories can interrelate concepts in such a way as to create a different way of looking at a particular phenomenon. Nursing is the focus of Orlando's work. Her theory views nursing as interacting with an individual in an immediate situation to relieve a sense of helplessness. She does relate concepts into a new and meaningful whole.

2. Theories must be logical in nature. Orlando's work does provide a reasonable and sequential process for nursing. Patient behavior initiates the nurse reaction. Exploration of this reaction with the patient leads to identification of a need and of an action to resolve that need. The nurse must react in a carefully prescribed manner to be certain she meets her goal of helping the patient. She must evaluate her action to be certain of its effectiveness. Thus, Orlando provides a logical rather than an intuitive approach to practice.

3. Theories should be relatively simple yet generalizable. Although Orlando's theory is simple in nature, it does generalize well to all of nursing practice. The theory remains simple by revolving around the nurse–patient interaction, the basic unit of nursing. This also makes the theory generalizable. This basic unit is applicable regardless of the setting of nursing care or the type of patient receiving care.

4. Theories can be the bases for hypotheses that can be tested. Orlando did derive hypotheses from her theory and tested them. Although her initial study was observational, she tested her ideas in a variety of nursing situations. In her second study, she developed criteria for the nurse's reaction that were specific enough for the development of hypotheses and statistical testing.

5. Theories contribute to and assist in increasing the general body of knowledge within the discipline through the research implemented to validate them. In testing her theory, Orlando added to the general body of nursing knowledge. She was able to test the effectiveness of her process discipline in a nurse's contacts with the patients, staff, and workers she supervises. Her findings showed a positive relationship between use of the process discipline and helpful outcomes of contacts. She also provided support for the idea that the process can be taught in a specified period of time.[40] Although her hypotheses need retesting, they provide a basis for other nurses to develop new theories. Other nursing theorists, such as Orem and Rogers, show consistency with, if not the influence of, aspects of Orlando's work.

6. Theories can be utilized by the practitioners to guide and improve their practice. Orlando has been quite successful in developing a theory useful to practice. Nurses can easily use her principles and process discipline in their interactions with patients and fellow workers. Using her theory, nurses are assured that they will not provide care in a way that is inappropriate for an individual patient. Orlando's theory is more easily applied to practice than that of some of the other nursing theorists. For example, Abdellah's twenty-one nursing problems lend themselves more easily to an educational than a practice setting.[41] If Orlando's theory was more consciously applied by nurses at all levels, collegiality within the profession would develop at a faster pace. Professional differences and alternative approaches could be shared and resolved in a constructive manner. Some institutions are attempting to change their nursing delivery systems to a more professional model, i.e., the case management system. When such a delivery system is used, there is less need for the invoking of hierarchial authority to resolve differences and enforce compliance to institutional policies and practices. Currently, within health care, much energy, time, and financial resources are being spent on teaching hospital personnel, including nurses, to communicate with patients, visitors, and each other. The goals of many of these programs are to teach people to listen to the needs expressed and to meet these needs. These programs encompass the essence of Orlando's theory. However, Orlando's theory does not guide all aspects of nursing practice. Areas for further study include long-term planning, dealing with family and community, and caring for patients who do not recognize that their health is endangered.

7. Theories must be consistent with other validated theories, laws, and principles but will leave open unanswered questions that need to be investigated. Orlando's theory does not conflict with other validated theories if it is viewed in the somewhat limited sense of a nurse–patient interaction. It is most consistent with interaction theory, but systems theory relates to it with difficulty. Orlando does discuss a "system of nursing practice."[42] This encompasses both the nurse–patient interaction and the relationship of nurses among themselves and with others in an organized work setting.

She does not, however, view the patient in relation to her subsystem and suprasystem. For this reason, Orlando's theory does not relate well to family theory. The family is mentioned only as a source of indirect data.

Thus, Orlando's work contains many of the characteristics of a theory. Despite her intent, however, it does not provide a comprehensive theory to guide nursing practice. Nonetheless, this deficit does not negate its usefulness in guiding nurse–patient interaction. Nor does it deny its value as a stimulus to other nurses to carry theory development further.

STRENGTHS AND LIMITATIONS

Orlando's theory has much to offer to nursing. The predominant strength of her work is its usefulness in nursing practice. It guides nurses through their interactions with patients. Use of her theory virtually assures that patients will be treated as individuals and that they will have an active and constant input into their own care. The nurse's focus must remain on the patient rather than on the demands of the work setting.

The nurse can keep Orlando in mind while applying the nursing process of today. Use of her theory prevents inaccurate diagnosis or ineffective plans because the nurse has to constantly explore her reactions with the patient. No nurse, following Orlando's principles, could fail to evaluate the care she has given.

Another of Orlando's strengths is her assertion of nursing's independence as a profession and her belief that this independence must be based on a sound theoretical framework. She bases this belief on her definition of nursing function. She believes that this clearly defined function will assist nursing in establishing its independence and in structuring the work setting so that nurses can effectively meet their patients' needs for help. The function of "finding out and meeting the patient's immediate needs for help" is broad enough to encompass nurses practicing in all settings and in all speciality areas.[43] It allows nursing to evolve over time by avoiding a rigid list of nursing activities.

Orlando guides the nurse to evaluate her care in terms of objectively observable patient outcomes. It is not the structure of the setting or the number of nurses on duty that determines effective care. Orlando has found a positive relationship between the use of her process and favorable outcomes of patient behavior. In planning to implement standards for nursing practice, the American Nurses' Association has described patient outcomes as "the ultimate indicators of quality patient care."[44] The immediate and interactive nature of her process does, however, make evaluation a time-consuming process.

As previously alluded to, the nursing profession's input into accreditation standards for health care organizations has placed great emphasis on the evaluation of interventions in terms of patient outcomes.

Consistent use of Orlando's theory by nurses could make evaluation a less time-consuming and more deliberate function, the results of which would be documented in patient charts. Such documentation of patient needs, planned interventions, and evaluation of interventions would provide data for analysis that would contribute to the general body of knowledge within the field of nursing.

Orlando's testing of her theory in the practice setting lends further support to its usefulness. Her first study, published in *The Dynamic Nurse–Patient Relationship*, provided a basis for future work. For a second study, described in *The Discipline and Teaching of the Nursing Process*, she developed specific criteria amenable to statistical testing. Nursing can pursue Orlando's work by retesting and further developing her work.

Although Orlando's ideas contain many of the characteristics of a theory, there are limitations. Her mental health background is probably responsible for the highly interactive nature of her theory. Although this interactive nature is one of the theory's strengths, it also provides limitation in her ideas. Nurses deal extensively with monitoring and controlling the physiological processes of patients to prevent illness and restore health. Orlando scarcely mentions this aspect of the nurse's role. The highly interactive nature of Orlando's theory makes it hard to include the highly technical and physical care that nurses give in certain settings such as intensive care units. Her theory does, however, prevent the nurse from forgetting the patient in her efforts to fulfill the technical aspects of her job.

Orlando's theory is also limited by its focus on interaction with an individual, whereas the patient should be viewed as a member of a family and within a community. Often it is vital to deal with the family as a whole to help the patient. Orlando does not deal with these areas.

Long-term care and planning are not applicable to Orlando's focus on the immediate situation. She only views long-term planning as related to adequate staffing within an institution. Orlando herself recognizes this problem. In *The Dynamic Nurse–Patient Relationship* she speculated that "repeated experiences of having been helped undoubtedly culminate over periods of time in greater degrees of improvement."[45] She also identified the cumulative effect of nursing as an area for further study.

In *The Discipline and Teaching of Nursing Process*, Orlando tried to define the entire nursing system. She described this as the "regularly, interacting parts of a nursing service."[46] This part of her theory attempts to incorporate nurses' relationships with other nurses and with members of different professions in the job setting. Her theory struggles with the authority derived from the function of the profession and that of the employing institution's commitment to the public. The same process is offered for dealing with others as for working with an individual patient. This part of her process is somewhat confusing. It appears to be more of a description of the administration of nursing services than a theory of nursing practice.

When a nurse-manager deals with staff, Orlando's theory provides a framework for an interaction that leads to a positive result. As the nurse executive listens to the needs of the staff, she must decide if deliberate action is needed; such action may take the form of a policy or procedure change, staffing variation, or institutional policy change. The nurse executive may need to influence another department, group, or level within the organization to effect a positive intervention with staff. On the administrative level, Orlando's theory is used, but the time span to complete all components varies depending on the situations. An organization that consistently and methodically uses Orlando's theory can positively respond to all issues that need to be confronted. In such an environment, needs can be met and emphasis placed on the present rather than the past or the way it is always done. Thus, the organization is able to maintain its competitive edge.

Orlando can be considered a nursing theorist who made a significant contribution to the advancement of nursing practice. She helped nurses to focus on the patient rather than on the disease or institutional demands. The nurse is firmly viewed as the handmaiden of the patient, not of the physician. Nurses must base their practice on logical thinking rather than on intuition. Orlando's nursing process continues to be useful to nurses in their interactions with patients.

SUMMARY

Orlando's nursing process is rooted in the interaction between a nurse and a patient at a specific time and place. A sequence of interchanges involving patient behavior and nurse reaction takes place until the patient's need for help, as he perceives it, is clarified. The nurse, then, decides on an appropriate action to resolve the need in cooperation with the patient. This action is evaluated after it is carried out. If the patient behavior improves, the action was successful and the process is completed. If there is no change or the behavior gets worse, the process recycles with new efforts to clarify the patient's behavior or the appropriate nursing action. Orlando summarizes her process as follows:

> A deliberative nursing process has elements of continuous reflection as the nurse tries to understand the meaning to the patient of the behavior she observes and what he needs from her in order to be helped. Responses comprising this process are stimulated by the nurse's unfolding awareness of the particulars of the individual situation.[47]

REFERENCES

1. Orlando, I.J. *The Dynamic Nurse–Patient Relationship: Function, Process and Principles*, New York: G.P. Putnam's Sons, 1961.

2. Orlando, I.J., *The Discipline and Teaching of Nursing Process*, New York: G.P. Putnam's Sons, 1972.
3. Orlando, *The Dynamic Nurse–Patient Relationship*.
4. Orlando, *The Discipline and Teaching*.
5. Orlando, *The Dynamic Nurse–Patient Relationship*, p. vii.
6. Ibid, viii.
7. Orlando, *The Discipline and Teaching*.
8. Orlando, *The Dynamic Nurse–Patient Relationship*, pp. 22–23.
9. Peplau, H. *Interpersonal Relations in Nursing*, New York: G.P. Putnam's Sons, 1952.
10. Harmer, B. & Henderson, V., *Textbook of the Principles and Practice of Nursing* (5th ed.), New York: Macmillan, Inc., 1955, p. 4.
11. Orlando, *The Dynamic Nurse–Patient Relationship*.
12. Ibid, 22.
13. Orlando, *The Discipline and Teaching*, p. 4.
14. Ibid, 12.
15. Pelletier, I.O. The Patient's Predicament and Nursing Function, *Psychiatric Opinion*, 1967, *4*, 28.
16. Orlando, *The Discipline and Teaching*, p. 12.
17. Orlando, *The Dynamic Nurse–Patient Relationship*, p. 5.
18. Rogers, M.E. Nursing: A Science of Unitary Man, in *Conceptual Models for Nursing Practice* (2nd ed), Riehl, J.P. & Roy, C. eds., New York: Appleton-Century-Crofts, 1980.
19. Orlando, *The Dynamic Nurse–Patient Relationship*, p. 4.
20. Orlando, *The Discipline and Teaching*, p. 29.
21. Ibid, 31.
22. Ibid, 24.
23. Orlando, *The Dynamic Nurse–Patient Relationship*, p. 40.
24. Ibid, 11.
25. Ibid, 37.
26. Ibid, 78.
27. Orlando, *The Discipline and Teaching*, p. 25.
28. Orlando, *The Dynamic Nurse–Patient Relationship*, p. 56.
29. Ibid, 35–36.
30. Orlando, *The Discipline and Teaching*, pp. 29–30.
31. Ibid, 114.
32. Orlando, *The Dynamic Nurse–Patient Relationship*, p. 60.
33. Ibid, 67.
34. Ibid, 60.
35. Orlando, *The Discipline and Teaching*, p. 16.
36. Orlando, *The Dynamic Nurse–Patient Relationship*, p. 70.
37. Joint Commission on Accreditation of Hospitals, *Accreditation Manual for Hospitals*, p. 146.
38. Orlando, *The Dynamic Nurse–Patient Relationship*, p. 31.
39. Ibid, 32.
40. Orlando, *The Discipline and Teaching*, p. viii.
41. Abdellah, F.G. and others, *Patient-Centered Approaches to Nursing*, New York: Macmillan, Inc., 1960.
42. Orlando, *The Discipline and Teaching*, p. 18.

43. Ibid, 20.
44. Congress of Nursing Practice, *A Plan for Implementation of the Standards of Nursing Practice*, Kansas City, Mo.: American Nurses' Association, 1975, p. 16.
45. Orlando, *The Dynamic Nurse–Patient Relationship*, p. 90.
46. Orlando, *The Discipline and Teaching*, p. 18.
47. Orlando, *The Dynamic Nurse–Patient Relationship*, p. 67.

CHAPTER 11

Ernestine Wiedenbach*

Agnes M. Bennett
Peggy Coldwell Foster

Ernestine Wiedenbach, a 1922 liberal arts graduate of Wellesley College, Wellesley, Massachusetts, received her nursing diploma from the Johns Hopkins School of Nursing, Baltimore, Maryland in 1925. Her master's degree in Public Health Nursing is from Teachers College, Columbia University, New York, in 1934. She also obtained a certificate in nurse midwifery from the Maternity Center Association in New York in 1946. She practiced as a nurse midwife and a public health nurse and has taught in a number of schools of nursing. She is an Associate Professor Emeritus from Yale University School of Nursing. She served as a visiting professor at California State University, Los Angeles and at the College of Nursing, University of Florida, Gainesville. In 1978, she received the Hattie Hemschemeyer award from the American College of Nurse Midwives for exceptional achievements in her professional life.

Ernestine Wiedenbach, a progressive nursing leader, began her nursing career in the 1920s. Wiedenbach first published *Family-Centered Maternity Nursing* in 1958.[1] It is of interest to note that in this book she recommended that babies be in hospital rooms with their mothers. This innovative concept was not widely implemented until twenty years later. In 1964, she wrote *Clinical Nursing—A Helping Art* in which she described her ideas about nursing as a "concept and philosophy" derived from forty years of nursing experience.[2] She credits Patricia James, James Dickoff, and Ida Orlando Pelletier as great influences in her nursing writing and theory development. In collaboration with Dickoff and James, she presented the symposium, "Theory in a Practice Discipline," in the late 1960s.[3a,3b] In 1970, Wiedenbach defined the essentials of her prescriptive theory in "Nurses' Wisdom in Nursing Theory."[4]

According to Ernestine Wiedenbach, nursing is nurturing and caring for someone in a motherly fashion. That care is given in the immediate present and can be given by any caring person. Nursing is a helping service

---

* Wiedenbach consistently uses the term *patient* and refers to the nurse as *her* in all her writings. This approach will be used in this chapter.

that is rendered with compassion, skill, and understanding to those in need of care, counsel, and confidence in the area of health.[5]

Nursing wisdom is acquired through meaningful experience. Sensitivity alerts the nurse to an awareness of inconsistencies in a situation that might signify a problem. It is a key factor in assisting the nurse to identify the patient's need for help.[6]

The nurse's beliefs and values regarding the significance of life, the worth of the individual, and the aspirations of each human being determine the quality of nursing care. The nurse's purpose in nursing represents a professional commitment.[7]

Wiedenbach states that the characteristics of a professional person that are essential for the professional nurse include: (1) *clarity* of purpose, (2) *mastery* of skills and knowledge essential for fulfilling her purpose, (3) *ability* to establish and sustain purposeful working relationships with others in the health care field, (4) *interest* in advancing knowledge in her area of interest and in researching new knowledge, and (5) *dedication* to furthering the good of man.[8]

The practice of nursing comprises a wide variety of services, each directed toward the attainment of one of its three components: (1) *identification* of the patient's need for help, (2) *ministration* of the help needed, and (3) *validation* that the help provided was indeed helpful to the patient.[9] Within Wiedenbach's "identification of the patient's need for help," she presents three principles of helping: (1) the principle of inconsistency/consistency, (2) the principle of purposeful perseverance, and (3) the principle of self-extension.[10] The *principle of inconsistency/consistency* refers to the assessment of the patient to determine some action, word, or appearance that is different than expected. That is, something out of the ordinary for this patient. It is important for the nurse to astutely observe the patient and then critically analyze these observations. The *principle of purposeful perseverance* is based on the nurse's sincere desire to help the patient. The nurse needs to strive to continue her helping efforts in spite of difficulties she encounters while seeking to effectively use her resources and capabilities. The *principle of self-extension* recognizes that each nurse has limitations that are both personal and situational. It is important that she recognizes when these limitations are reached and that she seek help from others.

WIEDENBACH'S PRESCRIPTIVE THEORY

Theory may be described as a system of conceptualizations invented to some purpose. Prescriptive theory (a situation-producing theory) may be described as one that conceptualizes both a desired situation and the prescription by which it is to be brought about. Thus, a prescriptive theory directs action toward an explicit goal. Wiedenbach's prescriptive theory is made up of three factors. These factors or concepts are[11]:

1. The *central purpose,* which the practitioner recognizes as essential to the particular discipline.
2. The *prescription* for the fulfillment of the central purpose.
3. The *realities in the immediate situation* that influence the fulfillment of the central purpose. See Figure 11–1.

The Central Purpose

The nurse's central purpose defines the quality of health she desires to effect or sustain in her patient and specifies what she recognizes to be her special responsibility in caring for him or her.[12] This central purpose (or commitment) is based on the individual nurse's philosophy. Wiedenbach states:

> Purpose and philosophy are, respectively, goal and guide of clinical nursing. . . . Purpose—that which the nurse wants to accomplish through what she does—is the overall goal toward which she is striving, and so is constant. It is her reason for being and doing. . . . Philosophy, an attitude toward life and reality that evolves from each nurse's beliefs and code of conduct, motivates the nurse to act, guides her thinking about what she is to do, and influences her decisions. It stems from both her culture and subculture and is an integral part of her. It is personal in character, unique to each nurse, and expressed in her way of nursing. Philosophy underlies purpose, and purpose reflects philosophy.[13]

Wiedenbach identifies three essential components for a nursing philosophy: (1) a reverence for the gift of life, (2) a respect for the dignity, worth, autonomy, and individuality of each human being, and (3) a resolu-

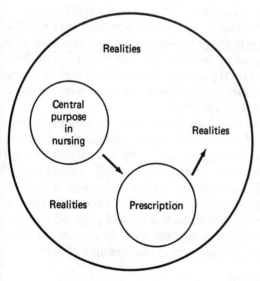

Figure   11–1. Wiedenbach's prescriptive theory. *(Adapted from Wiedenbach, E.* Meeting the Realities in Clinical Teaching, *New York: Springer Publishing Co., Inc., 1969, p. x.)*

tion to act dynamically in relation to one's beliefs.[14] Any of these concepts might be further developed. However, Wiedenbach emphasizes the second in her work.

Wiedenbach formulated the following beliefs about the individual[15]:

1. Each human being is endowed with unique potential to develop within himself the resources that enable him to maintain and sustain himself.
2. The human being basically strives toward self-direction and relative independence, and desires not only to make the best use of his capabilities and potentialities but to fulfill his responsibilities as well.
3. The human being needs stimulation in order to make the best use of his capabilities and realize his self-worth.
4. Whatever the individual does represents his best judgment at the moment of doing it.
5. Self-awareness and self-acceptance are essential to the individual's sense of integrity and self-worth.

Thus, the central purpose is a concept the nurse has thought through—one she has put into words, believes in, and accepts as a standard against which to measure the value of her action to the patient. It is based on her philosophy and suggests the nurse's reason for being, the mission she believes is hers to accomplish.[16]

The Prescription

Once the nurse has identified her own philosophy and recognizes that the patient has autonomy and individuality, she can work *with* the individual to develop a *prescription* or plan for his or her care.

A *prescription* is a directive to activity.[17] It "specifies both the *nature of the action* that will most likely lead to fulfillment of the nurse's central purpose and the *thinking process* that determines it."[18] A prescription may indicate the broad general action appropriate to implementation of the basic concepts as well as suggest the kind of behavior needed to carry out these actions in accordance with the central purpose. These actions may be voluntary or involuntary. Voluntary action is an intended response, whereas involuntary action is an unintended response.[19]

A prescription is a directive to at least three kinds of voluntary action: (1) *mutually understood and agreed upon* action (the practitioner has evidence that the recipient understands the implications of the intended action and is psychologically and physiologically receptive to it); (2) *recipient-directed* action (the recipient of the action essentially directs the way it is to be carried out); and (3) *practitioner-directed* action (the practitioner carries out the action).[19] Once the nurse has formulated a central purpose and has accepted it as a personal commitment she not only has established the prescription for her nursing but also is ready to implement it.[20]

The Realities

When the nurse has determined her central purpose and has developed the prescription, she must then consider the *realities* of the situation in which she is to provide nursing care. Realities consist of all factors—physical, physiological, psychological, emotional, and spiritual—that are at play in a situation in which nursing actions occur at any given moment.[20] Wiedenbach defines the five realities as: (1) the agent, (2) the recipient, (3) the goal, (4) the means, and (5) the framework.

The *agent* who is the practicing nurse or her delegate is characterized by personal attributes, capacities, capabilities, and most importantly, commitment and competence in nursing. As the agent, the nurse is the propelling force that moves her practice toward its goal. In the course of this goal-directed movement, she may engage in innumerable acts called forth by her encounter with actual or discrepant factors and situations within the realities of which she herself is a part.[21]

The agent or nurse has four basic responsibilities[22]:

1. To reconcile her assumptions about the realities . . . with her central purpose. . . .
2. To specify the objectives of her practice in terms of behavioral outcomes that are realistically attainable.
3. To practice nursing in accordance with her objectives.
4. To engage in related activities which contribute to her self realization and to the improvement of nursing practice.

The *recipient* is the patient who is characterized by personal attributes, problems, capacities, aspirations, and most importantly, the ability to cope with the concerns or problems being experienced. He or she is the recipient of the nurse's actions or the one on whose behalf the action is taken. The patient is vulnerable. he or she is dependent on others for help and risks losing his or her individuality, dignity, worth, and autonomy.[22]

The *goal* is the desired outcome the nurse wishes to achieve. The goal is the end result to be attained by nursing action. The stipulation of an activity's goal gives focus to the nurse's action and implies her reason for taking it.[23]

The *means* comprise the activities and devices through which the practitioner is enabled to attain her goal. The means include skills, techniques, procedures, and devices that may be used to facilitate nursing practice. The nurse's way of giving treatments, of expressing concern, of using the means available is individual and is determined by her central purpose and the prescription.[24]

The *framework* consists of the human, environmental, professional, and organizational facilities that not only make up the context within which nursing is practiced but also constitute its currently existing limits. The framework is composed of all the extraneous factors and facilities in the situation that affect the nurse's ability to obtain the desired results. It is a conglomerate of "objects, existing or missing, such as policies, setting, atmosphere, time of day, humans, and happenings that may be current, past, or anticipated."[25]

The realities offer uniqueness to every situation. The success of professional nursing practice is dependent on them. Unless the realities are recognized and dealt with, they may prevent the achievement of the goal.

The concepts of central purpose, prescription, and realities are interdependent in Wiedenbach's theory of nursing. The nurse develops a prescription for care, based on her central purpose, which is implemented in the realities of the situation.

In summary, the comparison of Wiedenbach's prescriptive theory, the practice of nursing, and the nursing process as outlined in Chapter 2 of this book is as follows: In the practice of nursing, a nurse with her unique personality, philosophy, education, and life experiences *assesses* the patient's individual health status and potential for development. She then identifies his or her need for help (makes a *nursing diagnosis*). She formulates a *plan* with the patient, setting goals that they will act upon (*implement*). This prescription and its implementation are affected by the realities, the strengths, and limitations of the situation (the *environment*). Their plan is implemented or the nurse provides the help needed. Validation is then obtained that the help provided was indeed helpful to the patient (*evaluation*).

WIEDENBACH'S CONCEPTUALIZATION OF NURSING PRACTICE AND PROCESS

According to Wiedenbach, nursing practice is an art in which the nursing action is based on the principles of helping. Nursing action may be thought of as consisting of four distinct kinds of actions[26]:

1. Reflex   (spontaneous)
2. Conditioned   (automatic)
3. Impulsive   (impulsive)
4. Deliberate   (responsible)

Nursing as a practice discipline is goal directed. The nature of the nursing act is based on thought. The nurse thinks through the kind of results she wants, gears her actions to obtain those results, then accepts responsibility for the acts and the outcome of those acts.[27] Since nursing requires thought, it can be considered a deliberate responsible action.

Nursing practice has three components[28]: (1) identification of the patient's need for help; (2) ministration of the help needed, and (3) validation that the action taken was helpful to the patient.[28] Within the identification component, there are four distinct steps. First, the nurse observes the patient, looking for an inconsistency between the expected behavior of the patient and the apparent behavior. Second, she attempts to clarify what the inconsistency means. Third, she determines the cause of the discomfort that she has ascertained the patient is experiencing. Finally, she validates with the patient that her help is needed.

The second component is the ministration of the help needed. In ministering to her patient, the nurse may give advice or information, make a referral, apply a comfort measure, or carry out a therapeutic procedure. Should the patient become uncomfortable with what is being done, the nurse will need to identify the cause and, if necessary, make an adjustment in the plan of action.

The third component is validation. After help has been ministered, the nurse validates that the actions were, indeed, helpful. Evidence must come from the patient that the purpose of the nursing actions has been fulfilled.[29]

Wiedenbach views the nursing process essentially as an internal personalized mechanism. As such, it is influenced by the nurse's culture, purpose in nursing, knowledge, wisdom, sensitivity, and concern.[30]

In Wiedenbach's nursing process (see Fig. 11–2), she identifies seven levels of awareness: sensation, perception, assumption, realization, insight, design, and decision.[31] Her nursing process begins with an activating situation. This situation exists among the realities and serves as a stimulus to arouse the nurse's consciousness. This consciousness leads to a subjective interpretation of the first three levels, which are defined as: *sensation* (experienced sensory impression), *perception* (the interpretation of a sensory impression), and *assumption* (the meaning the nurse attaches to the perception). These three levels of awareness are obtained through the focus of the nurse's attention on the stimulus; they are intuitive rather than cognitive and may initiate an involuntary response.

For example, a nurse enters a patient's room and states, "My, it's hot in here!" She immediately goes to the window and opens it. The *sensation* is: the room temperature. The *perception* is: "It feels hot." The *assumption* is: "If I am hot, then the patient must be hot." The involuntary response is to open the window.

Progressing from intuition to cognition, the nurse's actions become voluntary rather than involuntary. The next four levels of awareness occur in the voluntary phase. These are: *realization* (in which the nurse begins to validate the assumption previously made about the patient's behavior); *insight* (which includes joint planning and additional knowledge about the cause of the problem); *design* (the plan of action decided upon by the nurse and confirmed by the patient); and *decision* (the nurse's performance of a responsible action).[31]

To continue with the previous example: The nurse asks, "Are you too warm?" and the patient replies, "No, I'm not. I have felt cold since I washed my hair." The nurse responds, "I will close the window and get you a

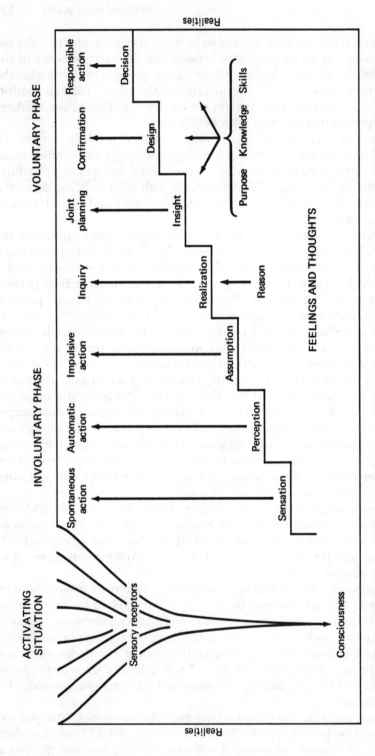

Figure 11–2. Conceptualization of the nursing process. *(Reproduced from Clausen, J.P. and others, Maternity Nursing Today, New York: McGraw-Hill Book Company, 1977, p. 43.)*

blanket." The patient agrees, "That would be fine." The nurse shuts the window and gets a blanket for the patient.

The *realization* is: the validation of the patient's perception of warmth. The *insight* is: the additional information that the patient had washed his or her hair. The *design* is: the plan to close the window and get a blanket as confirmed by the patient. The *decision* is: the nurse shuts the window and gets a blanket for the patient.

WIEDENBACH'S THEORY AND THE FOUR MAJOR CONCEPTS

Wiedenbach emphasizes that the human or *individual* possesses unique potential, strives toward self-direction, and needs stimulation. Whatever the individual does represents his or her best judgment at the moment. Self-awareness and self-acceptance are essential to the individual's sense of integrity and self-worth. Wiedenbach believes these characteristics require respect from the nurse.[32]

Wiedenbach does not define the concept of *health*. However, she supports the World Health Organization's definition of health as a state of complete physical, mental, and social well-being and not merely the absence of disease and infirmity.[33]

In Wiedenbach's work, she incorporates the *environment* within the realities—a major component of her theory. One element of the realities is the framework. According to Wiedenbach, the framework is a complex of extraneous factors and circumstances which are present in every nursing situation. The framework may include objects "such as policies, setting, atmosphere, time of day, humans, and happenings."[34]

According to Wiedenbach, *nursing*, a clinical discipline, is a practice discipline designed to produce explicit desired results.[35] The art of nursing is a goal-directed activity requiring the application of knowledge and skill toward meeting a need for help experienced by a patient.[36] It is a helping process that will extend or restore the patient's ability to cope with demands implicit in his or her situation.[37]

COMPARISON OF THE NURSING PROCESS WITH WIEDENBACH'S NURSING PROCESS AND NURSING PRACTICE

The comparison of the nursing process described in Chapter 2 and Wiedenbach's conceptualization of the nursing process and nursing practice yields some similarities and several significant differences (see Table 11–1). In Wiedenbach's nursing practice, the steps of (1) observation, (2) ministration of help, and (3) validation are comparable with the nursing process's phases of *assessment, implementation,* and *evaluation.*

Assessment, the first phase of the nursing process, considers the person

TABLE 11–1. COMPARISON OF THE NURSING PROCESS WITH WIEDENBACH'S NURSING PROCESS AND NURSING PRACTICE

Nursing Process	Wiedenbach's Nursing Process		Wiedenbach's Nursing Practice
1. Nursing assessment	***Stimulus***		1. Observation
	Involuntary 1. Sensation 2. Perception 3. Assumption	Voluntary	
1. (a) Analysis and synthesis 2. Nursing Diagnosis		4. Realization with reason —Inquiry	
3. (a) Goals and objectives 3. (b) Plans		5. Insight— Joint planning 6. Design— Confirmation	
	1. (a) Spontaneous Action 2. (a) Automatic action 3. (a) Impulsive action		2. Ministration of help
4. Implementation with scientific rationale		7. Decision with responsible action	
5. Nursing evaluation			3. Validation

holistically and requires extensive data collection. In Wiedenbach's model (see Fig. 11–3), there is a stimulus to which the nurse reacts. This stimulus produces a reaction of the level of sensation or perception. These levels are involuntary and intuitive. The nurse then makes an assumption about the situation and may act involuntarily. Such acts are spontaneous, automatic, or impulsive. They occur on the spur of the moment and are precipitated by unchecked, rampant thoughts and feelings. Occasionally in an emergency they may be lifesaving. However, these involuntary acts can frequently do more harm than good.[38]

If the nurse makes an assumption, she might act impulsively. However, Wiedenbach points out that the nurse needs to willfully apply a strategy brake (see Fig. 11–3). This provides time for her to assemble the resources necessary for disciplined thought to control her action.[38] This strategy brake then is applied just prior to Wiedenbach's realization level. At the realization level the process becomes voluntary as the nurse uses reason and inquiry.

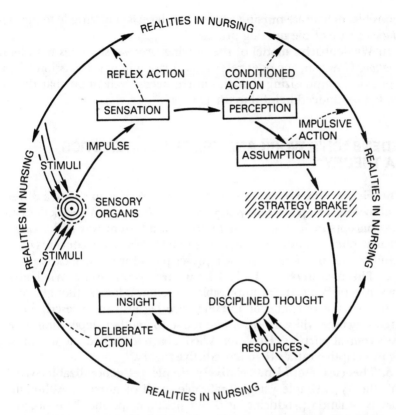

Figure 11-3. Genesis of nursing action. Diagrammatic presentation of how an impulse to act originates and how it is converted into action. Broken lines represent overt processes; solid lines represent covert processes. *(Reprinted by permission of G.P. Putnam's Sons from* Family-Centered Maternity Nursing *(2nd ed.) by Wiedenbach, E., 1967, G.P. Putnam's Sons.)*

Within the *assessment* phase of the nursing process (as presented in Chapter 2), components of *analysis* and *synthesis* require much conscious thought and deliberation about the corrected data before the nurse can make a *nursing diagnosis*. Once the nursing diagnosis has been determined, the nurse sets goals and objectives and *plans* the nursing care. This planning phase can be compared to Wiedenbach's levels of insight and design, which are part of her voluntary phase. The insight level of her nursing process model includes joint planning. This joint planning is between the nurse and the patient and does not involve other health care professionals.

Wiedenbach does not directly incorporate the concept of goal as part of the nursing process. However, the nurse's central purpose could be considered a goal.[39] On the design level the nurse plans a course of action. After the plan is decided on, the nurse confirms it with the patient. Once the plan has been decided on and confirmed, the nurse performs the responsible, deliberate nursing action. This level is comparable to the *implementation* phase of the nursing process.

In Wiedenbach's model of the nursing process, she does not identify *evaluation*. However, she does refer to evaluation in her discussion of nursing practice, emphasizing that the nurse needs "validation that the help provided was indeed helpful to the patient."[40]

WIEDENBACH'S WORK AND THE CHARACTERISTICS OF A THEORY

1. Theories can interrelate concepts in such a way as to create a different way of looking at a particular phenomenon. Wiedenbach's work does interrelate concepts in such a way as to create a different way of looking at a particular phenomenon. She defines and interrelates the concepts of realities and central purpose to devise a prescription for nursing care.

2. Theories must be logical in nature. When using Wiedenbach's theory, it is difficult, if not impossible, to follow a logical thought process and predict the outcome of nursing care because the prescription and desired outcome will vary from one nurse to another depending on each nurse's central purpose. However, Wiedenbach identified she was presenting a prescriptive rather than a predictive theory.[41]

3. Theories should be relatively simple yet generalizable. Wiedenbach's theory is simple yet generalizable to all of nursing. Although the theory is situation producing, it is not situation specific. The situation is produced by the nurse's central purpose and prescription within the existing realities. The situation is not site oriented and thus could be a hospital, a community setting, a school, or in the home.

4. Theories can be the bases for hypotheses that can be tested.

5. Theories contribute to and assist in increasing the general body of knowledge within the discipline through the research implemented to validate them. Although Wiedenbach's theory presents a philosophical approach that has not been tested, hypotheses can be formed. For example, how does the central purpose affect care when the realities and prescription remain fairly constant? That is, according to a patient or family survey, is there a perceived difference in the quality of nursing care between a group of nurses who work in a nursing care facility because it is close to their home and a group of nurses who chose to work in this setting because it has a specialized unit for patients with Alzheimer's disease?

6. Theories can be utilized by practitioners to guide and improve their practice. Wiedenbach's theory can be used to support, guide, and assist the nurse to fulfill her commitment to nursing. The nurse's commitment to nursing is her central purpose that will influence prescriptions within the situational realities. Thus the nurse whose central purpose is holistic support of the optimal development of the individual will develop prescriptions that deal with a multitude of aspects of the individual rather than focusing solely on the problem that led to initial contact.

7. Theories must be consistent with other validated theories, laws, and principles but should leave open unanswered questions that need to be investigated. Wiedenbach does not use theories or support her theory from other disciplines.

SUMMARY

Nursing is a helping art. The nurse renders compassionate care to those in need of help. Nursing requires a professional commitment and is based on the individual nurse's philosophy. For Wiedenbach, the concepts which epitomize the nurse's philosophy are the "reverence for the gift of life"; "respect for the dignity, worth, autonomy, and individuality of each human being"; and the "resolution to act dynamically in relation to one's beliefs."[41] The components of nursing practice are identification of the patient's need for help, ministration of help, and validation that help was beneficial.

Wiedenbach's theory for nursing, a prescriptive theory, contains three concepts: *central purpose, prescription,* and *realities.* The interrelationship of these three concepts would be as follows: Within the realities, the nurse develops a prescription for nursing care based on her central purpose. The central purpose is the nurse's philosophy for care; the prescription is the directive to activity; the realities are the matrix in which the action occurs. These concepts are all interdependent.

Wiedenbach identifies seven levels within her nursing process: sensation, perception, assumption, realization, insight, design, and decision. Sensation through realization involves involuntary action, insight through design involves voluntary action. With increased purpose, knowledge, and skill, the nurse moves from an involuntary response to voluntary action.

Wiedenbach's theory presents a philosophical, altruistic approach to nursing. The nurse is viewed as a loving, caring individual. The nurse's philosophy about the value and worth of the individual directs her care. Wiedenbach states: "Nursing [is] a service which ideally exemplifies man's humanity to man."[42]

The reader perceives that the nurse acts with a self-sacrificing commitment to nursing. If a nurse values the life and dignity of human beings, then she will provide quality nursing care.

Wiedenbach states that "although recognized as a humanitarian service, nursing in its entirety is hard to describe, and the nurse's responsibilities are hard to delineate."[43]

Wiedenbach's nursing process is different than the nursing process outlined in Chapter 2 in this text. She identifies the nursing process as being activated by a stimulus that may result in an involuntary response unless this reflexive action is halted by a strategy brake. This brake allows the nurse to think, gather more data, analyze, and then plan before a voluntary deliberate action is taken. The nursing process in Chapter 2 more closely parallels Wiedenbach's definition of nursing practice, that is, observation, ministration of help, and validation.

This theory is useful with an individual patient, but not with groups. With this theory, Wiedenbach recognizes that the "need for help" must be verified with the patient. This factor would require the patient to be coherent and responsive.

Wiedenbach's work occurred early in the development of the theoretical nursing models. Her prescriptive theory defines her concepts of central purpose, prescription, and realities. However, these concepts are broad, vary with each nurse, each patient, each situation, and are difficult to use in research.

Although Wiedenbach's work does not fulfill all the characteristics of a theory, it is innovative within the nursing profession. Her classic writings, as well as those written with Dickoff and James, serve as a basis for the development of nursing theory. Wiedenbach is a "mother" of nursing theory development.

REFERENCES

1. Wiedenbach, E. *Family-Centered Maternity Nursing,* New York: G.P. Putnam's Sons, 1958.
2. Wiedenbach, E. *Clinical Nursing—A Helping Art,* New York: Springer Publishing Company, Inc., 1964.
3.(a) Dickoff, J., James, P., & Wiedenbach, E. Theory in a Practice Discipline I: Practice-Orientated Research, *Nursing Research* 1968, *17,* 415–435.
3.(b) Dickoff, J., James, P., & Wiedenbach, E. Theory in a Practice Discipline II: Practice-Orientated Research, *Nursing Research,* 1968, *17,* 545–554.
4. Wiedenbach, E. Nurse's Wisdom in Nursing Theory, *American Journal of Nursing,* 1970, *70,* 1057–62.
5. Clausen, J.P., Flook, M.H., & Ford, B. *Maternity Nursing Today,* New York: McGraw-Hill, 1977, p. 39.
6. Wiedenbach, *Clinical Nursing,* p. 52.
7. Wiedenbach, Nurse's Wisdom, p. 1058.
8. Wiedenbach, *Clinical Nursing,* p. 2.
9. Clausen and others, *Maternity Nursing,* p. 39.
10. Wiedenbach, *Clinical Nursing,* pp. 48–52.
11. Wiedenbach, E. *Meeting the Realities in Clinical Teaching,* New York: Springer Publishing Co., 1969, p. 2.
12. Clausen and others, *Maternity Nursing,* p. 45.
13. Ibid, 13.
14. Wiedenbach, *Clinical Nursing,* p. 16.
15.(a) Ibid, 17.
15.(b) Wiedenbach, *Meeting the Realities,* pp. 9–10.
16. Wiedenbach, Nurse's Wisdom, p. 1058.

17.   Wiedenbach, *Meeting the Realities*, p. 3.
18.   Wiedenbach, Nurse's Wisdom, p. 1059.
19.   Wiedenbach, *Meeting the Realities*, p. 3.
20.   Wiedenbach, Nurse's Wisdom, p. 1060.
21.   Wiedenbach, *Family-Centered Maternity Nursing*, p. 6.
22.   Wiedenbach, Nurse's Wisdom, p. 1060.
23.   Ibid, 1061.
24.   Ibid, 1062.
25.   Ibid, 1061.
26.(a) Clausen and others, *Maternity Nursing*, p. 43.
26.(b) Wiedenbach, *Family-Centered Maternity Nursing*, p. 8.
27.   Wiedenbach, Nurse's Wisdom, p. 1059.
28.   Clausen and others, *Maternity Nursing*, p. 39.
29.   Wiedenbach, *Clinical Nursing*, pp. 57–58.
30.   Clausen and others, *Maternity Nursing*, p. 44.
31.   Ibid, 41–44.
32.   Wiedenbach, *Clinical Nursing*, p. 17
33.   Clausen and others, *Maternity Nursing*, p. 39.
34.   Wiedenbach, Nurse's Wisdom, p. 1061.
35.   Wiedenbach, *Meeting the Realities*, p. 2.
36.   Wiedenbach, Nurse's Wisdom, p. 1057.
37.   Wiedenbach, *Clinical Nursing*, p. 36.
38.   Clausen and others, *Maternity Nursing*, p. 42.
39.   Wiedenbach, *Clinical Nursing*, p. 13.
40.   Clausen and others, *Maternity Nursing*, p. 39.
41.   Wiedenbach, Nurse's Wisdom, p. 1058.
42.   Wiedenbach, *Family-Centered Maternity Nursing*, p. 5.
43.   Wiedenbach, *Clinical Nursing*, p. 1.

BIBLIOGRAPHY

Burst, H. V. Presentation of the Hattie Hemschemeyer Award, *Journal of Nurse-Midwifery*, 1979, *24*, 35–6.

Dickoff, J.J. Symposium in Theory Development in Nursing, Researching Research's Role in Theory Development, *Nursing Research*, 1968, *17*, 204–6.

Dickoff, J. J. and James, P. A. Symposium of Theory Development in Nursing: A Theory of Theories: A Position Paper, *Nursing Research*, 1968, *17*, 197–203.

Dunlop, M.J. Is a Science of Caring Possible? *Journal of Advanced Nursing*, 1986, *11*, 661–70.

Flaskerud, J.H. On Toward a Theory of Nursing Action: Skills and Competency in Nurse–Patient Interaction, *Nursing Research*, 1986, *35*, 250–52.

Wiedenbach, E. Childbirth as Mothers Say They Like It, *Public Health Nursing*, 1949, *51*, 417–21.

Wiedenbach, E. Nurse-Midwifery, Purpose, Practice and Opportunity, *Nursing Outlook*, 1960, *8*, 256.

Wiedenbach, E. The Helping Art of Nursing, *American Journal of Nursing*, 1963, *63*, 54–57.

Wiedenbach, E. Family Nurse Practitioner for Maternal and Child Care, *Nursing Outlook*, 1965, *13*, 50 ff.

Wiedenbach, E. Genetics and the Nurse, *Bulletin of the American College of Nurse Midwifery*, 1968, *13*, 8–13.

Wiedenbach, E. The Nurse's Role in Family Planning—A Conceptual Base for Practice, *Nursing Clinics of North America*, 1968, *3*, 355 ff.

Wiedenbach, E. Comment on Beliefs and Values: Basis for Curriculum Design, *Nursing Research*, 1970, *19*, 427.

Wiedenbach, E. and Falls, C. *Communication: Key to Effective Nursing*, New York: Tiresias Press, 1978.

CHAPTER 12

Myra Estrin Levine

Mary Kathryn Leonard*

Myra E. Levine (b. 1920) received her nursing education from Cook County School of Nursing, Chicago (1944); BS, University of Chicago (1949); and MSN, Wayne State University, Detroit, Michigan (1962). Her nursing experience includes staff nursing, administrative and teaching supervision, clinical instruction, and direction of nursing services. She was Chairman of the Department of Clinical Nursing at Cook County School of Nursing. She has also held positions as Associate Professor and Professor of Nursing, College of Nursing, University of Illinois, Chicago; faculty member at Loyola University School of Nursing, Chicago; and Director of Continuing Education, Evanston Hospital, Evanston, Illinois, and visiting professor at Tel Aviv University and Ben Gurion University of the Negev, Israel. Mrs. Levine is the author of a number of articles that have been published in nursing journals and of one book dealing with nursing (see references at end of chapter). In 1965, she presented a paper at the Regional Clinical Conferences sponsored by the American Nurses' Association. This paper, "Trophicognosis: An Alternative to Nursing Diagnosis," can be found in the American Nurses' Association publication Exploring Progress in Medical–Surgical Nursing Practice, New York, 1966, vol. 2. *In addition, Mrs. Levine has participated in a number of workshops and conferences. She is a member of Sigma Theta Tau (Alpha Beta Chapter, Loyola University), a Charter Fellow of the American Academy of Nursing, and an honorary member of the American Mental Health Aid to Israel. She is listed in* Who's Who of American Women *and received the Elizabeth Russell Belford Award for Education from Sigma Theta Tau in 1977.*

Within a framework of total patient care, Levine has developed four conservation principles that serve as the basis of her nursing theory. These principles seek to conserve energy, structural integrity, personal integrity, and social integrity. This theory focuses the nurse's intervention on the patient's adaptation and response to illness.†

This chapter will include a discussion of Levine's theory of nursing, its application to the nursing process, and the relationship of the concepts of

---

* Gratitude is expressed to Connie Hetrick Esposito for her contribution to this chapter in the first edition.

† The terms *intervention* and *patient* are consistent with Levine's terminology.

human being, society/environment, health, and nursing. A case study is included to demonstrate the application of this theory.

LEVINE'S THEORY OF NURSING

Levine views nursing as a dynamic, purposeful process. Her definition includes a description of what nursing is, how it accomplishes its purpose, and what its purpose is. She believes nursing is a *discipline,* the basis of which is people's dependence on their relationship with other people.[1] This discipline includes nursing interventions to support or promote the patient's adjustment.[2] Further, she states that the essence of nursing is human interaction.[3]

Assumptions

Levine's theory makes assumptions about: (1) the condition in which the patient enters the health care setting, (2) the responsibilities of the nurse in the situation and as each relates to nurse–patient interactions, and (3) the functions of the nurse in the situation. These assumptions provide structure and definition to this theory of nursing.

Condition. Levine has limited the focus of her theory to those patients entering the health care system in a state of illness or altered health. This limitation is consistent with her original intention to provide rationale for performing nursing activities.[4]

Responsibilities. The assumption regarding the responsibilities of the nurse interacting with a patient holds the nurse accountable for recognizing the patient's organismic response to an altered health state. Organismic response is change(s) in behavior or change(s) in level of functioning exhibited by the patient adapting or attempting to adapt to the environment.

The environment is viewed broadly by Levine and encompasses both internal environment and external environment. The internal environment deals with the body and its functioning and the external environment is composed of three dimensions: *perceptual,* referring to the five senses; *operational,* referring to forces, conditions, nonperceivable elements; and *conceptual,* encompassing thought processes, emotions, and social processes. While Levine does not make a direct connection, it would appear that in assessing the environment, conservation principles can be used to identify problems. The internal environment relates to the conservation of structural integrity and the external environment deals with the remaining three conservation principles. Levine identifies four levels of organismic response. These are: (1) response to fear, (2) inflammatory response, (3) response to stress, and (4) sensory response.[5]

Functions. The functions of the nurse include: (1) intervening to promote the patient's adaptation to the state of illness, and (2) evaluating the intervention as being supportive or therapeutic. *Supportive nursing interventions* help to maintain the patient's present state of altered health and to prevent further health deterioration. Nursing interventions that promote healing and restoration of health are referred to as *therapeutic interventions.*

Conservation Principles

Levine has identified four conservation principles that serve as the foundation for all nursing interventions. The goal of nursing, in this theory, is to maintain or restore a person to a state of health by conserving energy, structural integrity, personal integrity, and social integrity. The four conservation principles are: (1) *Conservation of energy* refers to balancing energy output and energy input to avoid excessive fatigue, i.e., adequate rest, nutrition, and exercise. (2) *Conservation of structural integrity* refers to maintaining or restoring the structure of the body, i.e., prevention of physical breakdown and the promotion of healing. (3) *Conservation of personal integrity* refers to maintenance or restoration of the patient's sense of identity and self-worth, i.e., acknowledgement of uniqueness. (4) *Conservation of social integrity* refers to the acknowledgment of the patient as a social being. It involves the recognition and presence of human interaction, particularly with the patient's significant others.[6] Conservation in Levine's theory means to keep together or maintain a proper balance.[7] The purpose of the conservation is to maintain the unity and integrity of the patient, and thus the health of the person.

Critical Components

A brief summary of the critical components of Levine's theory of nursing are: (1) the patient is in the predicament of illness, (2) the patient's environment includes the nurse, (3) the nurse must recognize the organismic manifestation of the patient's adaptation to illness, and (4) the nurse must make an intervention in the patient's environment based on the four conservation principles and must evaluate the intervention as therapeutic or supportive.[8] It appears that Levine suggests the good of the nurse and the patient should be facilitation of the patient's adaptation, since Levine views successful adaptation as necessary for sustaining life and health.[9]

The following is a simplified example of how Levine's theory could be used.

Situation. Mrs. H. is brought to the emergency room by her husband. She is experiencing severe chest pain, shortness of breath, nausea, and numbness in her left arm. Based on these data (organismic response), the nurse recognizes Mrs. H. is attempting to adjust to an altered state of health. Using the principles of conservation as the theoretical base, the nurse intervenes in Mrs. H.'s environment (see Table 12–1).

TABLE 12–1. APPLICATION OF LEVINE'S THEORY TO A GIVEN EXAMPLE

Intervention	Conservation Principle	Therapeutic/ Supportive	Rationale
1. Mrs. H. is put on a stretcher with her head elevated.	1. Energy	1. Supportive	1. Limit the expenditure of energy
2. Mrs. H. is given an injection of morphine.	2. (a) Energy (b) Structural integrity	2. (a) Supportive (b) Therapeutic	2. (a) To relieve pain and reduce energy expenditure (b) Decreased pain reduces the oxygen needs of the body, thereby reducing the work load demands on the heart
3. Mrs. H. is to receive oxygen. She is given a choice of how she prefers to receive it, by nasal cannula or face mask.	3. (a) Structural integrity (b) Personal integrity	3. (a) Supportive/ therapeutic (b) Supportive	3. (a) Maintain an adequate oxygen supply to reduce labored breathing (b) Maintain individuality and autonomy
4. Mrs. H.'s husband accompanies her to CCU.	4. Social integrity	4. Supportive	4. Provide Mrs. H. with a support system during transfer process

The nurse observes Mrs. H.'s response to the nursing interventions to determine how she is adjusting to her altered state of health. Mrs. H.'s chest pain is subsiding and her shortness of breath is relieved with the administration of oxygen via nasal cannula. Mrs. H. is settling into the coronary care unit (CCU) with her husband at her side. Based on these and other observations, the nurse decides what further nursing interventions are needed.[10]

LEVINE'S THEORY AND THE FOUR MAJOR CONCEPTS

In the first chapter of this book, the concepts basic to nursing are identified as the human being, society/environment, health, and nursing. Levine's theory of nursing relates to each of these concepts.

Levine stresses the need to view the *individual* holistically, which implies that the individual is a complex being. Her definition of nursing is based on the idea that the human being is dependent on his or her relationship with others. The dimensions of this dependence are implied in her delineation of the four conservation principles, i.e., energy needs and expenditures, structural integrity, social integrity, and personal integrity. Human beings are dependent to some extent on others for all aspects of survival: food, safety, recreation, and affiliation. Levine expects the nurse (1) to be aware of the complexities of these interactions, and (2) to support the maintenance or restoration of these relationships when the patient is in an altered state of health. The normal balance is disrupted by the illness, and the patient in an attempt to adjust to the stress of illness may exhibit behavior changes that alter his or her level of functioning. The nurse must assume responsibility in assisting the patient to adapt to these changes in a positive or health-fostering manner.

The *society/environment* implications in Levine's theory are important. The essence of Levine's definition of nursing is human interaction, and her use of the concepts of adaptation and organismic response are highly suggestive of a systems approach. In systems theory, environment is important. Levine explicitly states that the nurse is part of the patient's environment. Since Levine's theory is individual oriented, one could assume that the patient's family and significant others are also included in the patient's environment. Thus society is viewed broadly as being part of the external environment the patient experiences at any time. However, this theory is concerned with the patient entering or needing assistance in the health care system.

One can also assume that Levine's implied definition of *health* is the maintenance of the unity and integrity of the patient. The holistic view of the patient is essential to the application of this theory. An altered state of health is not restricted to just the impairment of physiological functioning (conservation of structural integrity), but can be viewed as an alteration or need related to any of the four conservation principles. Thus her theory applies only to individuals in an illness state, which restricts the focus of nursing care. Nursing care is directed toward the maintenance or restoration of health. Only in discussing the whole social system does Levine make reference to preventive health practices as being desirable or worth pursuing.[11] Therefore, one's health must be altered for the theory to apply.

Levine's theory relates to the concept of *nursing* in that it offers an approach to the giving of nursing care. Nursing is viewed as a discipline. A nurse must possess both skills and a theoretical and scientific knowledge base. Levine's theory is heavily grounded in the humanities and sciences; an underlying belief is that people are dependent on their relationships with other people. Nursing care is a process in which interventions are based on the assessment of the patient using the conservation principles, recognizing behavioral changes and changes in the level of functioning of the patient in his or her attempt to adapt to illness. Interventions are evaluated in terms of their impact on the health state of the patient.

LEVINE'S THEORY AND THE NURSING PROCESS

Levine's theory for nursing parallels many elements of the nursing process. According to Levine, the nurse must observe the patient, decide on an appropriate intervention, perform it, and then evaluate its usefulness in helping the patient. Levine's theory assumes the nurse and patient will participate together in the patient's care. However, the nursing process described in Chapter 2 emphasizes more mutuality between the patient and the nurse than is implied in Levine's theory.

In Levine's theory, the patient is assumed to be in a dependent position, which may restrict the patient's ability to participate in the data gathering, planning, implementation, or all three phases of the nursing process. As a result of this dependent position, the patient is in need of nursing assistance to help in adapting to a state of health. The nurse assumes responsibility for determining the extent to which the patient is able to participate in his or her care. The nursing process, on the other hand, does not necessarily assume the client is in a dependent position.

In the *assessment* phase, the patient is assessed using two methods: interviewing and observation. The focus is on the patient; the family, significant others, or both are only considered from the perspective of how they might help or interfere with the patient's well-being, and thus affect the patient through the external environment. The needs of the family, significant others, or both are not considered in relation to the patient. According to Levine, if a family member's needs are going to be dealt with, that person must become the target of the assessment.

In performing the holistic assessment, the nurse uses Levine's four conservation principles as an assessment guide. The nurse is concerned with the patient's balance of energy and maintenance of integrity. Thus, the nurse collects data about the patient's energy sources, i.e., nutrition, sleep–rest, leisure, coping patterns, significant relationships, medications, environment, and expenditures of energy, i.e., the functioning of various body systems, emotional and social stresses, and work patterns. In addition, data are collected about the patient's structural integrity, i.e., body defenses and physical body structure; personal integrity (patient's self-system), i.e., uniqueness, values, religious beliefs, and economic resources; and social integrity, i.e., decision-making processes of the patient, the patient's relationships with others, and his or her involvement in social and community affairs.

After the collection of all the data, the nurse critically analyzes the data to obtain a holistic view of the patient. This analysis reflects the patient's balance of strengths and weaknesses in each of the four assessment areas (conservation principles). The analysis also identifies areas needing further data collection. In the analysis, concepts and theories from other disciplines are also considered. Levine's theory has a close kinship to Selye's stress theory.[12] In Selye's stress theory, there is a stressor that stimulates a response as part of the general adaptation syndrome. In Levine's theory, illness is the stressor and the patient is continually trying to adapt to this changed state. This adaptation is manifested in the patient's organismic response, which includes changes in behavior or levels of functioning of the body.

Levine's theory also supports the work and beliefs of Florence Nightingale in relation to her concept of environment (see Chapter 3). Nursing has the responsibility of providing a supportive environment, one that is conducive to health and healing. In Levine's theory, the nurse is part of the patient's environment.

From the analysis, the nurse develops a *nursing diagnosis*. Levine suggests an alternate approach to the development of a nursing diagnosis and planning phase. Levine refers to the process of developing nursing care judgment(s) through the use of the scientific method as trophicognosis.[13] Since the patient is in a state of illness or altered health, the nursing diagnosis will reflect a problem or potential problem related to a deficit or a threatened deficit in one of the four areas of conservation. Levine's theory does not make provision for health promotion needs and teaching. The provision for health promotion is limited to areas directly related to the patient's present problem(s) associated with the illness or state of altered health. Therefore, it may be concluded that the nurse utilizing this theory has a time orientation in the present. Thus the nurse is not concerned with future planning except as it relates to the patient's present problem.

In the *planning* phase, which includes goal setting, the nursing process emphasizes the mutuality of this activity between nurse and patient. Levine, however, has not specifically indicated or stressed the need for mutual goal setting. It may be concluded that mutuality is not necessary initially for the application of this theory in the clinical setting. The bases of this assumption are: (1) the dependent position of the patient as a result of the state of illness or altered health with need for nursing assistance; and (2) the nurse's responsibility to monitor the patient's condition in order to regulate the balance between nursing intervention and patient participation in care. The nurse, as an individual, may include the patient in this activity based on the nurse's assessment of the patient's ability to participate in the goal-setting activity. In order for these goals to be workable, the nurse states the goal in behavioral terms so it is measurable. The goals reflect an attempt to help the patient adapt and reach a state of health.

In the *planning* phase, the nurse uses the goal (1) to determine the strategies to be used in the plan and (2) to determine the extent to which the plan must be developed to meet the goal. Levine indicated the nurse bases practice on knowledge. Thus, the steps of the nursing plan would be based on principles, laws, concepts, and theories from the sciences and humanities. In developing the plan, the nurse also considers the patient's ability to participate in the plan of care, and the patient's degree of participation is identified. During the planning phase, the nurse may consult with other health care team members.

As the plan of care is *implemented,* the nurse observes the patient for an organismic response. Data are collected for later use in the evaluation phase. During the implementation phase, the nurse is responsible for the care given to the patient. Levine's theory indicates that (1) the nurse is expected to possess the skill necessary to carry out the nursing interventions, and (2) the nursing interventions are aimed at supporting or promoting the patient's adaptation.

In the *evaluation* phase, the nurse considers the organismic response of the patient to the nursing action. The nurse uses the data collected about the patient's organismic response to determine if the nursing intervention was therapeutic or supportive. If the intervention was therapeutic, the patient is adapting and is progressing toward a state of health.

Levine's theory lends itself to use in the nursing process. However, one must remember that in using Levine's theory, the focus of the process is on one person, the time orientation is the present or short-term future, and the patient is in an altered or impaired state of health and in need of nursing intervention.

LEVINE'S WORK AND THE CHARACTERISTICS OF A THEORY

1. Theories can interrelate concepts in such a way as to create a different way of looking at a particular phenomenon. In considering Levine's ideas about nursing, the concepts of illness, adaptation, nursing interventions, and evaluation of nursing interventions are interrelated in just that way. They are combined to look at nursing care in a different way (perhaps a more comprehensive view incorporating total patient care) from previous times.

2. Theories must be logical in nature. Levine's ideas about nursing are organized in such a way as to be sequential and logical. They can be used to explain the consequences of nursing actions. There are no apparent contradictions in her ideas.

3. Theories should be relatively simple yet generalizable. Levine's theory is easy to use. Its major elements are easily comprehensible, and the relationships have the potential for being complex but are easily manageable. Perhaps certain isolated aspects of the theory are generalizable, i.e., those related to the conservation principles, but the interaction of these relationships are currently not generalizable. The major factor contributing to this lack of generalizability is the limited amount of research done using this theoretical base.

4. Theories can be the bases for hypotheses that can be tested. Levine's ideas can be tested. Hypotheses can be derived from them. The principles of conservation are specific enough to be testable. For example, it is possible to test if physiological structure is being supported or improved, thus testing the principle of conservation of structural integrity. However, more sophisticated research techniques would be needed to test if the patient's social integrity is being supported or ignored.

5. Theories contribute to and assist in increasing the general body of knowledge within the discipline through the research implemented to validate them. Since Levine's ideas have not yet been widely researched, it is hard to determine a contribution to the general body of knowledge within the discipline.

6. Theories can be utilized by the practitioners to guide and improve their practice. Levine's ideas can be used by practitioners to guide and improve their practice. Paula E. Crawford-Gamble successfully applied Levine's theory to a female patient undergoing surgery for the traumatic amputation of fingers.[14] These ideas lend themselves to use in practice, particularly in the acute care setting.

7. Theories must be consistent with other validated theories, laws, and principles but will leave open unanswered questions that need to be investigated. Levine's ideas seem to be consistent with other theories, laws, and principles, particularly those from the humanities and sciences, and many questions are left unanswered which would be worthy of investigation.

Since Levine's ideas meet four of the seven criteria for a theory, one might consider them as a framework of nursing. Levine herself does not refer to her ideas as either a theory or concepts.

CONCLUSIONS

Levine's theory for nursing focuses on one person—the patient. In utilizing this theory, the nurse is concerned with the patient's family and significant others only to the point that they influence or have an effect on the patient's progress. Thus, the utilization of this theory is limited. This theory could not be used in working with families, groups, or communities.

Levine's theory recognizes nursing as a professional practice based on scientific knowledge and skill. Her theory implies that nursing is considered as an independent practice profession. No mention is made about the relationship of nursing to the other health care professions. This theory does not make provisions for preventive teaching or anticipatory guidance, which are now considered to be nursing functions. These limitations may influence the collaboration with other health care team members. Continuity of care and long-range planning for the patient are limited in scope to helping the patient adapt. As mentioned before, provisions are made for anticipatory guidance and health teaching only as they relate to the patient's present illness.

Levine's theory for nursing is compatible with the practice of nursing in an acute care setting. The theory emphasizes the dependent position of the patient, the patient's impaired state of health, the patient's limited participation in his or her own care, and the increased responsibility of the nurse in directing and coordinating the patient's care. Thus, one might assume that these conditions are most likely to exist in an acute care setting or, possibly, in a home health setting.

Levine's theory of nursing is a significant contribution to the practice of nursing and its worth may become more obvious in the next few years. Levine's theory is capable of being used to direct nursing practice in the acute care setting. Its elements and their relationships to each other are relatively concise and straightforward enough to be taught by a hospital nursing inservice department to new staff during an orientation period. The theory provides inherent direction for the development of sound nursing judgments. Levine's theory is comprehensive in scope and its holistic orientation facilitates the delivery of total patient care. In our present health care environment, which is heavily regulated by various governmental agencies and licensing and accrediting bodies, the nurse is being required to assume more responsibilities. The use of the nursing process is mandated, and since Levine's theory parallels the nursing process it helps to promote efficiency and ease of use.

Home health care is another setting where Levine's theory could be used easily. The current Medicare guidelines indicate that the patient must be, for all intents and purposes, restricted to his or her home, and in need of professional nursing services. Nursing intervention would be needed until the point at which the patient in his or her environment, including the patient's family, had made the successful adaptation, and the patient could adequately function in this new environment. In the home health care setting, great emphasis is placed on the planning of nursing interventions, and this theory would facilitate an orderly use of the nursing process.

Levine's theory may offer some limitations when used in areas where the focus is on long-term care and rehabilitation. The time orientation is to the present or short-term future. A present-time orientation limits the attention that can be focused on health promotion and illness prevention. The practice of preventive health care and more specifically health promotion assume an interest in or a concern for anticipating future needs. Thus, in a program or course that is health oriented and concerned with health promotion with clients in a state of wellness, Levine's theory would be philosophically incompatible.

Levine's theory speaks to the patient's sense of personal integrity, i.e., autonomy and uniqueness. In the illness state, the patient is placed in a dependent position. This placement of the patient may clearly threaten the individual's sense of autonomy. In this theory, the nurse has the responsibility for determining the patient's ability to participate in the care given and for maintaining the balance between this participation and nursing intervention. If the perceptions of the nurse and the patient about the patient's ability to participate in care do not match, then this mismatch will be an area of conflict.

Finally, Levine's theory reflects current beliefs about the holistic nature of humanity. The utility of this theory for nursing practice is in an acute care setting, and possibly in home health.

SUMMARY

In Levine's theory of nursing, nursing is human interaction. This is based on the idea that people are dependent on their relationships with others. The nurse has the responsibility to intervene in the patient's situation after recognizing the patient's organismic response. Nursing interventions are supportive (maintain the status quo) or therapeutic (promote healing and restoration). The nurse's interventions are based on the four conservation principles. These are: (1) conservation of energy, (2) conservation of structural integrity, (3) conservation of personal integrity, and (4) conservation of social integrity. These conservation principles provide a guideline for viewing the individual in a holistic manner.

Levine's theory does relate to the concepts of individual, society/environment, health, nursing, and to the nursing process. Its major limitations relate to its focus on the individual in an illness state, and on the dependency of the patient.

REFERENCES

1. Levine, M.E. *Introduction to Clinical Nursing* (2nd ed.), Philadelphia: F.A. Davis Co., 1973, pp. 4–5.
2. Ibid, 13.
3. Ibid, 1.
4. Ibid, 7.
5. Levine, M.E. The Pursuit of Wholeness, *American Journal of Nursing*, 1969, *69*, 95–96.
6. Levine, *Introduction to Clinical Nursing*, pp. 14–18.
7. Ibid, 13–14.
8. Ibid, 1–3.
9. Ibid, 11.
10. Levine, M.E. Adaptation and Assessment: A Rationale for Nursing Intervention, *American Journal of Nursing*, 1966, *66*, 2452.
11. Levine, *Introduction to Clinical Nursing*, p. 18.
12. Selye, H. *The Stress of Life*, New York: McGraw-Hill, 1956, pp. 31–33.
13. Levine, M.E. Trophicognosis: An Alternative to Nursing Diagnosis, *American Nurses' Association Regional Clinical Conference*, Vol. 2, New York: American Nurses' Association, 1966.
14. Crawford-Gamble, P.E. An Application of Levine's Conceptual Model, *Perioperative Nursing Quarterly*, March 1986, 63–70.

BIBLIOGRAPHY

Hirschfeld, Miriam J. The Cognitively Impaired Older Adult, *American Journal of Nursing*, 1976, *76*, 1981–84.

Levine, Myra E. Adaptation and Assessment: A Rationale for Nursing Intervention, *American Journal of Nursing*, 1966, *66*, 2450–53.

Levine, M.E. Holistic Nursing, *Nursing Clinics of North America*, 1971, *6*, 253–64.

Levine, M.E. The Intransigent Patient, *American Journal of Nursing*, 1970, *70*, 2106–11.

Levine, M.E. The Four Conservation Principles of Nursing, *Nursing Forum*, 1967, *6*, 45–59.

Nursing Development Conference Group, *Concept Formalization in Nursing: Process and Product*, Boston: Little, Brown, 1973.

CHAPTER 13

Imogene M. King

Julia B. George

Imogene M. King (b. 1923) received her basic nursing education in 1946 from St. John's Hospital School of Nursing, St. Louis, Missouri. Her BS in Nursing Education (1948), MS in Nursing (1957) and EdD (1961) are from Teachers College, Columbia University, New York. King has had experience in nursing as an administrator, an educator, and a practitioner. Her positions in nursing education have included Director, School of Nursing, The Ohio State University, Columbus, Ohio; Professor of Nursing, Loyola University of Chicago, Chicago, Illinois; and Professor, College of Nursing, University of South Florida, Tampa, Florida.

Imogene M. King's *Toward a Theory for Nursing: General Concepts of Human Behavior* was published in 1971 and *A Theory for Nursing: Systems, Concepts, Process* in 1981.[1a,1b] These publications grew from King's thoughts about the vast amount of knowledge available to nurses and the difficulty this presents to the individual nurse in choosing the facts and concepts relevant to a given situation.[2] From the early 1960s the rapidity of scientific and technological advances has been having as great an impact on the profession of nursing as on other components of society. As emerging professionals, nurses have been identifying the knowledge base specific to nursing practice and to an expanding role for nurses.

In the preface to *Toward a Theory for Nursing*, King clearly states she was proposing a conceptual framework for nursing and not a nursing theory. As she denoted in the title, her purpose was to help move *toward* a theory for nursing.[3] In contrast, in the preface to *A Theory for Nursing*, she indicates she has expanded and built upon the original framework. In this second publication, she

> presents a conceptual framework by linking concepts essential to understanding nursing as a major system within health care systems ... offers one approach to developing concepts and applying knowledge in nursing ... [and] demonstrates one strategy for theory construction by presenting a theory of goal attainment derived from the conceptual framework.[4]

King identifies the conceptual framework as an open systems framework and the theory as one of goal attainment. As her extensive documentation indicates, she has drawn from a wide variety of sources in developing the framework and the theory.

Since the theory of goal attainment is derived from the open systems framework, the framework and its assumptions and concepts will be presented first, and then the goal attainment theory will be discussed.

KING'S OPEN SYSTEMS FRAMEWORK

King presents several assumptions that are basic to her conceptual framework. These include the assumptions that nursing's focus is the care of human beings, nursing's goal is "the health of individuals and health care for groups," and human beings are open systems in constant interaction with their environment.[5]

The conceptual framework is composed of three interacting systems; these are the personal systems, the interpersonal systems, and the social systems. Figure 13–1 presents a schematic diagram of these interacting systems. King summarizes the conceptual framework as follows:

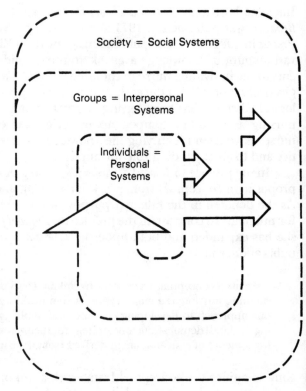

Society = Social Systems

Groups = Interpersonal Systems

Individuals = Personal Systems

Figure 13–1. Dynamic interacting systems. *(Adapted from King, I. M.* Toward a Theory for Nursing, *New York: Wiley, 1971, p. 20. Copyright © 1971, by John Wiley & Sons, Inc. Used with permission.)*

Individuals comprise one type of system in the environment called personal systems. Individuals interact to form dyads, triads, and small and large groups, which comprise another type of system called interpersonal systems. Groups with special interests and needs form organizations, which make up communities and societies and [these] are called social systems.[6]

She then identifies several concepts as relevant for each of these systems.

Personal Systems

Each individual is a personal system. For a personal system the relevant concepts are perception, self, growth and development, body image, space, and time.[7] *Perception* is presented as the major concept of a personal system, the concept that influences all behaviors or to which all other concepts are related. The characteristics of perception are that it is universal, or experienced by all; subjective or personal; and selective for each person, meaning that any given situation will be experienced in a unique manner by each individual involved. Perception is action oriented in the present and based on the information that is available. Perception is transactions; that is, individuals are active participants in situations and their identities are affected by their participation.[8] King further discusses perception as a process in which data obtained through the sense and from memory are organized, interpreted, and transformed. This process of human interaction with the environment influences behavior, provides meaning to experience, and represents the individual's image of reality.[9]

The characteristics of *self* are a dynamic individual, an open system, and goal orientation.[10] King accepts Jersild's definition of self:

> The self is a composite of thoughts and feelings which constitute a person's awareness of his individual existence, his conception of who and what he is. A person's self is the sum total of all he can call his. The self includes, among other things, a system of ideas, attitudes, values and commitments. The self is a person's total subjective environment. It is a distinctive center of experience and significance. The self constitutes a person's inner world as distinguished from the outer world consisting of all other people and things. The self is the individual as known to the individual. It is that to which we refer when we say "I."[11]

The characteristics of *growth and development* include cellular, molecular, and behavioral changes in human beings. These changes usually occur in an orderly manner, one that is predictable but has individual variations and is a function of genetic endowment, of meaningful and satisfying experiences, and of an environment conducive to helping individuals move toward maturity.[12] Growth and development can be defined as the processes in people's lives through which they move from a potential for achievement to actualization of self.[13] Theorists mentioned are Freud, Erikson, Piaget, Gesell, and Havinghurst; but no particular model, theory, or framework of growth and development is specifically selected.[14a–14e]

Body image is characterized as very personal and subjective, acquired or learned, dynamic and changing as the person redefines self, and part of each stage of growth and development. King defines body image as how one perceives both one's body and others' reactions to one's appearance.[15]

Space is characterized as universal because all people have some concept of it; personal or subjective; individual; situational and dependent on the relationships in the situation; dimensional as a function of volumes, area, distance, and time; and transactional or based on the individual's perception of the situation.[16] King's operational definition of space includes that space exists in all directions, is the same everywhere, and is defined by the physical area known as "territory" and by the behaviors of those who occupy it.[17]

Time is characterized as universal or inherent in life processes; relational or dependent on distance and the amount of information occurring; unidirectional or irreversible as it moves from past to future with a continuous flow of events; measurable; and subjective since it is based on perception.[18] King defines time as "a duration between one event and another as uniquely experienced by each human being; it is the relation of one event to another event."[19]

Perception, self, growth and development, body image, space, and time are the concepts of the personal system. When personal systems come in contact with each other, they form interpersonal systems.

Interpersonal Systems

Interpersonal systems are formed by human beings interacting. Two interacting individuals form a dyad, three form a triad, and four or more form small or large groups. As the number of interacting individuals increases, so does the complexity of the interactions. The relevant concepts for interpersonal systems are interaction, communication, transaction, role, and stress.[20]

Interaction is characterized by values; mechanisms for establishing human relationships; being universally experienced; being influenced by perceptions; reciprocity; being mutual or interdependent; containing verbal and nonverbal communication; learning occurring when communication is effective; unidirectionality; irreversibility; dynamism; and having a temporal–spatial dimension.[21] Interactions are defined as the observable behaviors of two or more persons in mutual presence.[21]

Characteristics of *communication* are that it is verbal; nonverbal; situational; perceptual; transactional; irreversible, or moving forward in time; personal; and dynamic.[22] Symbols for verbal communications are provided by language as such communication includes the spoken and written language that transmits ideas from one person to another. A very important aspect of nonverbal behavior is touch. Other aspects of nonverbal behavior are distance, posture, facial expression, physical appearance, and body movements.[22] King defines communication as "a process whereby information is given from one person to another either directly in face-to-face meeting or indirectly through telephone, television, or the written word."[22] Communication as a fundamental social process develops and maintains human relations and facilitates the ordered functioning of human groups and societies. As the information component of human interactions, communication occurs in all behaviors.[23]

Transactions, for this conceptual framework, are derived from cognition and perceptions and not from transactional analysis. The characteristics of transactions are that they are unique because each individual has a personal world of reality based on that individual's perceptions; they have temporal and spatial dimensions; and they are experience, or a series of events in time.[24] King defines transactions as "a process of interactions in which human beings communicate with environment to achieve goals that are valued . . . goal-directed human behaviors."[24]

The characteristics of *role* include reciprocity in that a person may be a giver at one time and a taker at another time, with a relationship between two or more individuals who are functioning in two or more roles; learned; social; complex; and situational.[25] There are three major elements to role. The first is that role consists of a set of expected behaviors of those who occupy a position in a social system. The second is a set of procedures or rules which define the obligations and rights associated with a position in an organization. The third is a relationship of two or more persons who are interacting for a purpose in a particular situation. The nurse's role can be defined as interacting with one or more others in a nursing situation in which the nurse, as a professional, uses those skills, knowledge, and values identified as nursing's to identify goals and help others achieve the goals.[26]

The characteristics of *stress* are that it is dynamic due to open systems being in continuous exchange with the environment; the intensity varies; there is a temporal–spatial dimension that is influenced by past experiences; it is individual, personal, and subjective, a response to life events that is uniquely personal.[27]

King derives a definition of stress to be "a dynamic state whereby a human being interacts with the environment to maintain balance for growth, development, and performance, which involves an exchange of energy and information between the person and the environment for regulation and control of stressors." In addition, stress involves objects, persons, and events as stressors which evoke an energy response from the person. Stress may be positive or negative, and may simultaneously help an individual to a peak of achievement and wear the individual down.[28]

The concepts of interpersonal systems are interaction, communication, transaction, role, and stress. Interpersonal systems join together to form larger systems known as social systems.

Social Systems

> A social system is defined as an organized boundary system of social roles, behaviors, and practices developed to maintain values and the mechanisms to regulate the practices and rules.[29]

Examples of social systems include families, religious groups, educational systems, work systems, and peer groups.[30] The concepts relevant to social systems are organization, authority, power, status, and decision making.[31] King proposes four parameters for *organization:*

> (1) human values, behavior patterns, needs, goals and expectations; (2) a natural environment in which material and human resources are essential for achieving goals; (3) employers and employees, or parents and children, who form the groups that collectively interact to achieve goals; (4) technology that facilitates goal attainment.[32]

Organization is characterized by structure that orders positions and activities and relates formal and informal arrangements of individuals and groups to achieve personal and organizational goals; functions that describe the roles, positions, and activities to be performed; goals or outcomes to be achieved; and resources. King defines organization as being made up of human beings who have prescribed roles and positions and who make use of resources to meet both personal and organizational goals.[33]

The characteristics of *authority* include that it is observable through provisions of order, guidance, and responsibility for actions; universal; essential in formal organizations; reciprocal because it requires cooperation; resides in a holder who must be perceived as legitimate; situational; essential to goal achievement; and associated with power.[34] Assumptions about authority include that it can be perceived by individuals and be legitimate; it can be associated with a position in which the position holder distributes rewards and sanctions; it can be held by professionals through their competence in using special knowledge and skills; and it can be exercised through group leadership by those with human relations skills. King defines authority as an active, reciprocal process of transaction in which the actors' backgrounds, perceptions, and values influence the definition, validation, and acceptance of those in organizational positions associated with authority.[35]

Power is characterized as universal; situational or not a personal attribute; essential in the organization; limited by resources in a situation; dynamic; and goal directed. Premises about power are that it is potential energy; is essential for order in society; enhances group cohesiveness; resides in positions in an organization; is directly related to authority; is a function of human interactions; and is a function of decision making.[36] King defines power in a variety of ways:

Power is the capacity to use resources in organizations to achieve goals . . . is the process whereby one or more persons influence other persons in a situation . . . is the capacity or ability of a person or a group to achieve goals . . . occurs in all aspects of life and each person has potential power determined by individual resources and the environmental forces encountered. Power is social force that organizes and maintains society. Power is the ability to use and to mobilize resources to achieve goals.[37]

Status is characterized as situational; position dependent; and reversible. King defines status as "the position of an individual in a group or a group in relation to other groups in an organization" and identifies that status is accompanied by "privileges, duties and obligations."[38]

Decision making is characterized as necessary to regulate each person's life and work; universal; individual; personal; subjective; situational; a continuous process; and goal directed. Decision making in organizations is defined as "a dynamic and systematic process by which goal-directed choice of perceived alternatives is made and acted upon by individuals or groups to answer a question and attain a goal."[39]

The major theses of King's conceptual framework are (1) that "each human being perceives the world as a total person in making transactions with individuals and things in the environment," and (2) that "transactions represent a life situation in which perceiver and thing perceived are encountered and in which each person enters the situation as an active participant and each is changed in the process of these experiences."[40] The concepts and systems of the framework are used as a base to develop a theory of goal attainment.

KING'S THEORY OF GOAL ATTAINMENT

The major elements of the theory of goal attainment are seen "in the interpersonal systems in which two people, who are usually strangers, come together in a health care organization to help and be helped to maintain a state of health that permits functioning in roles."[40] The concepts of the theory are interaction, perception, communication, transaction, self, role, stress, growth and development, time, and space. Although these terms have already been defined as concepts in the conceptual framework, they will be defined again here as part of the theory of goal attainment.

Interaction is defined as "a process of perception and communication between person and environment and between person and person, represented by verbal and nonverbal behaviors that are goal directed."[41] King diagrams interaction as seen in Figure 13–2. Each of the individuals involved in an interaction brings different ideas, attitudes, and perceptions to the exchange. The individuals come together for a purpose and perceive

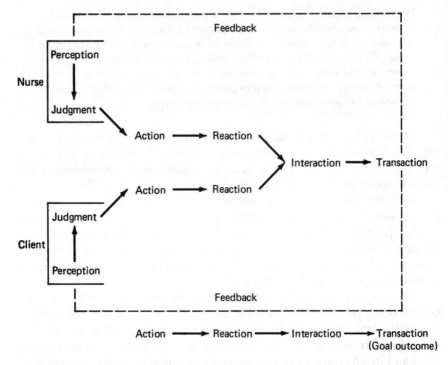

Figure 13–2. Interaction. *(Adapted from King, I. M.* Toward a Theory of Nursing: General Concepts of Human Behavior, *New York: Wiley, 1971, pp. 26, 92. Copyright © 1971 by John Wiley & Sons, Inc. Used with permission.)*

each other; each makes a judgment and takes mental action or decides to act. Then each reacts to the other and the situation (perception, judgment, action, reaction). King indicates that the interaction and transaction are directly observable.[42]

Perception is "each person's representation of reality."[42] The elements of perception are the importing of energy from the environment and organizing it by information; transforming energy; processing information; storing information; and exporting information in the form of overt behaviors.[42]

Communication is defined as "a process whereby information is given from one person to another either directly in face-to-face meetings or indirectly through telephone, television, or the written word."[42] Communication represents, and is involved in, the information component of interaction.

Transaction is defined as "observable behaviors of human beings interacting with their environment."[43] Transactions represent the valuation component of human interactions and involve bargaining, negotiating, and social exchange. When transactions occur between nurses and clients, goals are attained.[43]

Role is defined as "a set of behaviors expected of persons occupying a position in a social system; rules that define rights and obligations in a position; a relationship with one or more individuals interacting in specific situations for a purpose."[43] It is important that roles be understood and interpreted clearly to avoid conflict and confusion.

Stress is "a dynamic state whereby a human being interacts with the environment to maintain balance for growth, development, and performance . . . an energy response of an individual to persons, objects, and events called stressors."[43] Although stress may be positive or negative, too high a level of stress may decrease an individual's ability to interact and to attain goals.

Growth and development can be defined as the "continuous changes in individuals at the cellular, molecular, and behavioral levels of activities . . . the processes that take place in the life of individuals that help them move from potential capacity for achievement to self-actualization."[44]

Time is "a sequence of events moving onward to the future . . . a continuous flow of events in successive order that implies a change, a past and a future . . . a duration between one event and another as uniquely experienced by each human being . . . the relation of one event to another."[44]

Space exists in every direction and is the same in all directions. Space includes that physical area which is named territory. Space is defined by the behaviors of those individuals who occupy it.[44]

From the theory of goal attainment, King has developed eight predictive propositions, although she indicates that additional propositions may be generated. The eight propositions that she sets forth are as follows[45]:

1. If perceptual accuracy is present in nurse–client interactions, transactions will occur.
2. If nurse and client make transactions, goals will be attained.
3. If goals are attained, satisfactions will occur.
4. If goals are attained, effective nursing care will occur.
5. If transactions are made in nurse–client interactions, growth and development will be enhanced.
6. If role expectations and role performance as perceived by nurse and client are congruent, transactions will occur.
7. If role conflict is experienced by nurse or client or both, stress in nurse–client interactions will occur.
8. If nurses with special knowledge and skills communicate appropriate information to clients, mutual goal setting and goal attainment will occur.

In addition, King specifies internal and external boundary-determining criteria. Internal boundary criteria are derived from the characteristics of the concepts of the theory and speak to the theory itself. External boundary criteria speak to the area in which the theory is applicable. The internal boundary criteria for King's theory of goal attainment are listed below[46]:

1. Nurse and client do not know each other.
2. Nurse is licensed to practice professional nursing.

3. Client is in need of the services provided by the nurse.
4. Nurse and client are in a reciprocal relationship in that the nurse has special knowledge and skills to communicate appropriate information to help client set goals; client has information about self and perceptions of problems or concerns that when communicated to nurse will help in mutual goal setting.
5. Nurse and client are in mutual presence, purposefully interacting to achieve goals.

The external boundary criteria for King's theory of goal attainment are as follows[46]:

1. Interactions in a two-person group
2. Interactions limited to licensed professional nurse and to client in need of nursing care
3. Interactions taking place in natural environments

Thus, King is saying a professional nurse, with special knowledge and skills, and a client in need of nursing, with knowledge of self and perceptions of personal problems, meet as strangers in a natural environment. They interact mutually to identify the problems and to establish and achieve goals. The personal system of the nurse and the personal system of the client meet in the interaction with the interpersonal system of their dyad. Their interpersonal system is influenced by the social systems that surround them.

KING'S THEORY AND THE FOUR MAJOR CONCEPTS

In discussing her conceptual framework as an introduction to the presentation of her theory of goal attainment, King indicates that the abstract concepts of the framework are human beings, health, environment, and society.[47] Since the theory is presented as a theory for nursing, King also defines nursing. Thus the four major concepts of human beings, health, environment/society, and nursing are defined and discussed by King.

King identifies several assumptions about *human beings*. She describes human beings as social, sentient, rational, perceiving, controlling, purposeful, action oriented, and time oriented. From these beliefs about human beings, she has derived the following assumptions that are specific to nurse–client interaction[48]:

- Perceptions of nurse and of client influence the interaction process.
- Goals, needs, and values of nurse and client influence the interaction process.
- Individuals have a right to knowledge about themselves.
- Individuals have a right to participate in decisions that influence their life, their health, and community services.

- Health professionals have a responsibility to share information that helps individuals make informed decisions about their health care.
- Individuals have a right to accept or to reject health care.
- Goals of health professionals and goals of recipients of health care may be incongruent.

King further states that "nurses are concerned with human beings interacting with their environment in ways that lead to self-fulfillment and to maintenance of health."[49] Human beings have three fundamental health needs: (1) the need for health information that is usable at the time when it is needed and can be used, (2) the need for care that seeks to prevent illness, and (3) the need for care when human beings are unable to help themselves. She states, "nurses are in a position to assess what people know about their health, what they think about their health, how they feel about it, and how they act to maintain it."[50]

King defines *health* as "dynamic life experiences of a human being, which implies continuous adjustment to stressors in the internal and external environment through optimum use of one's resources to achieve maximum potential for daily living."[51] She discusses health as a functional state, and illness as an interference with that functional state. She then defines illness as "a deviation from normal, that is, an imbalance in a person's biological structure or in his psychological make-up, or a conflict in a person's social relationships."[51]

Environment and *society* are indicated as major concepts in King's framework but are not specifically defined in her work. Society may be viewed as the social systems portion of her open systems framework. Although her definition of health mentions both internal and external environment, the usual implication of the use of environment in *A Theory for Nursing* is that of external environment. Since she presents her material as based on open systems, it is assumed that a definition of external environment may be drawn from general system theory. Systems are considered to have boundaries that separate their internal components from the rest of the world. The external environment for a system is the portion of the world that exists outside of that boundary. Of particular interest as a system's external environment is the part of the world that is in direct exchange of energy and information with the system.[52a,52b]

Nursing is defined as "a process of action, reaction, and interaction whereby nurse and client share information about their perceptions in the nursing situation," and as "a process of human interactions between nurse and client whereby each perceives the other and the situation; and through communication, they set goals, explore means, and agree on means to achieve goals."[53] *Action* is defined as a sequence of behaviors involving mental and physical action. The sequence is first mental action to recognize the presenting conditions; then physical action to begin activities related to those conditions; and finally, mental action in an effort to exert control over the situation, combined with physical action seeking to achieve goals.[54] *Reaction* is not specifically defined but might be considered to be included in the sequence of behaviors described in action. *Interaction* has been previously discussed. Although King has altered her definition of nursing from that published in 1971, she has continued to refer to nursing as that which is done by nurses. This weakens her definition.

In addition to the above definition of nursing, King discusses the goal, domain, and function of the professional nurse. The goal of the nurse is "to help individuals maintain their health so they can function in their roles."[55] Nursing's domain includes promoting, maintaining, and restoring health, and caring for the sick, injured, and dying.[56] The function of the professional nurse is to interpret information in what is known as the nursing process to plan, implement, and evaluate nursing care.[57]

THEORY OF GOAL ATTAINMENT AND THE NURSING PROCESS

The basic assumption of the theory of goal attainment—that nurses and clients communicate information, set goals mutually, and then act to attain those goals—is also the basic assumption of the nursing process.

King indicates *assessment* will occur during the interaction of the nurse and client, who are likely to meet as strangers. The nurse brings to this meeting special knowledge and skills, whereas the client brings knowledge of self and perceptions of the problems that are of concern. Assessment, interviewing, and communication skills are needed by the nurse as is the ability to integrate knowledge of natural and behavioral sciences for application to a concrete situation.[57]

All concepts of the theory apply to assessment. Growth and development, knowledge of self and role, and the amount of stress influence perception and, in turn, influence communication, interaction, and transaction. In assessment, the nurse needs to collect data about the client's level of growth and development, view of self, perception of current health status, communication patterns, and role socialization, among other things. Factors influencing the client's perception include the functioning of the client's sensory system, age, development, sex, education, drug and diet history, and understanding of why contact with the health care system is occurring. The perceptions of the nurse are influenced by the cultural and socioeconomic background and age of the nurse and the diagnosis of the client.[58] Perception is the basis for gathering and interpreting data, thus the basis for assessment. Communication is necessary to verify the accuracy of perceptions. Without communication, interaction and transaction cannot occur.

The information shared during assessment is used to derive a *nursing diagnosis*, defined by King as a statement that "identifies the disturbances, problems, or concerns about which patients seek help."[59] The implication is that the nurse makes the nursing diagnosis as a result of the mutual sharing with the client during assessment. Stress may be a particularly important concept in relation to nursing diagnosis since stress, disturbance, and problem or concern may be closely connected.

After the nursing diagnosis is made, *planning* occurs. King describes planning as setting goals and making decisions about how to achieve these goals. This is part of transaction and again involves mutual exchange with the client. She specifies that clients are requested to participate in decision making about how the goals are to be met.[60] Although King indicates in her assumptions about nurse–client interactions that clients have the right to participate in decisions about their care, she does not say they have the responsibility. Thus, clients are requested to participate, not expected to do so.

Implementation occurs in the activities that seek to meet the goals. Implementation is a continuation of transaction in King's theory.

Evaluation involves descriptions of how the outcomes identified as goals are attained. In King's description, evaluation not only speaks to the attainment of the client's goals but also to the effectiveness of nursing care.[61]

Although all of the theory concepts apply throughout the nursing process, communication with perception, interaction, and transaction are vital for goal attainment and need to be apparent in each phase. King emphasizes the importance of mutual participation in interaction that focuses on the needs and welfare of the client and of verifying perceptions while planning and activities to achieve goals are carried out together. Although King emphasizes mutuality, she does not limit it to verbal communication, nor does she require the client's active physical participation in actions to achieve goal attainment.

In *A Theory for Nursing,* King presents an application of her theory of goal attainment that she identifies as the use of a goal-oriented nursing record. Her description of this goal-oriented nursing record closely parallels the steps of the nursing process.

KING'S WORK AND THE CHARACTERISTICS OF A THEORY

King has stated that she has derived a theory of goal attainment from her open system framework of personal, interpersonal, and social systems. How her work compares with the characteristics of a theory presented in Chapter 1 will be discussed below.

1. Theories can interrelate concepts in such a way as to create a different way of looking at a particular phenomenon. King has interrelated the concepts of interaction, perception, communication, transaction, self, role, stress, growth and development, time, and space into a theory of goal attainment. Her theory deals with a nurse–client dyad, a relationship to which each person brings personal perceptions of self, role, and personal levels of growth and development. The nurse and client communicate, first in interaction and then in transaction, to attain mutually set goals. The relationship takes place in space identified by their behaviors and occurs in forward moving time. In particular, the specification of transaction as dealing with mutual goal attainment is a different way of looking at the phenomenon of nurse–client relationships.

2. Theories must be logical in nature. King's theory of goal attainment does describe a logical sequence of events. The concepts are clearly defined. However, a major inconsistency within her writing is the lack of a clear definition of environment, which is identified as a basic concept for the framework from which she derives her theory. In addition, she indicates that nurses are concerned about the health care of groups but defines nursing as occurring in a dyadic relationship. Thus the theory essentially draws on only two of the three systems described in the conceptual framework. The social systems portion of the framework is not clearly connected to the theory of goal attainment. The definition of stress indicates that it is both negative and positive, but discussion of stress always implies that it is negative. Finally, King indicates that the nurse and client are strangers, yet she speaks of their working together for goal attainment and of the importance of health maintenance. Attainment of long-term goals, such as those concerning health maintenance, is not consistent with not knowing each other.

3. Theories should be relatively simple yet generalizable. Although the presentation appears to be complex, King's theory of goal attainment is relatively simple. Ten concepts are identified, defined, and their relationships considered. Even though King indicates many of the concepts are situation dependent, they are not situation specific; that is, they are influenced by the situation but may occur in many different situations. The theory of goal attainment is limited in setting only in regard to "natural environments" and, with growth and development as a major concept, is certainly not limited in age. The theory of goal attainment is generalizable to any nursing situation. The emphasis on mutuality would initially appear to limit the theory to dealing with those clients who can verbally interact with the nurse and physically participate in implementations to meet goals. However, King points to observable behaviors and to both verbal and nonverbal communication. Indeed, the comatose individual has observable behaviors in the form of vital signs and does communicate nonverbally. The major limitation in relation to this characteristic is the effort required of the reader to sift through the presentation of a conceptual framework and a theory with repeated definitions to find the basic concepts.

4. Theories can be the bases for hypotheses that can be tested. King presents the following hypotheses that she has derived from her theory of goal attainment[62]:

1. Perceptual accuracy in nurse–patient interactions increases mutual goal setting.
2. Communication increases mutual goal setting between nurses and patients and leads to satisfactions.
3. Satisfactions in nurses and patients increase goal attainment.
4. Goal attainment decreases stress and anxiety in nursing situations.
5. Goal attainment increases patient learning and coping ability in nursing situations.
6. Role conflict experienced by patients, nurses, or both, decreases transactions in nurse–patient interactions.
7. Congruence in role expectations and role performance increases transactions in nurse–patient interactions.

These and other hypotheses could be used to test the theory.

5. Theories contribute to and assist in increasing the general body of knowledge within the discipline through the research implemented to validate them. King reports the results of a descriptive study conducted to test the theory of goal attainment. The study resulted in a classification system to analyze nurse–patient interactions and identified that goal attainment is facilitated when the nurse and patient have accurate perceptions, adequate communication, and set goals mutually.[63] This is one example of a contribution to the general body of knowledge. The theory of goal attainment needs to be tested further. Such testing will expand the theory's contribution to the discipline.

6. Theories can be utilized by the practitioners to guide and improve their practice. As demonstrated in the discussion of nursing process, King's theory of goal attainment can be used to guide and improve practice. Even though this theory in itself can be used as a guide to practice, King has also developed the goal-oriented nursing record in an effort to assist the practice of nursing. She presents the goal-oriented nursing record as an application of the theory of goal attainment in nursing.

7. Theories must be consistent with other validated theories, laws, and principles but will leave open unanswered questions that need to be investigated. King's theory of goal attainment is not in apparent conflict with other validated theories, laws, and principles. She has clearly documented the sources on which she has based her characteristics and definitions of concepts, and she states that "the major technique used in developing concepts . . . has been a review of the literature in nursing and related fields to identify characteristics of the concept. From this information, an operational definition of the concept is formulated."[64] Using the review of the literature as a base has helped to avoid being in conflict with others. King shares many similarities with other nursing theorists. As does Peplau, King indicates the nurse and client usually enter the relationship as strangers when the client has a need.[65] King's basic assumptions about human beings as thinking, sentient decision makers who have a right to information and to participate in decisions about themselves has a humanistic base similar to that of Paterson and Zderad.[66] The emphasis on the right to participate in decisions is similar to that of Orlando, among others.[67a,67b]

Throughout *A Theory for Nursing,* King identifies those theories from other fields that support what she is saying. Although there is no apparent conflict, there are many questions open for exploration. A few of these are discussed in the hypotheses presented earlier in this chapter.

SUMMARY

Imogene King has presented an open systems framework from which she derived a theory of goal attainment. The framework consists of three systems—personal, interpersonal, and social—all of which are in continuous exchange with their environments. The concepts of the personal systems are perception, self, body image, growth and development, time, and space. The concepts of the interpersonal systems are role, interaction, communication, transaction, and stress. Social systems concepts are organization, power, authority, status, decision making, and role.

From these systems, and their abstract concepts of human beings, health, environment, and society, she derives a theory of goal attainment. The major concepts of the theory of goal attainment are interaction, perception, communication, transaction, role, stress, and growth and development. Each of these are defined, and overall propositions and criteria for determining internal and external boundaries of the theory are presented.

Imogene King has developed a theory of goal attainment that is based on a philosophy of human beings and an open systems framework. She presents the results of one descriptive research study to test the theory and proposes an application of the theory in the form of a goal-oriented nursing record.

The theory is useful, testable, and applicable to nursing practice. Although it is not the "perfect theory," it is widely generalizable and not situation specific. As with her previous writing, Dr. King's work is solidly based in the literature and provides the reader with a rich set of resources for further study.

References

1.(a) King, I.M. *Toward a Theory for Nursing: General Concepts of Human Behavior,* New York: John Wiley & Sons, Inc., 1971.
1.(b) King, I.M. *A Theory for Nursing: Systems, Concepts, Process,* New York: Wiley, 1981.
2.   King, *A Theory for Nursing,* p. 9.

3.   King, *Toward a Theory*, p. x.
4.   King, *A Theory for Nursing*, p. vii.
5.   Ibid, 10.
6.   Ibid, 141.
7.   Ibid, 10.
8.   Ibid, 23.
9.   Ibid, 24.
10.   Ibid, 26–27.
11.   Jersild, A.T. *In Search of Self*, New York: Columbia University Teachers College Press, 1952, pp. 9–10.
12.   King, *A Theory for Nursing*, pp. 30–31.
13.   Ibid, 31.
14.(a) Freud, S., *Introductory Lectures on Psychoanalysis*, translated by J. Strachey, New York: W. W. Norton & Co., Inc., 1966.
14.(b) Erikson, E. *Childhood and Society*, New York: W. W. Norton & Co., Inc., 1950.
14.(c) Inhelder, B.F. & Piaget, J. *The Early Growth of Logic in the Child*, New York: W. W. Norton & Co., Inc., 1964.
14.(d) Gesell, A. *Infant Development*, New York: Harper & Row, 1952.
14.(e) Havinghurst, R. *Human Development and Education*, New York: David McKay Co., Inc., 1953.
15.   King, *A Theory for Nursing*, p. 33.
16.   Ibid, 36–37.
17.   Ibid, 37–38.
18.   Ibid, 42–44.
19.   Ibid, 45.
20.   Ibid, 59.
21.   Ibid, 84–85.
22.   Ibid, 69–74.
23.   Ibid, 79–80.
24.   Ibid, 82.
25.   Ibid, 91–92.
26.   Ibid, 93.
27.   Ibid, 96.
28.   Ibid, 98–99.
29.   Ibid, 115.
30.   Ibid, 113.
31.   Ibid, 114.
32.   Ibid, 116.
33.   Ibid, 119.
34.   Ibid, 123.
35.   Ibid, 124.
36.   Ibid, 127.
37.   Ibid, 127–28.
38.   Ibid, 129–30.
39.   Ibid, 132.
40.   Ibid, 141, 142.
41.   Ibid, 145.
42.   Ibid, 145–46.
43.   Ibid, 147.

44.   Ibid, 148.
45.   Ibid, 149.
46.   Ibid, 150.
47.   Ibid, 141.
48.   Ibid, 143–44.
49.   Ibid, 3.
50.   Ibid, 8.
51.   Ibid, 5.
52.(a) Bertrand, A.L., *Social Organization,* Philadelphia: F.A. Davis Co., 1972.
52.(b) Katz, D. & Kahn, R., *The Social Psychology of Organizations,* New York: Wiley, 1966.
53.   King, *A Theory for Nursing,* pp. 2, 144.
54.   Ibid, 60.
55.   Ibid, 3–4.
56.   Ibid, 4.
57.   Ibid, 9.
58.   Ibid, 24.
59.   Ibid, 177.
60.   Ibid, 176.
61.   Ibid, 177.
62.   Ibid, 156.
63.   Ibid, 155.
64.   Ibid, 22.
65.   Peplau, H.E., *Interpersonal Relations in Nursing,* New York: G. P. Putnam's Sons, 1952.
66.   Paterson, J. & Zderad, L., *Humanistic Nursing,* New York: Wiley, 1976.
67.(a) Orlando, I.J., *The Dynamic Nurse–Patient Relationship: Function, Process and Principles,* New York: G. P. Putnam's Sons, 1961.
67.(b) Orlando, I.J., *The Discipline and Teaching of Nursing Process,* New York: G. P. Putnam's Sons, 1972.

Bibliography

Daubenmire, M. J. and King, I. M. Nursing Process Model: A Systems Approach, *Nursing Outlook,* 1973, 21 (8) 512–17.

King, I. M. A Conceptual Frame of Reference for Nursing, *Nursing Research,* 1968, 17(1) 27–31.

King, I. M. The Health Care System: Nursing Intervention Subsystem, in Werley, W. H. et al., eds., *Health Research: The Systems Approach,* New York: Springer Publishing Co., Inc., 1976.

King, I. M. Nursing Theory-Problems and Prospects, *Nursing Science,* October 1964, 394–403.

King, I. M. Planning for Change, *Ohio Nurses Review,* 1970, 4–7.

King, I. M. *Curriculum and Instruction in Nursing,* Englewood Cliffs, N.J.: Prentice-Hall, 1986.

CHAPTER 14

Martha E. Rogers

Suzanne M. Falco
Marie L. Lobo

Martha E. Rogers was born in Dallas, Texas, May 12, 1914, the eldest of four children. Her family heritage includes many active women suffragists and a strong belief in the necessity of a college education. Before entering the Knoxville General Hospital School of Nursing, she attended the University of Tennessee in Knoxville from 1931 to 1933. She received her diploma in 1936, a BS in public health nursing from George Peabody College, Nashville, Tennessee, in 1937; an MA in public health nursing supervision from Teachers College, Columbia University, New York, in 1945; and an MPH in 1952 and a ScD in 1954, both from Johns Hopkins University.

Following numerous leadership and staff positions in community health nursing, she moved into higher education as a visiting lecturer and then as a research associate. For twenty-one years, Dr. Rogers was Professor and Head of the Division of Nurse Education at New York University. Since 1975 she has continued to teach at the University and is Professor Emeritus there.

Dr. Rogers has been active in numerous professional organizations, has received many awards and honors, and has published extensively in numerous nursing journals. She has authored several books.

As "a humanistic science dedicated to compassionate concern for maintaining and promoting health, preventing illness, and caring for and rehabilitating the sick and disabled", nursing historically has meant service to humanity.[1] Throughout nursing's evolution, from the earliest ages to the present, nurturance of the human race has been an ever-present and central concern.[2] Over the years, the scientific extension of people's centuries-long interest in life and its many manifestations have become integral components of nursing. Thus, the history of humanity is reflected in the evolutionary development of nursing. Consequently, Martha Rogers believes that knowledge of the past is a necessary foundation for the present understanding of nursing, and for evolving the theories and principles that must guide nursing practice.[3]

The concept that human life is valuable did not develop until people had begun to band together into tribes, villages, and towns. Such communal living allowed for sharing of work and responsibility and the provision of mutual support. This more settled life style made it possible for mothers to keep their newborns and care for more children.[4] Thus, partly out of love and partly out of need, human beings began to develop strong feelings about and concern for fellow human beings.

As culture developed and more complex concepts in economic, political, and social structures increased, the value of human life increased. Science, art, and religion brought a growing awareness of one's fellow human beings. The Hebrews developed a monotheistic faith, while the Greeks contributed philosophy, politics, and government. Humanism was becoming strongly entrenched in culture. Following the rise of Christianity, the medieval world was dominated by the Christian religions whose members assumed the responsibility for nursing. With the Dark Ages came a decline in religious, cultural, and political life. The end of this period led to the beginning of modern science.[5]

As modern science evolved, new ideas mushroomed into new discoveries. The nature of the universe was explored. Descartes established the basis of modern philosophy. Einstein's theory of relativity brought a fourth dimension in the coordinate of space-time to man's previously three-dimensional world. Space research has multiplied scientific knowledge and has altered life style. The reality of these evolutionary changes is reflected in man's growing complexity.

As a result of these factors, the rate at which society has been storing up useful knowledge about humanity and the universe has been spiraling upward for the past 10,000 years.[6] This vast storehouse of knowledge coupled with a high degree of humanism and value for life has made advancement of nursing through scientific means and theoretical development a reality.

ROGERS' DEFINITION OF NURSING

Capitalizing on the knowledge base gained from anthropology, sociology, astronomy, religion, philosophy, history, and mythology, Rogers, in 1970, developed a conceptual framework for nursing. Since human beings are at the center of nursing's purpose, this conceptual framework for nursing looks at the total individual and is strongly based in general system theory. *Nursing*, then, is a humanistic and a humanitarian science directed toward describing and explaining the human being in synergistic wholeness and in developing the hypothetical generalizations and predictive principles basic to knowledgeable practice. The science of nursing is a science of humanity— the study of the nature and direction of human development.[7]

BASIC ASSUMPTIONS

Underlying the conceptual framework developed by Rogers are five assumptions about human beings.[8] First, the human being is a unified whole possessing an individual integrity and manifesting characteristics that are more than and different from the sum of the parts. The distinctive properties of the whole are also significantly different from those of its parts. Extensive knowledge of the subsystems is ineffective in enabling one to determine the properties of the living system—the human being. The human being is visible only when particulars disappear from view. Because of this wholeness, the individual's life process is a dynamic course that is continuous, creative, evolutionary, and uncertain, resulting in highly variable and constantly changing patterning.

Second, it is assumed that the individual and the environment are continuously exchanging matter and energy with each other. Environment for any individual is defined as the patterned wholeness of all that is external to a given individual. This constant interchange of materials and energy between the individual and the environment characterizes each of them as open systems.

The third assumption holds that the life process of human beings evolves irreversibly and unidirectionally along a space-time continuum. Consequently, the individual can never go backwards or be something he or she previously was. At any given point in time, then, the individual is the expression of the totality of events present at that given time.

Identifying individuals and reflecting their wholeness are life's patterns. These patterns allow for self-regulation, rhythmicity, and dynamism. They give unity to diversity and reflect a dynamic and creative universe. Thus, the fourth assumption is that pattern identifies individuals and reflects their innovative wholeness.

Finally, the fifth assumption is that the human being is characterized by the capacity for abstraction and imagery, language and thought, sensation and emotion. Of all the earth's life forms, only the human is a sentient thinking being who perceives and ponders the vastness of the cosmos.

Based on these assumptions are the four building blocks identified by Rogers—energy fields, openness, pattern, and four dimensionality.[9] A unifying concept for both animate and inanimate environments, *energy fields* have no boundaries; they are indivisible and extend to infinity, they are dynamic. Thus, these fields are *open,* allowing exchange with other fields. The interchange between and among energy fields has *pattern* that is perceived as a single wave; these patterns are not fixed but change as situations require. The interchanges occur at different points in the *four dimensionality* of space-time. With these building blocks as the base, *unitary humans* are defined as irreducible four-dimensional, negentropic energy fields identified by pattern and manifesting characteristics and behaviors that are different from those of the parts and which cannot be predicted from knowledge of the parts, with the *environment* being an irreducible four-dimensional, negentropic energy field identified by pattern and manifesting characteristics different from the person. (See Fig. 14-1.)[10a,10b]

There is a strong parallel between Rogers' basic assumptions and general system theory. According to von Bertalanffy, a system is a set of ele-

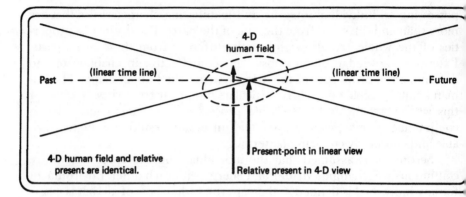

Figure 14–1. 4-D Environmental field. *(Adapted from Rogers, M.E. Nursing: A Science of Unitary Man, in* Conceptual Models for Nursing Practice *(2nd ed.), Riehl, J.P. & Roy, C., eds., New York: Appleton-Century-Crofts, 1980, p. 332.)*

ments that are interrelated.[11] The interrelated elements in this conceptual model are human beings and their environments. As a living system and energy field, the individual is capable of taking in energy and information from the environment, and releasing energy and information to the environment.[12] Because of this exchange, the individual is an open system—an underlying assumption and building block.

General system theory is a general science of wholeness. It is concerned with the problems of organization, phenomena that are not resolvable to individual events, and dynamic interactions manifested in the difference of the behavior of the parts when isolated. As a result, order and behavior are not understandable by investigation of the respective parts in isolation.[13] Thus, the assumption of wholeness and the building block of pattern result.

The principle of hierarchial order is applicable.[14] The individual as an open system attempts to move toward a higher order by progressive differentiation, as for example, the differentiation of the cells of the zygote to form a human being. Within the order of the universe, the human being is of a higher order than other two-legged animals. Characteristic of this is Rogers' fifth assumption of human beings as sentient thinking beings, and congruent with this is the building block of pattern.

Using these five assumptions and building blocks as a base, the life process in human beings becomes a phenomenon of wholeness, of continuity, of dynamic and creative change. It possesses its own unity. It is inseparable from the environment and occurs in four dimensionality. Since the individual is the recipient of nursing services, life processes of humanity are the *core* around which nursing revolves. According to Rogers, the science of nursing is directed toward describing the life process of humanity, and toward explaining and predicting the nature and direction of its development.[15]

ROGERS' THEORY: PRINCIPLES OF HOMEODYNAMICS

Although Rogers offers no theoretical statement, she grounded her *principles of homeodynamics* in the five basic assumptions and four building blocks as discussed above. The principles of homeodynamics are composed of three separate principles—integrality, helicy, and resonancy.[16a,16b] By combining the principles of homeodynamics with the concept of humanity from her definition of nursing, a theoretical statement can be postulated. Using the definition that a theory interrelates concepts in such a way as to create a different way of looking at a particular phenomenon, an appropriate theoretical statement might be that nursing is the use of the principles of homeodynamics for the service of humanity.

Integrality
The first principle is that of *integrality*. Because of the inseparability of human beings and their environment, sequential changes in the life process are continuous revisions occurring from the interactions between human beings and their environment. Between the two entities, there is a constant mutual interaction and mutual change whereby simultaneous molding is taking place in both at the same time. Thus, integrality is the continuous, mutual, simultaneous interaction process between human and environmental fields.

Resonancy
The next principle, *resonancy*, speaks to the nature of the change occurring between human and environmental fields. The change in the pattern of human beings and environments is propagated by waves that move from lower frequency longer waves to higher frequency shorter waves. The life process in human beings is a symphony of rhythmical vibrations oscillating at various frequencies. Human beings experience their environments as a resonating wave of complex symmetry uniting them with the rest of the world. Resonancy, then, is the identification of the human field and the environmental field by wave patterns manifesting continuous change from lower frequency longer waves to higher frequency shorter waves.

Helicy
Finally, the principle of *helicy* states that the nature and direction of human and environmental change are continuous, innovative, probabilistic, and characterized by the increasing diversity of human field and environmental field pattern emerging out of the continuous, mutual, simultaneous interaction between the human and environmental fields and manifesting non-repeating rhythmicities. Because the life process is a constantly evolving series of change in which the past has been incorporated and out of which new patterns have emerged, it is a becoming, a dynamic repatterning, a growing complexity, a unidirectional phenomenon, a probabilistic goal di-

rectedness. The concepts of rhythmicality, evolutionary emergence, and the unitary nature of the human-environmental field relationship are encompassed. Therefore, helicy postulates the direction of the change occurring between the human and environmental fields.

Consequently, the principles of homeodynamics are a way of viewing human beings in their wholeness. Changes in the life process of humanity are irreversible, nonrepeatable, rhythmical in nature, and evidence of the growing complexity of pattern. Change proceeds by continuous repatterning of both human and environmental fields by resonating oscillations of lower frequency longer waves to higher frequency shorter waves, and reflects the mutual simultaneous interaction between the two fields at any given point in space-time.

COMPARISON WITH OTHER THEORIES

The principles of homeodynamics are closely aligned to selected principles of general system theory. The homeodynamic principle of helicy can be compared to the principles of equifinality and negentropy. *Equifinality* means that an open system may attain a time-independent state independent of initial conditions and determined only by the system parameters. Thus, the system has a goal.[17] The *negentropic* principle provides that open systems have mechanisms that can slow down or arrest the process of movement toward less efficiency and growth.[18] Environmental exchange can provide support for such mechanisms.

For example, growth and development in the individual are equifinal. The same final state can be reached from different initial states and by means of different pathways. The various phases or stages along the way are maintained for an interval until spontaneous transition toward a higher order evokes new developments. The evolution toward an increase of order and organization at a higher level is made possible by negentropy.[19] Thus, growing complexity and evolutionary emergence are made possible.

Consider the case of identical twins Susie and Joanie. Shortly after their two-month birthday, one of the twins, Susie, spent six weeks in bilateral leg casts to correct a congenital deformity. As a result of this experience, Susie is maintained at a developmental plateau, while Joanie continues to develop along the sequential axis. Consequently, Susie experiences an altered developmental pattern, the extent of which is depicted in figure 14–2. At four months, the difference in development between the twins is substantial, whereas at eight months the difference has been greatly reduced. The equifinal state of this development will be achieved despite the increased time required.

Because of the evolutionary nature of this framework, many developmental theories are consistent with it. Infants are born with many capabili-

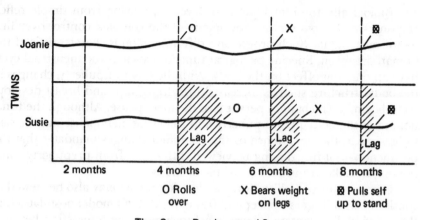

Figure 14–2. Pictorial representation of the altered developmental pattern experienced by one twin, Susie, as a result of leg-casting for six weeks following her second-month birthday.

ties. They have a repertoire of reflexes and behaviors with which they communicate with the world. The fetus evolves from a complex of cells into an organism which cues and responds to the environment, both inanimate and animate. Developmental theorists have demonstrated that the innate competence of the infant evolves through time.

For example, Erikson's psychosocial stages of development beginning with trust versus mistrust, and autonomy versus shame and doubt, through generativity versus self-absorption, and ego integrity versus despair, profess a forward growth of an increasingly complex individual.[20] Havinghurst's developmental tasks support the same philosophy of growth and development as Erikson.[21] Development is an ongoing process from learning the first basic tasks of walking, eating, and talking to control of bodily functions to adjusting to retirement or death of a spouse.

Another example is Piaget's concepts of intellectual development.[22] From sensorimotor to preoperational to concrete operational to formal operational thought, a nonreversible growth occurs. Kohlberg validates Piaget's work in his findings that moral development begins when thought processes shift from preoperational to concrete operations.[23] Again, Kohlberg found males develop through a series of stages, from a premoral punishment and obedience orientation to a principled morality and a universal ethical principle orientation. Gilligan has challenged the developmental theorists and their exclusion of women's thought and development in the presentations of their work.[24] Gilligan's thought-provoking observations are supportive of Rogers' conceptual model of the uniqueness of unitary man. In all these developmental theories, what has happened in the past in the individual's life will always affect the future.

Biologically, the individual also develops, moving from simple reflex responses and gross motor movements to the complex control over fine motor movements. Such progressive differentiation is characteristic of the human organism. Specific biological functions such as the menstrual cycle have an ongoing effect on the body. With the onset of puberty, changes in the body structure such as increased breadth of hips and breast development begin. Such changes persist past the menopause. Although the functioning of the body before puberty and following menopause may be said to be similar, the persistence of the identified changes mandates that the postmenopausal functioning be viewed differently from prepuberty functioning, thus illustrating the principle of helicy.

Components of Callista Roy's adaptation model may also be viewed as consistent with Rogers' conceptual framework. Roy's model postulates that the individual's adaptation level is a function of the interaction between adaptation mechanisms and the environment.[25] The physiological adaptation to the environmental stimulus of altitude change such as that experienced by mountain climbers demonstrates the mutual interaction between the individual and the environment. The simultaneous change in the mountain climber and in the altitude is consistent with the principle of integrality.

According to Roy, the individual's adaptation of self-concept is affected by social experience, which reflects the external stimuli that surround the person, and the processes of perception and social learning.[26]

Rogers' principle of helicy postulates that each new mutual interaction will promote continuous innovative changes. For example, a woman who is a wife and mother had developed a self-concept that is consistent with her perceptions of her interactions with husband and children. When that same woman then becomes a college student, interactions with faculty, students, and the college environment will promote changes and adaptations in her self-concept.

This mother–wife–student will have a change in her environment and therefore a change in her interaction with that environment. This is representative of integrality. The new environment of a university will include new faculty, new peers, new books, and new learning experiences in laboratories; and the new environment will cause changes in the old environment—the home—and how the woman interacts with the environment there. At specified points in time the changes caused by the new environment create changes in the life pattern in which she has been functioning.

As the mother–wife–student grows and changes because of her interaction with faculty, peers, and the college environment, she will integrate the material presented and will adapt—emerging from the program as a different woman. This adaptation will affect the rhythms that have related to her former life style. Before entering the program, the mother of the family always cooked the meals; after she enters the program, another member of the family may assume the cooking role, thus changing the rhythms of family functioning. Rogers's principle of helicy can be used in the changes of rhythms occurring because of the change in the environment.

Resonancy examines the variations occurring during the life process of the "whole" person. The experiences as a student mandate changes in the wife–mother. Because of the progression in space-time, the wife–mother–student can never return to the wife–mother unaffected by the experience of being a student.

ROGERS' THEORY AND THE FOUR MAJOR CONCEPTS

Martha Rogers speaks to the four major concepts. She presents five assumptions about *human beings*. Each human is assumed to be a *unified* being with individuality. The human is in continuous exchange of energy with the environment. The life processes of a human evolve irreversibly and unidirectionally in space and time. There is pattern to life. Finally, the human is capable of abstraction, imagery, language, thought, sensation, and emotion. Humans are four-dimensional, negentropic energy fields identified by pattern and manifesting characteristics and behaviors that are different from those of the parts and which cannot be predicted from knowledge of the parts.[27]

Environment consists of the totality of patterns existing external to the individual. Both the individual and the environment are considered to be open systems. Environment is a four-dimensional, negentropic energy field identified by pattern and integral with the human field.[27]

Nursing is an art and science that is humanistic and humanitarian. It is directed toward the unitary human and its concerned with the nature and direction of human development.

Health is not specifically addressed and indeed, if viewed as a state, is not appropriate to Rogers' theory. Malinski quoted personal communication with Rogers where Rogers stated she viewed health as a value term.[28] This communication confirms previous inferences that disease, pathology, and health were value terms. Value terms change and, when discussed in terms of the dynamics of the behaviors manifested by the human field, need to be individually defined.[28]

USE OF ROGERS' PRINCIPLES IN THE NURSING PROCESS

If the profession of nursing is viewed as concerned with unitary human beings, the principles of homeodynamics provide guidelines for predicting the nature and direction of the individual's development as responses to health-related problems are made. Using these guidelines, the professional practice of nursing would then seek to promote symphonic integration of human beings and their environments, to strengthen the coherence and integrity of the human field, and to direct and redirect patterning of the human and environmental fields for the realization of maximum health.[29a, 29b] These goals would be reflected in the nursing process.

To successfully utilize the principles of homeodynamics, there needs to be a consideration of the nurse and an involvement of both the nurse and the client in the nursing process. If anything or anyone external to the individual is part of the environment, then the nurse would be part of the client's environment. Because of the mutual interaction of the individual and the environment, it is implied that the client is a willing, integral partici- pant in the nursing process. Consequently, individualized nursing care re- sults, which Rogers maintains is necessary if the client is to achieve maxi- mum potential in a positive fashion.[30] Nursing, then, is working *with* the client, not *to* or *for* the client. This involvement in the nursing process by the nurse demonstrates concern for the total person, rather than one aspect, one problem, or a limited segment of need fulfillment.[31]

In the nursing assessment phase of the nursing process, all facts and opinions about the individual and the environment are collected. Because of our limited measuring devices and data-collection tools, the information collected in the assessment is frequently of an isolate or particulate nature. However, to implement the guidelines, the analysis of the data must be in such a fashion as to reflect wholeness. This may be done by asking several questions and seeking the responses from the collected data.

The first series of questions reflect the principle of integrality. What is the interaction between the person and the environment? How has one adjusted to the other? Are there any maladjustment factors present? Are they able to work together? What factors support or undermine this work- ing relationship? If the individual is in an environment that is not the normal one, how are the two environments different? Based on the differ- ences, what kind of predictions can be made about the individual's interac- tion with this new environment?

The next series of questions would reflect the principle of resonancy. How has the life process of the individual progressed? What kind of varia- tions have occurred during the course of this life process? What factors have influenced these variations? What role has the environment played in these variations? How would a strange environment affect the individual's life process?

The last series of questions would be influenced by the principle of helicy. What kinds of rhythms are reflected in the collected data? How com- plex are these rhythms? Are they old established rhythms or new emerging ones? How does the environment support these rhythms? If the individual is in a strange environment, how will these rhythms be affected by the new environment? What sequential stages of development has the individual passed through? What were the effects? How has the environment sup- ported or retarded the progress of the individual? How will a new environ- ment affect this progress? What kinds of goals does the individual have?

How have these goals affected development? Where do the individuals wish to go as reflected by their goals? What kinds of new vistas are sought?

To reflect the idea of patterning, additional questions for the principle of helicy would be considered. What kinds of patterns characterize the individual? How have the patterns developed? What kinds of past experience have influenced the development of specified patterns? How has the environment promoted certain patterns? How complex are the patterns? How has time affected the patterns? Although these questions may be answered, it must be remembered that the responses reflect a specific point in space-time. Consequently, the identified patterns are not static but rather ever-changing, reflecting both a change in time and additional new past experiences.

By no means are these questions all inclusive, but using them as a reference will help provide the nurse with a view of the whole individual. It will identify individual differences and the sequential cross-sectional patterning in the life process. It will also show the total pattern of events for the person at any given point in space-time.[32] The nursing assessment, then, is an assessment of the whole human being and not an assessment of only physical or mental status. It is an assessment of health and health potential for the individual and not an assessment of an illness or a disease process. As a result, the individual is paramount, not the disease.

As a result of the nursing assessment, a conclusion is drawn about the individual. This conclusion is the nursing diagnosis, the second step in the nursing process, and it will reflect the principles of homeodynamics. Rhythms, patterns, complexity, interactions, and life-process variations would become evident. The nursing diagnosis seeks to identify sequential, cross-sectional patterns in the life process and encompasses man–environment relationships.[33] Such a nursing diagnosis would not be consistent with the problem-oriented system for providing care. In the problem-oriented system, a problem would be identified that would be stated as a symptom, finding, or (medical) diagnosis.[34] As such, the problem would reflect a piece of the individual and not the whole human being. Although also imperfect, the nursing diagnoses based on Gordon's functional health patterns have a greater potential for usefulness with Rogers' framework because they tend to reflect a more unitary view of the individual.[35]

The purpose of the nursing diagnosis is to provide a framework within which the nursing intervention is planned and implemented. Consequently, the thrust of the nursing intervention will depend on the focus of the nursing diagnosis. The focus on integrality will require implementation within the environment as well as within the individual. It can be expected that change in one will cause simultaneous change in the other. Because of the individual's integration with the environment, health problems cannot be separated from the world's social ills. Therefore, these problems cannot be dealt with effectively by means of the commonly accepted transitional, disease-oriented measures.[36] Creativity and imagination become essential.

Resonancy requires that the nursing plan be geared toward supporting or modifying variations in the life process of the whole human being. Because the human life process is a unidirectional phenomenon, the intervention cannot be aimed at returning the individual to a former level of existence; rather, the nurse helps the individual move forward to a higher, more complex level of existence.

Nursing planning in the area of helicy requires an acceptance of individual differences as an expression of evolutionary emergence. The strategies are geared at supporting or modifying rhythms and life goals. To do this requires the informed and active participation of the client in the nursing process. The concept of the unitary human and a recognition of the human being's capacity to feel and to reason will enable the nurse to assist the individual in the resolution of the health problem and in the setting of goals directed toward achieving health.[36] Health will not be achieved by promoting homeostasis and equilibrium, but rather by taking steps to enhance dynamism and complexity within the individual.

Additionally, helicy requires that the nursing plan be geared toward promoting dynamic repatterning of the whole human being. This repatterning includes the individual's relationship to self and to the environment so that the total potential as a human being can be developed. This repatterning is aimed at assisting people to develop patterns of living that coordinate with environmental changes rather than conflict with them.[37] Although the pattern may be altered or maintained, it must be remembered that this is an evolving, ever-changing pattern rather than a static, constant phenomenon.

Regardless of the focus, the aim of the nursing plan is the attainment of an optimum state of health for the individual. This state of health may not be the ideal but will be the maximum health that is potentially possible for the individual.[38] Generally, implementation strategies will seek to strengthen the integrity of the individual–environment relationship and to give direction to humanity's struggle to achieve new levels of well-being. By assisting individuals to mobilize their resources, consciously and unconsciously, their integrity will be heightened.[39]

If attainment of an optimum state of health is the aim of the nursing plan, then it becomes the focus for nursing evaluation, the final phase of the nursing process. Has the integrity of the individual–environment relationship been strengthened? Have resources been mobilized? Has the patterning of the human and environmental fields been directed toward the realization of maximum health potential? Only when the nursing goal of the highest possible health state has been realized can nursing interventions be evaluated as effective.

A schematic representation of the relationship between the principles of homeodynamics and the elements of the nursing process is presented in Table 14–1. As can be seen, there is no absolute distinction between the areas covered by the various principles. Table 14–2 attempts to apply the

TABLE 14–1. RELATIONSHIP OF THE PRINCIPLES OF HOMEODYNAMICS TO THE NURSING PROCESS

Components of the Nursing Process	Principles of Homeodynamics		
	Integrality	Resonancy	Helicy
Nursing assessment component	Look at the interaction of the individual and the environment—how they work together rather than what they are like in isolation.	Look at the variations occuring during the life process of the whole human being.	Look at the rhythmic life patterns of the individual and the environment. Progression of time of necessity creates change in the rhythmic life patterns of the whole human being. Look at life goals. Be aware of growing complexity of the whole human being.
Nursing diagnosis component	Reflects integration of the individual and environmental fields.	Reflects the variations in the life process of the whole individual.	Reflects the rhythmic pattern of the individual and environmental fields.
Nursing plan for implementation component	Intervene in the environment as well as in the individual. Change promoted in one area will cause simultaneous change in the other—simultaneous molding.	Support or modify variations in the life process of the whole individual.	Promote dynamic rhythmic repatterning of both the individual and the environment. Accept differences as an expression of evolutionary emergence. Promote dynamism and complexity rather than homeostasis and equilibrium. Support or modify life goals.
Nursing evaluation component	Evaluate changes in the integration that have occurred.	Evaluate the modification made in the variations of the life process of the whole human being.	Evaluate rhythmic repatterning of the individual and the environment. Evaluate goal-directedness. Evaluate relationship of goal to the whole individual.

TABLE 14–2. RELATIONSHIP OF THE PRINCIPLES OF HOMEODYNAMICS IN THE NURSING PROCESS FOR JANIE

Components of the Nursing Process	Principles of Homeodynamics		
	Integrality	Resonancy	Helicy
Nursing assessment component	1. How does Janie see her environment? 2. What kind of differences are there between the hospital and her home? 3. How is she reacting to the changes in her environment? 4. How do her health problem and the environment affect each other?	1. What is Janie's past history? 2. What kinds of deviations from the expected norms have there been? 3. Were these deviations individually or environmentally related? 4. What is the reason for the hospitalization? 5. How will this affect her life?	1. What are Janie's normal behavior patterns and routines? 2. Were the behaviors or routines undergoing a change prior to her admission? 3. What kinds of activities can she perform? 4. What kinds of past experiences has she had? 5. How might those experiences influence her current situation? 6. What is Janie's developmental level? 7. Will the hospital environment support or retard developmental progress? 8. What are Janie's goals?
Nursing diagnosis component	1. What is the nature of the interaction between Janie and the hospital?	1. What is the interference this hospitalization will make in Janie's life?	1. What are the rhythmic patterns that are being exhibited?

Nursing plan for implementation component

1. How can the hospital environment be modified to reduce the differences identified?
2. How can Janie be helped to understand the differences that cannot be eliminated?
3. How can her health potential be improved by manipulating the environment?

1. How can Janie's normal development be promoted?
2. How can the effects of the interferences be minimized?

1. How can Janie's normal behavioral patterns and routines be promoted in the hospital?
2. What kind of modifications can be made to promote her normal behavioral patterns and routines?
3. What kind of provisions can be made to promote her normal growth and development?
4. How can Janie be helped to develop successful rhythmic behavioral patterns within the hospital environment?
5. How can Janie be helped to reach her goals?

Nursing evaluation component

1. Has Janie's behavior changed as a result of environmental modification?
2. What kind of new reactions are now taking place?

1. Is Janie developing normally, based on theories?
2. Has the interference with development been minimized?

1. What kind of rhythmic repatterning has taken place?
2. Is Janie's development being supported?
3. Is she moving toward her goals?

generalities to the specific situation of Janie who is hospitalized. In no way is either figure designed to be all inclusive. Rather, they are offered as an attempt to make abstract ideas more concrete and operational.

While the examples given focus on the individual, the Rogerian model can also be applied to families. An "irreducible, four-dimensional, negentropic family energy field becomes the focus of study" or practice.[40] The definition of the family can be left open to the situation at hand. Families may include nuclear families, extended families, homosexual families, single person families, or any other structure that the client regards as family.

Johnston has taken Rogers a step further than family care by using Rogerian theory as an approach for family therapy intervention.[41] Health and family health are viewed as manifestations of family and environment. The interrelationships between the family and environmental fields preclude looking at family members as individual units and their actions in isolation. Changes occur in the entire family, which is viewed as an energy field.

LIMITATIONS OF ROGERS' PRINCIPLES OF HOMEODYNAMICS

Although the principles of homeodynamics are consistent with the universally accepted aims and goals of nursing, there are major limitations to the universal implementation of the principles. Many persons will have difficulty understanding the principles. Even though basic assumptions are provided and the principles are defined, the framework remains an abstract phenomenon. Terms have not been sufficiently operationalized to provide for clear understanding.[42] By "operationalizing terms" is meant the description of a set of physical procedures that must be carried out in order to assign to every case a value for the concept.[43] For example, to operationalize the concept of width is to place an instrument consisting of the units of inches or centimeters along the edge of the item to be measured and then count the units. Difficulties with operationalizations of the concepts as well as with bringing the abstractness of the concepts and the relationships to an empirical level for testing are plaguing many nurse scientists.[44]

Because of the lack of operational definitions, research done to support or verify the principles provides questionable results. Operational definitions are needed for the development of hypotheses that test the theoretical concepts, and for the selection of instruments that will adequately measure the concepts involved.[45] Without such definitions just what was confirmed or not confirmed by these studies is in doubt.[46]

At this stage in the development of nursing science, instruments that will adequately assess human beings in their totality are nonexistent. For example, it is difficult to measure the individual as a unity or measure energy fields and wave patterns.[47] The issue of measurement is at a critical juncture, and indepth discussions of ways to address this issue are greatly needed.[48] Without such instruments, the ability to utilize or test the framework successfully is virtually impossible. Furthermore, the inability to adequately utilize or test the framework makes successful nursing implementation difficult. Thus, utilization of principles of homeodynamics in its totality is limited. At best, varying aspects of the principles can be applied to nursing practice in a very limited fashion.

ROGERS' WORK AND THE CHARACTERISTICS OF A THEORY

1. Theories can interrelate concepts in such a way as to create a different way of looking at a particular phenomenon. Rogers' framework clearly creates an alternative view of people and their world. The theoretical statement that nursing is the use of the principles of homeodynamics for the service of humanity compels one to look at nursing in a very different way. An excellent example is the principle of helicy with its emphasis on pattern and rhythmicity.

2. Theories must be logical in nature. There is definitely a logical development of the major constructs. This logical development proceeds from the identification of assumptions, through the building blocks, to the principles of homeodynamics.

3. Theories should be relatively simple yet generalizable. The theory is generalizable since it is not dependent on any given setting. It has been stated that Rogers' conception of man is elegant in its simplicity.[49] However, the theory is far from simple in that its level of abstraction and the nature of the terminology contribute to difficulties in understanding. In addition, the theory is based on the use of open systems that are inherently complex.

4. Theories can be the bases for hypotheses that can be tested.

5. Theories contribute to and assist in increasing the general body of knowledge within the discipline through the research implemented to validate them. It is clear that the abstract level of the framework leads to the generation of a plethora of research questions. Rogers, Malinski, and Madrid and Winstead-Fry all cite numerous studies ostensibly designed to test this framework.[50a-50c] However, research is hampered by the lack of simplicity, operational definitions, and valid instruments to measure outcomes. The complex interrelationships involved in the framework contribute to these difficulties. Qualitative research approaches have been suggested as an effective method for minimizing these problems.[51a,51b] These and other efforts designed to minimize these research problems need to be continued so that nursing can truly benefit from Rogers' framework.

6. Theories can be utilized by the practitioners to guide and improve their practice. Rogers' ideas can be applied to practice. When these ideas are applied to nursing practice, the understanding of the client's behavior takes on new dimensions. Such dimensions include accepting diversity as the norm, empowering both nurse and client, viewing change as positive, and accepting the integral connectedness of life.[52] This changed understanding results in alterations in the focus of nursing actions. The case study of Jamie presented in this chapter provides an example. In addition, nursing interventions such as therapeutic touch and the use of light, color, music, and movement have been derived from Rogers' tenets.[52] However, evidence of positive effects of nursing interventions derived from this model is needed.[53]

7. Theories must be consistent with other validated theories, laws, and principles but will leave open unanswered questions that need to be investigated. Rogers' work is consistent with other validated theories, laws, and principles. The abstract nature of the framework provides great potential for generating questions for further study and deriving interventions for nursing practice. Rogers' framework has also been instrumental in the development of other theories. Newman's and Parse's frameworks are two such examples.[54a,54b]

SUMMARY

Building on a broad theoretical base from a variety of disciplines, Rogers developed the principles of homeodynamics. Inherent in the principles are five basic assumptions: (1) the human being is a unified whole, possessing individual integrity and manifesting characteristics that are more than and different from the sum of the parts; (2) the individual and the environment are continuously exchanging matter and energy with each other; (3) the life process of human beings evolves irreversibly and unidirectionally along a space–time continuum; (4) patterns identify human beings and reflect their innovative wholeness; and (5) the individual is characterized by the capacity for abstraction and imagery, language and thought, sensation and emotion. The principles of integrality, helicy, and resonancy are compared to general system theory, developmental theories, and adaptation theories. Ways to use the principles in the nursing process are explored. The difficulty in understanding the principles, the lack of operational definitions, and inadequate instruments for measurement are the major limitations to the effective use of this theory.

REFERENCES

1. Rogers, M.E. An Introduction, *The Theoretical Basis of Nursing*, Philadelphia: F. A. Davis Co., 1970, pp. vii, ix.
2. Ibid, ix.
3. Ibid, 4.
4. Ibid, 6–8.
5. Ibid, 12–14.

6.   Toffler, A. *Future Shock,* New York: Bantam Books, Inc., 1970, p. 30.
7.   Rogers, M.E. Accountability, Convention address, University of Utah College of Nursing, June 5, 1971, p. 3.
8.   Rogers, *The Theoretical Basis of Nursing,* pp. 43–73.
9.   Rogers, M.E. Science of Unitary Human Beings: A Paradigm for Nursing, paper presented at International Nurse Theorist Conference, Edmonton, Alberta, May 2, 1984.
10.(a) Ibid.
10.(b) Malinski, V.M. ed., *Explorations on Martha Rogers' Science of Unitary Human Beings,* Norwalk, CT.: Appleton-Century-Crofts, 1986, p. 5.
11.   von Bertalanffy, L. *General System Theory,* New York: George Braziller, Inc., 1968, p. 38.
12.   Hazzard, M.E. An Overview of Systems Theory, *Nursing Clinics of North America,* 1971, *6,* 385.
13.   von Bertalanffy, *General System Theory,* p. 37.
14.   Ibid, 27–28.
15.   Rogers, *The Theoretical Basis of Nursing,* pp. vii, 84–85.
16.(a) Ibid, 97–102.
16.(b) Rogers, Science of Unitary Human Beings.
16.(c) Malinski, *Explorations on Martha Rogers,* p. 6.
17.   Hazzard, An Overview of Systems Theory, pp. 389–90.
18.   Bertrand, A.L. *Social Organization,* Philadelphia: F.A. Davis Co., 1972, p. 99.
19.   Hazzard, An Overview of Systems Theory, p. 390.
20.   Erikson, E. *Childhood and Society* (2nd ed.), New York: W.W. Norton & Co., Inc., 1963, pp. 247–74.
21.   Havinghurst, R. *Developmental Tasks and Education* (3rd ed.) New York: David McKay Co., Inc., 1972.
22.   Paiget, J. & Inhelder, R. *The Psychology of the Child,* New York: Basic Books, Inc., 1969.
23.   Kohlberg, L. *Collected Papers on Moral Development and Moral Education,* Cambridge, Mass.: Moral Education and Research Foundation, 1973.
24.   Gilligan, C. *In a Different Voice: Psychological Theory and Women's Development,* Cambridge, MA.: Harvard University Press, 1982.
25.   Roy, C. & Roberts, S. *Theory Construction in Nursing: An Adaptation Model,* Englewood Cliffs, N.J.: Prentice Hall, 1981, pp. 45, 59.
26.   Ibid, 251.
27.   Rogers, Science of Unitary Human Beings.
28.   Malinski, *Explorations on Martha Rogers,* p. 26.
29.(a) Rogers, *The Theoretical Basis of Nursing,* p. 122.
29.(b) Rogers, Science of Unitary Human Beings.
30.   Fawcett, J. *Analysis and Evaluation of Conceptual Models,* Philadelphia: F.A. Davis Co., 1984, p. 222.
31.   LaMonica, E.L. *The Humanistic Nursing Process,* Monterey, CA.: Wadsworth Health Science Division, 1985, pp. 1–2.
32.   Roy, C. Rogers' Theoretical Basis of Nursing, in *Conceptual Models for Nursing Practice,* Riehl, J.P. & Roy, C., eds., New York: Appleton-Century-Crofts, 1974, pp. 98–99.
33.   Fawcett, *Analysis and Evaluation,* p. 223.
34.   Berni, R. & Readey, H. *Problem-Oriented Medical Record Implementation,* St. Louis, Mo.: C.V. Mosby, 1975.

35. Bircher, A.U. Nursing Diagnosis: Where Does the Conceptual Framework Fit? in *Classification of Nursing Diagnoses*, Hurley, M.E. ed., St. Louis: C.V. Mosby, 1975.

36. Rogers, *The Theoretical Basis of Nursing*, p. 134.

37. Ibid, 123.

38. Roy, Rogers' Theoretical Basis of Nursing, pp. 97, 99.

39. Rogers, *The Theoretical Basis of Nursing*, pp. 134, 139.

40. Rogers, M.E. Science of Unitary Human Beings: A Paradigm for Nursing, in *Family Health: A Theoretical Approach to Nursing Care*, Clements, I.W. & Roberts, F.B., eds., New York: Wiley Medical, 1983, p. 226.

41. Johnston, R.L. Approaching Family Intervention Through Rogers' Conceptual Model, in *Family Therapy Theory for Nursing: Four Approaches*, Whall, A.L., ed., Norwalk, CT.: Appleton-Century-Crofts, 1986.

42. King, I. *Toward a Theory for Nursing*, New York: Wiley, 1971, p. 18.

43. Hardy, M.E. Theories: Components, Development, Evaluation, *Nursing Research*, 1974, *23*, 101.

44. Kim, H.S. *The Nature of Theoretical Thinking in Nursing*, Norwalk, CT.: Appleton-Century-Crofts, 1986.

45. Hardy, Theories: Components, Development, Evaluation, p. 105.

46. Rogers, *The Theoretical Basis of Nursing*, pp. 103–28.

47. Burns, N. & Grove, S.K. *The Practice of Nursing Research: Conduct, Critique, and Utilization*, Philadelphia: Saunders, 1987, p. 168.

48. Parse, R.R. *Nursing Science: Major Paradigms, Theories, and Critiques*, Philadelphia: Saunders, 1987, p. 157.

49. Fawcett, *Analysis and Evaluation*, p. 237.

50.(a) Rogers, *The Theoretical Basis of Nursing.*

50.(b) Malinski, *Explorations on Martha Rogers.*

50.(c) Madrid, M. & Winstead-Fry, P. Rogers's Conceptual Model, in *Case Studies in Nursing Theory*, Winstead-Fry, P., ed., New York: National League for Nursing, 1986, pp. 73–102.

51.(a) Wilson, L.M. & Fitzpatrick, J.J. Dialectic Thinking as a Means of Understanding Systems-in-Development: Relevance to Rogers's Principles, *Advances in Nursing Science*, 1984, *6*, 24–41.

51.(b) Reeder, F. Philosophical Issues in the Rogerian Science of Unitary Human Beings, *Advances in Nursing Science*, 1984, *6*, 14–23.

52. Malinski, *Explorations on Martha Rogers*, pp. 28–30.

53. Fawcett, *Analysis and Evaluation*, p. 231.

54.(a) Newman, M. *Theory Development in Nursing*, Philadelphia: F.A. Davis Co., 1979.

54.(b) Parse, R.R. *Man–Living–Health: A Theory of Nursing*, New York: Wiley, 1981.

BIBLIOGRAPHY

Meleis, A. I. *Theoretical Nursing: Development and Progress*, Philadelphia: Lippincott, 1985.

Safier, G. *Contemporary American Leaders in Nursing*, New York: McGraw-Hill, 1977.

Sarter, B., *The Stream of Becoming: A Study of Martha Rogers's Theory*, New York: National League for Nursing, 1988.

CHAPTER 15

Sister Callista Roy

Julia Gallagher Galbreath

Sister Callista Roy, RN, PhD (b. 1939) is nurse theorist, Boston College, Massachusetts. Previous to this appointment, Roy was a Post-Doctoral Fellow and Robert Wood Johnson Clinical Nurse Scholar at the University of California, San Francisco. Roy has served in many positions including Chair of the Department of Nursing, Mount Saint Mary's College, Los Angeles; Adjunct Professor, Graduate Program, School of Nursing, University of Portland; and Acting Director and Nurse Consultant, Saint Mary's Hospital, Tucson, Arizona. Roy earned her BS in nursing in 1963 from Mount Saint Mary's College, Los Angeles; her MS in nursing in 1966 and doctorate in sociology in 1977 from the University of California, Los Angeles. She is a Fellow of the American Academy of Nursing and active in many nursing organizations including Sigma Theta Tau and the North American Nurses Diagnosis Association (NANDA). She is the author or co-author of a number of works including Introduction to Nursing: An Adaptation Model, Essentials of the Roy Adaptation Model, *and* Theory Construction in Nursing: An Adaptation Model.[1a–1d]

The Roy Adaptation Model has evoked much interest and respect since its inception in 1964 by Roy as part of her graduate work at the University of California, Los Angeles, under the guidance of Dorothy E. Johnson. In 1970, the faculty of Mount Saint Mary's College in Los Angeles adopted the Roy Adaptation Model as the conceptual framework of the undergraduate nursing curriculum. A text was written by Roy and fellow faculty describing the Roy Adaptation Model and presenting nursing assessment and intervention reflective of the distinctive focus of the mode. In 1984, an extensively revised edition of *Introduction to Nursing: An Adaptation Model* was published.[2] Further, Roy and Roberts wrote *Theory Construction in Nursing: An Adaptation Model* to discuss the use of the Roy Model to construct nursing theory.[3] The reader who is excited by the model will find that a rich response has been made and continues to be made by nurse practitioners, educators, and researchers in the analysis, testing, and application of the model for nursing.[4a–4c]

ELEMENTS OF THE ROY ADAPTATION MODEL

There are five essential elements of the Roy Adaptation Model. They are[5]:

1. The person who is the recipient of nursing care
2. The goal of nursing
3. The concept of health
4. The concept of environment
5. The direction of nursing activities

The model presents concepts related to the above areas clarifying each and defining their interrelationships.

The Person

The first area of concern is the identity of the recipient of nursing care. Roy states that the recipient of nursing care may be the person, a family, a group, a community, or a society. Each is considered by the nurse as a holistic adaptive system.[6] The idea of an adaptive system combines the concepts of adaptation and system.

First, consider the concept of a system as applied to an individual. Roy conceptualizes the person in a holistic perspective. Individual aspects of parts act together to form a unified being. Additionally, persons, as living systems, are in constant interaction with their environments. Between the system and the environment occurs an exchange of information, matter, and energy. This characteristic of a living system is called openness. Dunn, a system theorist, calls our attention to the smallest unit of life, the cell. The cell is a living open system. The cell has its inner and outer worlds. From its outer world, it must draw forth the substances it needs to survive. Within itself, the cell must maintain order over its vast numbers of molecules.[7] System openness, therefore, implies the constant exchanging of information, matter, and energy between the system and the environment. These system qualities are held by the person. The constant interaction of persons with their environment is characterized by both internal and external changes. Within this changing world persons must maintain their own integrity; that is, each person continuously adapts. Hence, the person is viewed as a holistic adaptive system.

Figure 15–1 is used by Roy to represent the adaptive system of a person. The adaptive system has input coming from the external environment as well as input coming internally from the person. Roy identifies inputs as stimuli. A stimulus is a unit of information, matter, or energy from the environment or from within the person that elicits a response.

Along with stimuli, the adaptation level of the person acts as input to that person as an adaptive system. The adaptation level is the range of stimuli to which the person can adaptively respond with ordinary effort.[8] This range of response is unique to the individual. Each person's adaptation level is a constantly changing aspect which is influenced by the coping mechanisms of that person. Roy uses Helson's work to develop this construct. It will be presented later in this chapter when the goal of nursing, as defined by the model, is discussed.

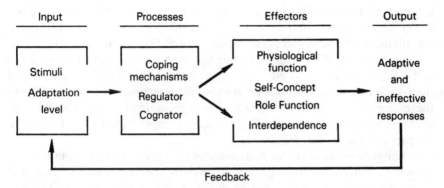

Figure 15–1. The person as an adaptive system *(From Roy, Sr. C.* Introduction to Nursing: An Adaptation Model, *(2nd ed.), Englewood Cliffs, N.J.: Prentice-Hall, 1984, p. 30. Used with permission).*

Outputs of the person as a system are the behaviors of the person. (See Fig. 15–1.) Output behaviors can be both external and internal. Thus, these behaviors may be observed, measured, or subjectively reported. Output behaviors become feedback to the system. Roy has categorized outputs of the system as either adaptive responses or ineffective responses. *Adaptive responses* are those that promote the integrity of the person. The person's integrity or wholeness is behaviorally demonstrated when the person is able to meet the goals in terms of survival, growth, reproduction, and mastery. *Ineffective responses* do not support these goals.[9]

Roy has used the term *coping mechanisms* to describe the control processes of the person as an adaptive system. Some coping mechanisms are inherited or genetic, such as the white blood cell defense system against bacteria seeking to invade the body. Other mechanisms are learned, such as the use of antiseptics to cleanse a wound. Roy presents a unique nursing science concept of control mechanisms. These mechanisms are called the *regulator* and the *cognator.* Roy's model considers the regulator and cognator coping mechanisms as subsystems of the person as an adaptive system (see Fig. 15–1).

The *regulator subsystem* has the system of components of input, internal process, and output. Input stimuli may originate externally or internally to the person. The transmitters of the regulator system are chemical, neural, or endocrine in nature. Autonomic reflexes, which are neural responses originating in the brain stem and spinal cord, are generated as output behaviors of the regulator subsystem. Target organs and tissues under endocrine control also produce regulator output behaviors. Finally, Roy presents psychomotor responses originating from the central nervous system as regulator subsystem behaviors.[10] Many physiological processes can be viewed as regulator subsystem behaviors. For example, several regulatory feedback mechanisms of respiration have been identified. One of these is increased carbon dioxide, the end product of metabolism, which stimulates chemoreceptors in the medulla to increase the respiratory rate. Strong stimulation of these centers can increase ventilation six to sevenfold.[11]

An example of a regulator process is when a noxious external stimulus is visualized and transmitted via the optic nerve to higher brain centers and then to lower brain autonomic centers. The sympathetic neurons from these origins have multiple visceral effects, including increased blood pressure and increased heart rate. Roy's schematic representation of the regulator processes is seen in Figure 15–2.

The other control subsystem original to the Roy model is the *cognator subsystem*. Stimuli to the cognator subsystem are also both external and internal in origin. Output behavior of the regulator subsystem can be feedback stimuli to the cognator subsystem. Cognator control processes are related to the higher brain functions of perception or information processing, judgment, and emotion. Perception or information processing is related to the internal process of selective attention, coding, and memory. Learning is correlated to the processes of imitation, reinforcement, and insight. Problem solving and decision making are the internal processes related to judgment; and finally, emotion has the processes of defense to seek relief, affective appraisal, and attachment.[12] A schematic presentation by Roy of the cognator subsystem is presented in Figure 15–3.

In maintaining the integrity of the person, the regulator and cognator are postulated as frequently acting together. The adaptation level of the person as an adaptive system is influenced by the individual's development and use of these coping mechanisms. Maximal use of coping mechanisms broadens the adaptation level of the person and increases the range of stimuli to which the person can positively respond.

Situation. A decrease in the oxygen supply to Albert Smith's heart muscle stimulates pain receptors that transmit the message of pain along sympathetic afferent nerve fibers to his central nervous system. The autonomic centers of his lower brain then stimulate the sympathetic efferent nerve fibers, and there is an increase in heart and respiratory rates. The result is an increase in the oxygen supply to the heart muscle. This can be viewed as regulator subsystem action.

The cognator subsystem also receives the internal pain stimuli as input. Mr. Smith has learned from past experiences that the left chest and arm pain is related to his heart. His judgment is activated in deciding what action to take. He decides to go inside to air conditioning, to sit with his legs elevated, and to take slow, deep breaths. He also decides not to call for emergency help. Certainly, he believes an adaptive response secondary to these actions will occur. However, he may be increasingly alert for further regulator subsystem output behaviors that might change his decision. This represents the cognator process of selective attention and coding. Following the episode of pain, Mr. Smith may attempt to gain further insight into the

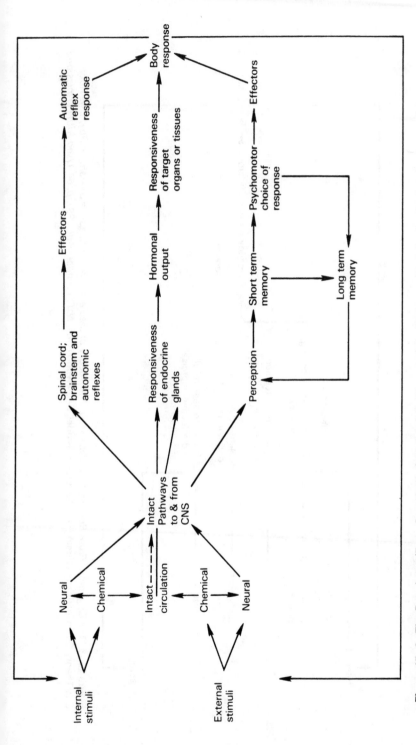

Figure 15–2. The Regulator *(From Roy, Sr. C. & McLeod, D. Theory of the Person as an Adaptive System, in Roy, C. & Roberts, S.L. Theory Construction in Nursing: An Adaptation Model, Englewood Cliffs, N.J.: Prentice-Hall, 1984, p. 61. Used with permission.)*

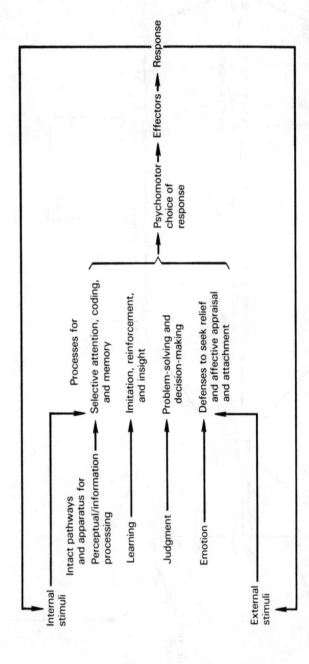

Figure 15–3. The Cognator. *(From Roy, Sr. C. & McLeod, D. The Theory of the Person as an Adaptive System, in Roy, C. & Roberts, S.L. Theory Construction in Nursing: An Adaptation Model, Englewood Cliffs, N.J.: Prentice-Hall, 1981, p. 64. Used with permission.)*

cause of the episode. He may decide that the 90°F weather was causal and remember to limit his activities during extreme heat. In this example, Mr. Smith used the cognator subsystem processes of perception, learning, and judgment.

Roy does not limit the concept of control processes to the regulator and cognator subsystems. She identifies the development of these concepts as a step towards greater understanding of human behavior. Hence, knowledge of the control processes of the person as an adaptive system is open to research and development.

In further delineation of the internal processes of the person as an adaptive system, Roy defines the system effectors. The four effectors or *adaptive modes* are physiological function, self-concept, role function, and interdependence. The regulator and cognator mechanisms are viewed as acting within these modes.[13] Behavior related to the modes is the manifestation of the person's adaptive level and reflects the use of coping mechanisms. By observing the person's behavior in relation to the adaptive modes, the nurse can identify adaptive or ineffective responses in situations of health and illness.

The four adaptive modes require further explanation. The physiological function mode is as follows:

- *Oxygenation:* Describes the pattern of oxygen use related to respiration and circulation[14]
- *Nutrition:* Describes patterns of nutrient use for body repair and development[15]
- *Elimination:* Describes patterns of elimination of waste products[16]
- *Activity and Rest:* Describes patterns of exercise, activity, rest, and sleep[17]
- *Skin Integrity:* Describes patterns of the physiological function of the skin[18]
- *Senses:* Describes the sensory–perceptual functions related to obtaining visual, auditory, kinesthetic, gustatory, tactile, and olfactory information[19]
- *Fluids and Electrolytes:* Describes patterns of physiological use of fluids and electrolytes[20]
- *Neurological function:* Describes the neural patterns of control, regulation, and intellect[21]
- *Endocrine function:* Describes patterns of control and regulation including the stress response and the reproduction system[22]

The self-concept mode identifies patterns of values, beliefs, and emotions as related to one's idea of self. Attention is given to the realm of physical self, personal self, and moral–ethical self.[23]

The role function mode identifies the patterns of social interaction of the person in relation to others reflected by primary, secondary, and tertiary roles. Selected areas of focus include the process of role identity and role mastery.[24]

Strongly reflective of the humanistic values held by Roy, the interdependence mode identifies patterns of human value, affection, love, and affirmation. These processes occur through interpersonal relationships on both individual and group levels.[25]

The concept of the above four adaptive modes came early in Roy's work in an effort to answer the question, How do people adapt to the changes they incur? These four modes are the channels through which the person adapts to internal and external changes. Response to change by the person may be processed predominately in a single adaptive mode. More often, the response is processed simultaneously in more than one mode.

Goal of Nursing

Roy defines the goal of nursing as the promotion of adaptive responses in relation to the four adaptive modes.[26] *Adaptive responses* are those that positively affect health. Helson's work is cited by Roy as useful in understanding the concept of adaptation in relation to the holistic qualities of the person. Helson views the person's adaptation to change as dependent upon the stimuli that are input for the person and the person's adaptation level.[27a, 27b]

Internal and external changes, that is, input stimuli, interface with the person's state of coping, the other significant element in the adaptation process. The condition of the person or the individual's state of coping is that person's *adaptation level*. The person's adaptation level will determine whether a postive response to internal or external stimuli will be elicited. The person's adaptation level is determined by focal, contextual, and residual stimuli. The stimuli immediately confronting the person are the *focal stimuli*. The focal stimuli normally constitute the greatest degree of change impacting upon the person. *Contextual stimuli* are all other stimuli of the person's internal and external world that influence the situation and are observable, measureable, or subjectively reported by the person. *Residual stimuli* are those make-up characteristics of the person that are present and relevant to the situation but are elusive or difficult to measure objectively.[28]

In the example of the person experiencing chest pain, the stimulus immediately confronting Mr. Smith, the focal stimulus, is the deficit of oxygen supply to his heart muscle. The contextual stimuli include the 90°F temperature, the sensation of pain, Mr. Smith's age, weight, blood sugar level, and degree of coronary artery patency. The residual stimuli include his history of cigarette smoking and work-related stress.

The degree of change facing the person is equated to the focal stimulus. If the person's adaptation level is viewed as a line, the zone of adaptation is the distance above and below that line that sets the limit of the person's adaptation capacity. When the total stimuli (focal, contextual, and residual) fall within the person's zone of adaptation, an adaptive response or output results. However, when the total stimuli fall outside the individual's zone of adaptation, ineffective output behavior or responses occur. Nursing seeks to reduce ineffective responses and promote adaptive responses as output behavior of the person.[29] Figure 15–4 depicts this conceptualization.

In the example of Mr. Smith, the total stimuli had fallen outside his adaptation zone. The resulting deficit of oxygen to his heart, indicated by chest pain, was an ineffective response. This response became feedback to the system and a focal stimulus. Mr. Smith used the cognator mechanism to adjust the total stimuli by going indoors to a cooler room and decreasing his oxygen needs by sitting down and elevating his legs. After the adjustment of the stimuli, the oxygen needs of his heart muscle were met, and the pain stopped.

A person's ability to cope varies with the state of the person at different times. For example, the person who has suffered major trauma has a narrowed zone of adaptation and may not survive exposure to a bacterial infection. That same person prior to the injury may have tolerated exposure to the same bacteria without developing any symptoms of illness.

Humanistic values of the Roy Adaptation Model are linked to its definition of the specific purpose or goal of nursing. Human existence is viewed as dynamic and purposeful. The person is respected as creative and active in use of his or her coping processes and as an active participant in his or her care.[30] Nursing's aim of promoting adaptation is contributory to the health of the person and to the unity and solidarity of the person within himself or herself and in relation to others.[31]

Nursing Activities
Nursing activities are delineated by the model as those that promote adaptive responses in situations of health and illness. As a rule, these approaches

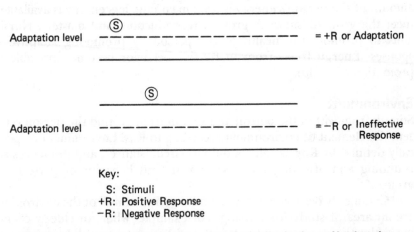

Key:
    S: Stimuli
   +R: Positive Response
   −R: Negative Response

Figure 15–4. Adaptation level. *(From Roy, Sr. C.* Introduction to Nursing: An Adaptation Model *(2nd ed.), Englewood Cliffs, N.J.: Prentice-Hall, 1984, p. 38. Used with permission.)*

are identified as actions taken by the nurse to manipulate the focal, contextual, or residual stimuli impinging on the person.[31] By making these adjustments, the total stimuli fall within the adaptive zone of the person. Whenever possible, the focal stimulus, that which represents the greatest degree of change, is manipulated. For a person with chest pain, the focal stimulus is the imbalance between the demand for oxygen by the body and the supply of oxygen that the heart can provide. To alter the focal stimuli, the nurse manipulates the stimuli of demand so that an adaptive response can be made. In turn, when focal stimuli cannot be altered, the nurse promotes an adaptive response by manipulating contextual and residual stimuli.

Additionally, the nurse may anticipate that the person has a potential for ineffective responses secondary to stimuli likely to be present in a particular situation. The nurse acts to prepare the person for the anticipated changes through strengthening regulator, cognator, or other coping mechanisms. Plans that broaden the person's adaptation level correlate with the ideas of health promotion currently found in the literature. Finally, nursing actions suggested by the model include approaches aimed at maintaining adaptive responses thus supporting the person's efforts to creatively use his or her coping mechanisms.

Health

Previously, the Roy model defined health as a continuum from death to high-level wellness. This is no longer used in the present model. Instead, Roy presently defines health as "a state and a process of being and becoming an integrated and whole person."[32] The integrity of the person is expressed as the ability to meet the goals of survival, growth, reproduction, and mastery. The nurse using Roy's model uses the concept of health as the goal point for the person's behavior. When a disproportionate amount of the person's energy is used in coping, less energy is available to meet the goals of survival, growth, reproduction, and mastery. Nursing aims to promote the health of the person by promoting adaptive responses. Energy freed from ineffective behavior becomes available for promotion of health.

Environment

Stimuli from within the person and stimuli from around the person represent the element of environment according to Roy. Environment is specifically defined by Roy as "all conditions, circumstances, and influences surrounding and affecting the development and behavior of persons and groups."[33]

Commonly occurring internal and external stimuli of the environment are an area of study for nursing. For example, when an elderly client is institutionalized, significant external environmental stimuli have impinged upon him or her. The study of this environmental condition aids nurses in promoting adaptation to this change or, perhaps more ideally, defining interventions that minimize the risk of institutionalization for the elderly. Similarly, nurses are increasing their involvement in the institutions of our nations: health, education, industry, and politics. By their involvement, they are altering the environmental stimuli related to situations of health and illness in a broad and often far-reaching manner at a community system level.

THE NURSING PROCESS

The Roy adaptation model offers guidelines to the nurse in developing the nursing process. The elements of the Roy nursing process include first and second level assessment, diagnosis, goal setting, intervention, and evaluation.[33] If first and second level assessments are considered subparts of the same element, the five elements of Roy's nursing process parallel the five phases of the nursing process identified in Chapter 2.

First Level Assessment

First level assessment is considered the gathering of output behaviors of the person as an adaptive system in relation to each of the four adaptive modes: physiological function, self-concept, role function, and interdependence. First level assessment is referred to as *behavioral assessment.*[34]

Assessment of the client in each of the four adaptive modes enhances a systematic and holistic approach. Such assessment clarifies the focus that the nurse or nursing team will take in caring for the client. Ideally, thoroughly conducted and recorded nursing assessment in the four adaptive modes sets the tone of understanding the particular situation of a client for an entire health care team. Figure 15–5 presents a Nursing History/ Assessment developed by the nurses at Upper Valley Medical Center in Piqua, Ohio. This form uses the four adaptive modes of the Roy model. Guide questions related to each adaptive mode can be developed to reflect the age or acuity of the client population being assessed. Information collected includes subjective, objective, and measurement data.

Second Level Assessment

After a first-level assessment, the nurse analyzes the emerging themes and patterns of client behavior to identify ineffective responses or adaptive responses requiring nurse support. When ineffective behaviors or adaptive behaviors requiring support are present, the nurse conducts a second level assessment. In this phase of assessment, the nurse collects data about the focal, contextual, and residual stimuli impacting on the client. This process clarifies the etiology of the problem and identifies significant contextual and residual factors. Martinez identified "genetic make-up, sex, developmental stage, drugs, alcohol, tobacco, self-concept, role functions, interdependence, social interaction patterns, coping mechanisms and styles, physical and emo-

INSTRUCTIONS: Check all boxes or circle answers that apply.
White area donotes P.A.T.   *See Nurse's Note/Care Plan
Grey area denotes day of admission.

Date	Time	Received From: ☐ ER ☐ w/c ☐ admitting ☐ doctor's office	V/A ☐ w/c ☐ ambulatory ☐ cart				
Temp.	Apical Pulse	Regular Irregular	Resp.	BP(LA)	BP(RA)	Height	Weight

History and present status of chief complaint:

Pain Present: ☐ no ☐ yes/location	Intensity Scale 1 (mild)-10 (severe)	When did pain start?	How was pain managed at home?

Allergies: ☐ none ☐ food
☐ medications (list drug reaction)

Allergy nand on ☐

Patient/Family History: (circle and explain in comments)
1. Diabetes
2. Cancer
3. Hypertension
4. Stroke
5. Heart Disease
6. Seizures
7. Kidney Disease
8. Respiratory Disease
9. Alcoholism/Drug Abuse
10. Mental Illness
11. Liver Disease (Hepatitis, Mono)
12. Communicable Disease (T.B., S.T.D.)
13. Blood Disorder
14. Blood Transfusion
15. Other

Comments

Past Surgery/Hospitalizations/X-rays:

INTERDEPENDENCE
ROLE FUNCTION–SELF-CONCEPT

Figure 15–5. Upper Valley Medical Center admission nursing assessment. *Developed for testing by Frantz, Mikolajewski, Meiring, Ely, Garber, and Boyer. Used with permission.*

Medications: (prescription & O.T.C.) include dose and frequency. ☐ none

_____

_____

_____

Are medications taken as prescribed: ☐ yes ☐ no ☐ n/a | Last dose of medications taken:

Social History: (education, religion, social support-community agency use, coping mechanisms)

_____

Home Situation: (family/significant others, living environment-stairs, apt., etc.)

_____

Job Situation:

_____

Personal Concerns:

_____

Is someone available after discharge to care for you if needed: ☐ no ☐ yes _____

Reaction to hospitalization/patient behavior:

_____

NEUROLOGICAL

Level of consciousness:
☐ alert ☐ oriented ☐ disoriented ☐ restless ☐ drowsy ☐ comatose ☐ _____ ☐ comment:

Speech
☐ clear ☐ slurred ☐ confused ☐ aphasic ☐ hoarse ☐ foreign language:

Pupil Size

2 3 4 5 6 7 8 9

Right Eye: _____ mm-Reaction ☐ Brisk ☐ Sluggish ☐ None
Left eye: _____ mm-Reaction ☐ Brisk ☐ Sluggish ☐ None
Comments:

Ability to move extremities to command
0 (no movement) 1 (weak) 2(strong)
RA: LA: RL: LL:

(continued)

SEN-SES

| N/A ☐ | glasses/contacts ☐ | artificial eye ☐ | cataracts ☐ | glaucoma ☐ | blind ☐ r ☐ l |
| N/A ☐ | hearing impairment ☐ | partial deaf ☐ r ☐ l | total deaf ☐ r ☐ l | hearing aid ☐ r ☐ l |

ACTIVITY/REST

Activities of daily living
☐ independent   ☐ dependent: explain

Ambulation aids, prosthesis: ☐ no   ☐ yes/list:

Sleep (usual time of day and hours)
Sleep problems:
☐ no   ☐ yes/explain:

OXYGENATION

Skin lesions (mark location of skin lesions by number on diagram)
☐ none   ☐ scar (1)   ☐ rash (2)   ☐ wound or open area (3)   ☐ bruise (4)
☐ incision (5)   ☐ sutures, staples (6)   ☐ abrasions (7)   ☐ discolorations (8)
☐ other (9)   Description _____   Skin risk factor: _____

Dressings: ☐ no   ☐ yes, location _____
Respirations: ☐ normal   ☐ dyspnea   ☐ irregular ☐ _____

Smoker: ☐ no   ☐ yes
_____ pkg/day   x ____ years

Breath sounds:

Cough ☐ no   ☐ yes   ☐ non-productive   ☐ productive/color:

Oxygen: ☐ no   ☐ yes-method-amt.

ELIMINATION

Abdomen: ☐ soft   ☐ firm   ☐ distended   ☐ tender/location

Bowel sounds: ☐ present   ☐ absent   Last bm/color/character:

Bowel   ☐ no problem   ☐ constipation   ☐ laxative/enema   Normal bowel pattern
        ☐ diarrhea   ☐ incontinence

Bladder   ☐ no problem   ☐ burning discomfort   ☐ nocturia (# times/night _____)
          ☐ incontinence   ☐ hematuria   ☐ difficulty starting flow

Drainage Tubes: ☐ none   ☐ foley/urine (1)   ☐ n/g (2)   ☐ G-tube (3)   Describe Drainage _____
☐ chest tube (4)   ☐ T-tube (5)   ☐ penrose (6)   _____
☐ ostomy _____ (7)   ☐ other _____ (8)

Figure 15–5. (Continued)

244

LYTES-NUTRITION	Current diet/restrictions:	Is diet followed: ☐ yes ☐ no
		GI disorder ☐ none ☐ nausea ☐ emesis ☐ vicer
	Appetite weight change ☐ no ☐ yes	Fluid intake: ☐ Caffeine: Amt. _____ ☐ Alcohol: Amt. _____
	Dentures: ☐ no Upper: ☐ full ☐ partial ☐ Bridge work ☐ yes Lower: ☐ full ☐ partial ☐ Caps	
	IV: ☐ no ☐ yes-solution-rate-site-cath #	☐ heparin lock ☐ vascular access device
ENDOCRINE	Last menstrual period	Problems: ☐ none ☐ abnormal bleeding ☐ vaginal drainage ☐ other
	Would you like to discuss any sexual concerns with a health professional-sometimes medication or illness may cause problems and we may assist you in finding the answers. ☐ no ☐ yes	
	Pap smear requested during hospitalization: ☐ no ☐ yes* ☐ n/a	
	Breast/testicular self-exam: ☐ done ☐ not done	

Signature admitting nurse   Signature P.A.T. nurse   Date   Time
(if applicable)

Are you interested in Anatomical Gift donation? ☐ no ☐ yes

I certify that the information in the white area given by me is current and correct to the best of my knowledge.

Patient's Signature   Date

Admission Nursing Assessment

245

tional stress, cultural orientation, religion, and physical environment"[35] as contextual stimuli which influence the adaptive modes.

The science of this decision-making process is still in the developmental phase for nursing. Often additional theories, laws, and principles of the arts and sciences are used to validate the presence of an adaptation problem. Adaptation problems are indicated when the survival, growth, reproduction, or mastery goals of the person are impeded or, in other words, when the integrity of the person is threatened.[36] For example, laws of science indicate that body pH must remain above certain levels to support cellular function. Hence, a low pH clearly indicates an ineffective response requiring further assessment and intervention to maintain the survival of the person. Further validation may be gained by reviewing the defining characteristics and etiologies related to nursing diagnosis developed by the North American Nursing Diagnosis Association (NANDA).

Nursing Diagnosis

Roy describes three methods of making a nursing diagnosis.[37] One method is to use a typology of diagnoses developed by Roy and related to the four adaptive modes. Table 15–1 is a list of common adaptation problems using this typology. In applying this method of diagnosis to the example of Mr. Smith, the diagnosis would be: "Hypoxia."

The second method is to make a diagnosis by stating the observed behavior along with the most influencing stimuli. Using this method, a diagnosis for Mr. Smith could be stated as: "Chest pain caused by a deficit of oxygen to the heart muscle associated with an overexposure to hot weather."

The third method summarizes behaviors in one or more adaptive modes related to the same stimuli. For example, if the person experiencing chest pain is a farmer, working outside in hot weather is necessary for success in his or her work. In this case, an appropriate diagnosis might be: "Role failure associated with limited physical (myocardial) ability to work in hot weather."

On the other hand, a nursing diagnosis using any of the above methods can also be a statement of adaptive behaviors that the nurse wishes to support. For example, if Mr. Smith is seeking help through vocational counseling to adapt to his physical limitation, the nurse may diagnose a need to support this behavior. In this case, an appropriate diagnosis would be: "Adaptation to role failure by seeking an alternative career."

Many nurses are familiar with the work of NANDA and the list of nursing diagnoses that have been accepted for testing through their seven conferences. In the second edition of *Introduction to Nursing: An Adaptation Model,* chapter authors began to identify NANDA diagnoses related to each adaptive mode. As the second edition predates the most recent NANDA taxonomy,[38] a correlation of adaptive modes and the NANDA list has not been published by Roy or her co-authors. However, following trends developed by Roy and others, Table 15–2 has been developed.

TABLE 15–1. WORKING TYPOLOGY OF COMMON ADAPTATION PROBLEMS (Revised)

A. Physiologic Mode	B. Self-Concept Mode	C. Role Function Mode	D. Interdependence Mode
1. *Oxygenation* Hypoxia Shock Overload	1. *Physical self* Decreased sexual self-concept Aggressive sexual behavior Loss	Role transition Role distance Role conflict Role failure	Separation anxiety Loneliness
2. *Nutrition* Malnutrition Nausea Vomiting	2. *Personal self* Anxiety Powerlessness Guilt Low self-esteem		
3. *Elimination* Constipation Diarrhea Flatulence Incontinence Urinary retention			
4. *Activity and rest* Inadequate physical activity Potential disuse consequences Inadequate rest Insomnia Sleep deprivation Excessive rest			
5. *Skin integrity* Itching Dry skin Pressure sores			

Source: Roy, Sr. C. Introduction to Nursing: An Adaptation Model (2nd ed.), Englewood Cliffs, N.J.: Prentice-Hall, 1984, p. 56. Used with permission.

TABLE 15–2. ROY'S ADAPTIVE MODES AND NANDA NURSING DIAGNOSES

Adaptive Mode	NANDA Nursing Diagnoses
Physiological Mode	
Activity and rest	Mobility: Impaired physical
	Self-care deficit: Feeding
	Self-care deficit: Bathing–hygiene
	Self-care deficit: Dressing–grooming
	Self-care deficit: Toileting
	Potential for infection
	Diversional activity deficit
	Sleep Pattern Disturbance
	Activity intolerance
	Potential activity intolerance
	Impaired home maintenance management
	Altered growth and development
Elimination	Altered urinary elimination pattern
	Urinary retention
	Functional incontinence
	Reflex incontinence
	Stress incontinence
	Urge incontinence
	Total incontinence
	Alteration in bowel elimination: Constipation
	Alteration in bowel elimination: Diarrhea
	Alteration in bowel elimination: Incontinence
Endocrine function	Sexual dysfunction
	Rape trauma syndrome
	Rape trauma syndrome: Compound reaction
	Rape trauma syndrome: Silent reaction
	Altered sexuality patterns
Fluid and electrolytes	Potential volume deficit
	Fluid volume excess
	Actual fluid volume deficit
	Potential fluid volume deficit
Neurological function	Altered thought processes
	Knowledge deficit (specify)
	Ineffective thermoregulation
	Hyperthermia
	Hypothermia
Nutrition	Alteration in oral mucous membrane
	Alteration in nutrition: Potential for more than body requirements
	Alteration in nutrition: Less than body requirements
	Alteration in nutrition: More than body requirements
	Impaired swallowing
	Potential alteration in body temperature
Oxygenation	Alteration in tissue perfusion: Renal, cerebral, cardiopulmonary, gastrointestinal, peripheral
	Ineffective airway clearage
	Ineffective breathing pattern
	Impaired gas exchange
	Altered cardiac output: Decreased

TABLE 15–2. (Continued)

Adaptive Mode	NANDA Nursing Diagnoses
Physiological Mode	
Senses	Alteration in comfort: Pain
	Alteration in comfort: Chronic pain
	Sensory perceptual alteration: Visual, auditory, kinesthetic, gustatory, tactile, olfactory
	Unilateral neglect
Skin integrity	Impaired skin integrity
	Potential impairment of skin integrity or potential skin breakdown
	Potential for infection
	Potential for injury
	Potential for injury: Trauma
	Potential for injury: Poisoning
	Potential for injury: Suffocation
	Impaired tissue integrity
Self-Concept Mode	Self-esteem disturbance in self-concept
	Personal identity disturbance in self-concept
	Anxiety
	Body image disturbance in self-concept
	Ineffective individual coping
	Depression, reactive (situational)
	Fear
	Alteration in health maintenance
	Impaired adjustment
	Identity confusion, personal
	Powerlessness
	Spiritual distress
	Noncompliance (specify)
	Disturbance in self-concept: Disturbance in role performance
	Hopelessness
	Personal identity confusion
	Post-trauma response
Role Function Mode	Alterations in family process
	Family coping: Potential for growth
	Ineffective family coping: Compromised
	Ineffective family coping: Disabled
	Potential alteration in parenting
	Actual alteration in parenting
	Impaired verbal communication
Interdependence Mode	Anticipatory grieving
	Dysfunctional grieving
	Translocation syndrome
	Social isolation
	Potential for violence: Self-directed or directed at others
	Impaired social interaction
	Spiritual distress (distress of human spirit)

Goal Setting

Goals are the end point behaviors that the person is to achieve. They are recorded as client behaviors indicative of resolution of the adaptation problem. Long-term goals would reflect resolution of adaptive problems and the availability of energy to meet other goals (survival, growth, reproduction, and mastery). Short-term goals identify expected client behaviors after manipulation of focal, contextual, or residual stimuli, as well as, state client behaviors that indicate cognator or regulator coping. Goals, whenever possible, are set mutually with the person. Mutual goal setting respects the privileges and rights of the person.

Plans for Implementation

Nursing implementations are planned with the purpose of altering or manipulating the focal, contextual, or residual stimuli. Implementation may also focus on broadening the person's coping ability, or adaptation zone, so that the total stimuli fall within that person's ability to adapt.[39]

Evaluation

The nursing process is completed by evaluation. Goal behaviors are compared to the person's output behaviors and movement toward or away from goal achievement is determined. Readjustments to goals and interventions are made, based on evaluation data.[40]

The Roy Nursing Process Applied to Nursing in a Recovery Room

The Roy model can be applied to nursing assessment and intervention within various clinical situations. In the following case study, the Roy model will be applied to a person during the period of immediate recovery from surgery and anesthesia.

First level assessment focuses on the physiological mode behaviors during the first hour of recovery time after a person experiences surgery and general anesthesia. Applying the Roy model, significant behaviors can be conceptualized as regulator output behaviors. Increased sympathetic or parasympathetic system activity can signal regulator system activity. Regulator output behaviors that vary from baseline values determined for the person may be the first warning of an ineffective response to postoperative stimuli. Key baseline values are the person's presurgery measures of heart rate, blood pressure, and respiratory rate. Immediately upon observation of changes from the baseline, second level assessment is done. Goals are set with the basic survival of the person as a priority. Interventions are taken so that focal and contextual stimuli are altered and adaptation is promoted. The evaluation of goal achievement is made, and further actions are taken as necessary.

Situation. Mrs. Reed is received from surgery after a major abdominal operation. Before surgery, her baseline vital signs were: heart rate, 80 beats per minute; blood pressure, 120/80 mm Hg; and respiratory rate, 16 per minute. After 45 minutes in recovery, her vital signs are: heart rate, 150 beats per minute; blood pressure, 90/60 mm Hg; respiratory rate, 32 per minute. Increased regulator output behavior is signaled by sympathetic nervous system stimulation of the heart in response to decreased blood pressure. The nurse decides that an ineffective response is occurring for Mrs. Reed. Therefore second level assessment is done.

The focal stimulus is a decrease of arterial blood pressure secondary to an unknown underlying cause. The contextual stimuli are: age 45 years, cool extremities, poor nail blanching, no food or drink for 12 hours, intravenous infusion (IV) of dextrose 5 percent in water with lactated Ringer's solution at 100 cc per hour. Also, contextual stimuli include 200 cc of IV fluids infused during surgery, 10 cc of urine excreted during the first 45 minutes in recovery, 1 ½ hours of general anesthesia, estimated blood loss of 500 cc during surgery, no operative site bleeding, and level of consciousness slow to respond to tactile stimuli after 45 minutes in recovery. The residual stimuli include history of renal infections.

The nursing diagnosis of a decreased arterial blood pressure secondary to fluid volume deficit is made. A fluid volume loss is suggested both by the contextual data and by the changes in the baseline heart rate, blood pressure, and urine output. The nurse then intervenes by altering contextual stimuli so that an adaptive response is promoted. The goal of a circulatory volume adequate to maintain a blood pressure of plus or minus 20 mm Hg of baseline levels within 15 minutes is set. The nurse plans and then takes the following intervention steps. The IV rate is increased to 300 cc per hour. The foot of the bed is elevated to increase venous return. Forty percent oxygen is given by mask. Mrs. Reed is verbally and tactilely stimulated and told to take slow deep breaths. The nurse prepares vasopressor medications for immediate use and applies an external continuous blood pressure cuff for constant blood pressure monitoring. The nurse also consults with other team members as to Mrs. Reed's clinical presentation.

A constant evaluation as to the effectiveness of the nursing actions is made. The nurse holds Mrs. Reed in recovery until the behavior goal of adequate circulation volume is met. Evaluation criteria would include urine output greater than 30 cc per hour, mental alertness, rapid nail bed blanching, blood pressure plus or minus 20 mm Hg of presurgery levels, pulse plus or minus 20 beats per minute of baseline, and respirations plus or minus 5 per minute of presurgery levels.

This concludes the discussion of the nursing process for the individual client. Before leaving the area of application of the model, let us consider briefly some additional uses. Use of the model to organize curriculum has been demonstrated by the faculty of Mount Saint Mary's College in Los Angeles. Similarly, extensive use of the model as well as pictorial representations of it have been made by the faculty and students of the Royal Alexander Hospitals School of Nursing.[41] Use of the model for the care of various client populations is exemplified by the works of Janelli, Farkas, and Giger, Bower, and Miller.[42a–42c] Research studies examining the use of the model in nursing practice include the work of Limandri and Hoch.[43a,43b]

ROY'S WORK AND THE CHARACTERISTICS OF A THEORY

1. Theories can interrelate concepts in such a way as to create a different way of looking at a particular phenomenon. The Roy model does interrelate concepts in such a way as to present a new view of the phenomenon being studied. It identifies the key concepts relevant to nursing: the person, environment, health, and the goal of nursing. The person is viewed as constantly interacting with internal and external stimuli. The person is active and reactive to these stimuli. Stimuli are defined as focal, that which invokes the greatest degree of change; contextual; and residual. Adaptation is a positive response made by the person to the experience being encountered. Adaptation is facilitated by the use of the regulator and cognator coping mechanisms. The adaptation level represents the range of stimuli that the person can tolerate and maintain an adaptive response. The areas of behavior where the effects of coping are evidenced include the four adaptive modes: physiological, self-concept, role function, and interdependence. Thus, by a quick review of the concept of the person who is the recipient of nursing care, one sees that a very specific perspective or image has been defined by the Roy Model. Beginning work in the development of theory related to these concepts has been done by Roy, Roberts, and others.[44] The view suggests a holistic framework as opposed to a view of the ill person as a biological entity with a disease process. It reflects a view of nursing that is concerned with many aspects of the person, physiological, self-concept, role function, and interdependence.

2. Theories must be logical in nature. The sequence of concepts of the Roy model follow logically. In the presentation of each of the key concepts, there is the recurring idea of adaptation to maintain integrity. The definition of health is based on the idea of integrity which in turn is operationalized to mean behaviors which meet the person's goals of survival, growth, reproduction, and mastery. Promoting adaptive responses in situations of health and illness is the goal of nursing. The person is conceptualized as a holistic, adaptive system. In fact, Figure 15–1 demonstrates the logic of the model.

3. Theories should be relatively simple yet generalizable. The concepts of the model are stated in relatively simple terms. However, the concept of the person as an adaptive system does present a challenging use of specific terms including cognator and regulator mechanisms and adaptation level. The four adaptive modes may be the first aspect of the model that the student or nurse is able to assimilate. Based upon nursing tradition, assessment of fluid and electrolytes, elimination, oxygenation, roles, and such evoke familiar images. As one nurse studying the theory stated, "It's what we've always done. I don't know what the big deal is!" Perhaps, she failed to realize that such a statement was complimentary of the simplicity of the model.

Let us also consider the generalizability of the model in various settings. Literature cited throughout this chapter speaks positively to the generalizability of the model to various client populations. Use in curriculum development also demonstrates generalizability.

4. Theories can be the bases for hypotheses that can be tested, and

5. Theories contribute to and assist in increasing the general body of knowledge of a discipline through the research implemented to validate them. The testing of a theory in practice is the basis for scientific development of a profession. Because Roy presents her work as a model, subtheorizing is present when application of the model is made for predictive understanding in a clinical situation. The model must be able to clearly identify the connecting relationships between underlying theories. Testable hypotheses are thus generated. Hill and Roberts discuss "relevant theory derivations," in their study of nursing interventions to promote the health of children with birth defects who are in need of habilitation. Developmental and social learning concepts are related to the Roy premises and hypotheses for testing are proposed (see Table 15–3).[45] Multiple examples of hypotheses for testing are generated by Roy and Roberts.[46] Because the model is an umbrella that is capable of linking theories, its contributions in the future to the body of nursing knowledge may be considerable.

6. Theories can be utilized by the practitioners to guide and improve their practice. Perhaps the most important aspect of a theory is its usefulness in practice. How does application of the Roy model guide and improve the work of the practitioner? A major strength of the model is that it guides nurses to utilize observation and interviewing skills in doing an individualized assessment of each person. Behavior related to the four adaptive modes is collected during first level assessment. In considering all the adaptive modes—physiological function, self-concept, role function, and interdependence—the nurse is likely to have a comprehensive view of the person.

The concepts of the model are applicable within many practice settings of nursing. Literature cited throughout this chapter reflects application of the model by nurse educators, practitioners, and researchers in a variety of educational and clinical settings.

The use of the model may demand a change in the allocation of time and resources. Painstaking application of the model would require significant input of time and effort. The benefit to the client of complete assessment and implementations in areas of concern, however, justifies the effort and allocation of resources. Even in practice settings which require quick action, the elements of the model are still compatible with quality care.

TABLE 15–3. RELEVANT THEORY DERIVATIONS

Roy's Premises	Developmental Unit—Child Habilitation	Social Learning Unit—Maternal Locus of Control
Man is an adaptive being.	Habilitation is an adaptation problem.	Generalized expectancy of control is directional towards internality or externality.
If man is an adaptive being, he has an adaptation level. The adaptation level is a function of the interaction between adaptation mechanisms and the environment.	The greater the adaptation level, the greater the habilitation level. The habilitation level is a function of the interaction between adaptation mechanisms and the environment.	
	The greater the deficits in habilitation, the greater the impairment of adaptation level. The greater the impairment of adaptation level, the greater the impairment in activities of daily living.	
	The greater the impairment of adaptation level, the greater the significance of the environment.	A significant stimulus in a child's environment is the mother.
		The greater the maternal internal locus of control, the greater the parenting patterns fostering independence of a child.
		The greater the maternal external locus of control, the less the parenting patterns fostering independence of a child.
Nursing intervention is directed towards manipulation of the environment.	The less the habilitation level of the child, the greater the need for nursing intervention.	The less the parenting patterns fostering independence of a child, the less the habilitation level of the child.

(From Roy. Sr. C. & Roberts, S.L. Theory Construction in Nursing: An Adaptation Model, Englewood Cliffs, N.J.: Prentice-Hall, pp. 36–37. Used with permission.)

Especially useful is the second level assessment guide to identification of focal, contextual, and residual stimuli. The development by Roy of a typology of nursing diagnoses of common adaptation problems is an exciting outflow of the model. Further integration of Roy's work with that of NANDA is yet to be seen. Even at this point, however, compatibility of the model to the work related to nursing diagnosis by NANDA is obvious.

Goal setting and achievement in nursing are likely to be facilitated by application of commonly defined concepts and direction of focus. The model, because it encourages identification of the focal, contextual, and residual stimuli within a situation, immediately indicates the course of nursing action. Nursing actions are geared to altering these stimuli. This aspect of the model helps the practitioner in making specific decisions about what actions to take. In another way, practitioners can see the importance of their actions in influencing the adaptation of the person. For example, the nurse can view nursing actions such as maintaining bed rest or relieving pain or fears as significant in maintaining an adaptive response for the person.

7. Theories must be consistent with other validated theories, laws, and principles but will leave open unanswered questions that need to be investigated. The model, by its structure, requires the integration of further theorizing for explanatory and predictive information in clinical situations. The concept of adaptation as developed by the model appears to have good linkage qualities. Theory development has been undertaken by Roy, her co-authors, and others as cited throughout this chapter. Future nursing research and field application will continue to validate and adjust the Roy model.

SUMMARY

The Roy model consists of the five elements of person, goal of nursing, nursing activities, health, and environment. Persons are viewed as living adaptive systems whose behaviors may be classified as adaptive responses or ineffective responses. These behaviors are derived from the regulator and cognator mechanisms. These mechanisms work within the four adaptive modes of physiological function, self-concept, role function, and interdependence. The goal of nursing is to promote adaptive responses in relation to the four adaptive modes, using information about the person's adaptation level, and focal, contextual, and residual stimuli. Nursing activities involve the manipulation of these stimuli to promote adaptive responses. Health is a process of becoming integrated and able to meet the goals of survival, growth, reproduction, and mastery. The environment consists of the person's internal and external stimuli.

These elements are in a nursing process that consists of first and second level assessments, diagnosis, goal setting, intervention, and evaluation.

First level assessment, or behavioral assessment, deals with the four adaptive modes, whereas second level assessment focuses on the three areas of stimuli. Diagnosis consists of stating the problem. Goals are set in relation to the problem and are written in behavioral terms. Interventions are planned to manipulate the stimuli, and evaluation compares the person's output behaviors with the desired behaviors established in the goals.

Roy's model is seen as applicable in the nursing process presented in Chapter 2. The characteristics of a theory are also met. There is need for continued research that centers on hypotheses generated by the model.

REFERENCES

1.(a) Roy, C. *Introduction to Nursing: An Adaptation Model,* Englewood Cliffs, N.J.: Prentice-Hall, Inc., 1976.

1.(b) Roy, C. *Introduction to Nursing: An Adaptation Model* (2nd ed.), Englewood Cliffs, N.J.: Prentice-Hall, 1984.

1.(c) Andrews, H.A., & Roy, C. *Essentials of the Roy Adaptation Model,* Norwalk, CT.: Appleton-Century-Crofts, 1986.

1.(d) Roy, C. & Roberts, S. *Theory Construction in Nursing: An Adaptation Model,* Englewood Cliffs, N.J.: Prentice-Hall, 1981.

2.   Roy, *Introduction to Nursing* (2nd ed.).

3.   Roy and Roberts, *Theory Construction.*

4.(a) Randell, B., Tedrow, M.P., & Van Landingham, J. *Adaptation Nursing: The Roy Conceptual Model Applied,* St. Louis: C.V. Mosby, 1982.

4.(b) Rambo, B. *Adaptation Nursing: Assessment and Intervention,* Philadelphia: Saunders, 1983.

4.(c) Riehl, J.P., & Roy, C. *Conceptual Models for Nursing Practice* (2nd ed.), New York: Appleton-Century-Crofts, 1980.

5.   Roy, *Introduction to Nursing* (2nd ed.), p. 8.

6.   Ibid, 28.

7.   Dunn, H.L. *High Level Wellness,* Arlington, VA.: R.W. Beatty, 1971.

8.   Roy, *Introduction to Nursing* (2nd ed.), p. 30.

9.   Ibid, 35.

10.   Roy and Roberts, *Theory Construction,* pp. 60–62.

11.   Guyton, A.C. *Basic Human Physiology: Normal Function and Mechanisms of Disease,* Philadelphia: Saunders, 1971, p. 353.

12.   Roy and Roberts, *Theory Construction,* pp. 63–66.

13.   Roy, *Introduction to Nursing* (2nd ed.), p. 33.

14.   Vavio, S.A. Oxygenation, in Roy, C. *Introduction to Nursing: An Adaptation Model* (2nd ed.), Englewood Cliffs, N.J.: Prentice-Hall, 1984, pp. 91–109.

15.   Servonsky, J. Elimination, in Roy, C. *Introduction to Nursing: An Adaptation Model* (2nd ed.), Englewood Cliffs, N.J.: Prentice-Hall, 1984, pp. 125–137.

16.   Servonsky, J. Elimination, in Roy, C. *Introduction to Nursing: An Adaptation Model* (2nd ed.), Englewood Cliffs, N.J.: Prentice-Hall, 1984, pp. 125–137.

17.   Cho, J.S. Activity and Rest, in Roy, C. *Introduction to Nursing: An Adaptation Model* (2nd ed.), Englewood Cliffs, N.J.: Prentice-Hall, 1984, pp. 138–158.

18.   Sato, M.K. Skin Integrity, in Roy, C. *Introduction to Nursing: an Adaptation Model* (2nd ed.), Englewood Cliffs, N.J.: Prentice-Hall, 1984, pp. 159–167.

19.   Driscoll, S. The Senses, in Roy, C. *Introduction to Nursing: An Adaptation Model* (2nd ed.), Englewood Cliffs, N.J.: Prentice-Hall, 1984, pp. 168–188.

20.   Perley, N.Z. Fluid and Electrolytes, in Roy, C. *Introduction to Nursing: An Adaptation Model* (2nd ed.), Englewood Cliffs, N.J.: Prentice-Hall, 1984, pp. 189–210.

21.   Robertson, M.M. Neurological Function, in Roy. C. *Introduction to Nursing: An Adaptation Model* (2nd ed.), Englewood Cliffs, N.J.: Prentice-Hall, 1984, pp. 211–237.

22.   Howard, M. & Valentine, S. Endocrine Function, in Roy, C. *Introduction to Nursing: An Adaptation Model* (2nd ed.), Englewood Cliffs, N.J.: Prentice-Hall, 1984, pp. 238–252.

23.   Buck, M.H. Self-Concept: Theory and Development, in Roy, C. *Introduction to Nursing: An Adaptation Model* (2nd ed.), Englewood Cliffs, N.J.: Prentice-Hall, 1984, pp. 255–283.

24.   Nuwayhid, K.A. Role Function: Theory and Development, in Roy, C. *Introduction to Nursing: An Adaptation Model* (2nd ed.), Englewood Cliffs, N.J.: Prentice-Hall, 1984, pp. 284–305.

25.   Tedrow, M.P. Interdependence: Theory and Development, in Roy, C. *Introduction to Nursing: An Adaptation Model* (2nd ed.), Englewood Cliffs, N.J.: Prentice-Hall, 1984, pp. 306–322.

26.   Roy, *Introduction to Nursing* (2nd ed.), p. 12.

27.(a) Helson, H. *Adaptation Level Theory*, New York: Harper & Row, 1966.

27.(b) Roy, C. *Introduction to Nursing* (2nd ed.), pp. 37–38.

28.   Roy, *Introduction to Nursing* (2nd ed.), p. 37.

29.   Ibid, 38.

30.   Roy and Roberts, *Theory Construction*, p. 47.

31.   Roy, *Introduction to Nursing* (2nd ed.), p. 39.

32.   Ibid, 38.

33.   Ibid, 39.

34.   Ibid, 45–51.

35.   Martinez, C. Nursing Assessment Based on Roy Adaptation Model, in Roy, C. *Introduction to Nursing: An Adaptation Model*, Englewood Cliffs, N.J.: Prentice-Hall, 1976, pp. 379–385.

36.   Roy. *Introduction to Nursing* (2nd ed.), p. 53.

37.   Ibid, 55–57.

38.   North American Nursing Diagnosis Association, *Taxonomy I with Complete Diagnosis*, St. Louis: St. Louis University School of Nursing, 1987.

39.   Roy, *Introduction to Nursing* (2nd ed.), pp. 59–60.

40.   Ibid, 61.

41.   Andrews & Roy, *Essentials of the Roy Adaptation Model*, p. xi.

42.(a) Janelli, L.M. Utilizing Roy's Adaptation Model from a Gerontological Perspective, *Journal of Gerontological Nursing* 1980, *6*, 140–150.

42.(b) Farkas, L. Adaptation Problems with Nursing Home Application for Elderly Persons: An Application of the Roy Adaptation Nursing Model, *Journal of Advanced Nursing* 1981, *6*, 363–368.

42.(c) Giger, J.A., Bower, C.A., & Miller, S.W. Roy Adaptation Model: ICU Adaptation Model: ICU Application, *Dimensions of Critical Care Nursing* 1987, *6*, 215–224.

43.(a) Limandri, B.J. Research and Practice with Abused Women: Use of the Roy Adaptation Model as an Explanatory Framework, *Advances in Nursing Science* 1986, *8*, 52–61.

43.(b) Hoch, C.C. Assessing Delivery of Nursing Care, *Journal of Gerontological Nursing* 1987, *13*, 10–17.

44.   Roy & Roberts, *Theory Construction.*

45.   Hill, B.J. & Roberts, C.S. Formal Theory Construction: An Example of the Process, in Roy, C. & Roberts, S.L. *Theory Construction in Nursing: An Adaptation Model,* Englewood Cliffs, N.J.: Prentice-Hall, 1981, pp. 30–39.

46.   Roy & Roberts, *Theory Construction.*

CHAPTER 16

Betty Neuman

Joanne R. Cross

Betty Neuman was born on a farm in Lowell, Ohio, in 1924. Her first nursing education was completed at Peoples Hospital, (now called General Hospital) School of Nursing in Akron, Ohio, in 1947, and she received her BS in Nursing in 1957 and her MS in Mental Health, Public Health Consultation, from UCLA in 1966. She holds a PhD in clinical psychology.

Since 1966, her area of practice has been mental health consultation and counseling. A broad background in nursing includes public health school, industrial, and hospital settings. She has been active in family therapy, continuing education, and curriculum consultation. Her teaching experience includes mental health, consultation and organization, leadership, and counseling. She was a pioneer in the community mental health movement in the late 1960s. During her UCLA work in organization and planning with the community mental health movement, she developed her nursing model of the "whole person approach" based on a systems adaptation framework.

Betty Neuman's theoretical approach to nursing is exemplified in a holistic approach to her own life. She has a great zest for life and a keen sense of using time creatively and usefully. She actively maintains a wellness program for herself and jointly practices marriage and family counseling with her husband. She continues to act as consultant to university schools of nursing, hospitals, and community settings that wish to adopt and implement her theoretical framework into their curriculum and patient care delivery.[1]

Betty Neuman began developing her health systems model while a lecturer in community health nursing at the University of California, Los Angeles. The model was initially developed in response to graduate nursing students' expression of a need for course content that would expose them to a breadth of nursing problems prior to focusing on specific nursing problem areas.[2]

The model was published in 1972 as "A Model for Teaching Total Person Approach to Patient Problems," in *Nursing Research*.[2] It was refined and subsequently published in the first edition of *Conceptual Models for Nursing Practice*, 1974, and in the second edition in 1980.[3] The most recent refinement, along with numerous examples for application to curriculum, nursing practice, and administration, is in her 1989 publication, *The Neuman Systems Model*.[4]

Although the Neuman conceptual model was initially developed in a curricular context, and she asserted that she "had no intention of creating a specific conceptual model for the nursing community,"[5] it is important to note that the works of several other nursing theorists (e.g., Martha Rogers, Dorothea Orem, and Imogene King) were being published at the time of her initial publication.[6a–6c] Indeed, it was in the early 1970s that the National League for Nursing (NLN) emphasized the importance of conceptual models for nursing education and that conceptual frameworks became a major emphasis of the NLN criteria for accreditation.[7]

Neuman describes her model as comprehensive and dynamic. The model is a multidimensional view of individuals, groups (families), and communities who are in constant interaction with environmental stressors. Essentially, the model focuses on the client's reaction to stress and the factors of reconstitution or adaptation. It is considered an appropriate model not only for nursing but also for all health care professions.

DEVELOPMENT OF THE MODEL

Neuman's conceptual approach is the result of synthesis of knowledge from several theoretical sources, including de Chardin,[8] Marx,[9] Gestalt,[10] Selye,[11] von Bertalanffy,[12] and Caplan.[13]

From these theoretical influences, interaction in the Neuman model may be summarized as follows:

Gestalt and field theories emphasize the person's perceptual field as a state of dynamic equilibrium. Tension in the field is created by a problem, which then results in a disturbance of equilibrium. The disequilibrium is seen to serve as a source of motivation for interaction with the environment. Field and systems theories describe the interrelationship and interdependence of the component parts of the individual or society. . . . it is the stressors in the environment that produce the stimuli (tension) that cause the individual (whole) to interact with his environment.[14]

In comparing a systems model with nursing actions, Neuman postulates that although both are goal directed, a systems model is general in nature. In contrast, nursing actions have very specific goals for vigorously controlling those variables that affect nursing care. Such goals might include general improvement in the client, performance or pattern of behavior change, or a specific improvement in self-care skills. Since nursing is increasingly focusing on primary prevention, Neuman sets forth a description of how primary prevention variables interface with those of secondary and tertiary prevention.

Although this model was initially developed for use by all health care professionals, Neuman states that nurses can uniquely use it to assist individuals, families, and other groups to attain and maintain maximum levels of total wellness by purposeful interventions.[15] She uses the term *intervention* for the phase of the nursing process described in this book as *implementation*. When discussing her work, the term *intervention* will be used. The interventions are aimed at the reduction of stress factors and adverse conditions that are potential or actual in any given clinical situation.[16a,16b]

Basic Assumptions

There are ten basic assumptions underlying Neuman's conceptual framework[17]:

1. Though each individual client or group as a client system is unique, each system is a composite of common known factors or innate characteristics within a normal, given range of response contained within a basic structure.
2. Many known, unknown, and universal environmental stressors exist. Each differs in its potential for disturbing a client's usual stability level, or normal line of defense. The particular interrelationships of client variables—physiological, psychological, sociocultural, developmental, and spiritual—at any point in time can affect the degree to which a client is protected by the flexible line of defense against possible reaction to a single stressor or a combination of stressors.
3. Each individual client/client system, over time, has evolved a normal range of response to the environment that is referred to as a normal line of defense, or usual wellness/stability state.
4. When the cushioning, accordionlike effect of the flexible line of defense is no longer capable of protecting the client/client system against an environmental stressor, the stressor breaks through the normal line of defense. The interrelationships of variables—physiological, psychological, sociocultural, developmental, and spiritual—determine the nature and degree of the system reaction or possible reaction to the stressor.
5. The client, whether in a state of wellness or illness, is a dynamic composite of the interrelationships of variables—physiological, psychological, sociocultural, developmental, and spiritual. Wellness is on a continuum of available energy to support the system in its optimal state.
6. Implicit within each client system is a set of internal resistance factors known as lines of resistance, which function to stabilize and return the client to the usual wellness state (normal line of defense) or possibly to a higher level of stability following an environmental stressor reaction.
7. Primary prevention relates to general knowledge that is applied in client assessment and intervention in identification and reduction or mitigation of risk factors associated with environmental stressors to prevent possible reaction.

8. Secondary prevention relates to symptomatology following a reaction to stressors, appropriate ranking of intervention priorities, and treatment to reduce their noxious effects.
9. Tertiary prevention relates to the adjustive processes taking place as reconstitution begins and maintenance factors move the client back in a circular manner toward primary prevention.
10. The client is in dynamic constant energy exchange with the environment.[18]

The Systems Model

Neuman's framework is basically an open systems model with the major components of stressors, reaction to stressors, and the "person"* (represented by a series of concentric circles in Neuman's diagram—see Fig. 16–1) interacting with the environment. This organizing framework enables the nurse to intervene appropriately with health promotion (primary prevention), corrective (secondary prevention), or rehabilitative (tertiary prevention) nursing actions to maintain or restore equilibrium to the system.[19]

Note in Figure 16–1 that the series of concentric rings surrounding the basic core structure of human being, family, or community (labeled "basic structure, energy resources") vary in size and distance from the reactor. They represent the *lines of resistance,* the internal factors defending against stressors. The *normal line of defense* is essentially what the person becomes over a lifetime—the normal state of wellness, or steady state—and is composed of physiological–psychological–sociocultural–developmental–spiritual skills that the system uses to deal with stressors. This line of defense is considered to be dynamic since it relates to the way a system is stabilized over time. The *flexible line of defense* (outer broken line) is "accordianlike" in nature and acts as a buffer to the normal line of defense when the environment is actively stressful, and as a "filter when the environment offers support and serves as a positive force to facilitate growth and development."[20] It is also dynamic and can be altered rapidly over a short period of time. Its effectiveness can be reduced by such changes as loss of sleep, malnutrition, or any alterations in activities of daily living.

Stressors

More than one stressor can occur at a time as[21]:

1. *Extrapersonal*—forces that occur outside the system, e.g., unemployment (outside force) influenced by peer acceptability (socio-cultural force), personal feelings about present and past unemployment (psychological), ability to perform the job (biological–developmental–psychological).

---

* *Person* refers to the client system, which can be an individual person, family, other group, or community.

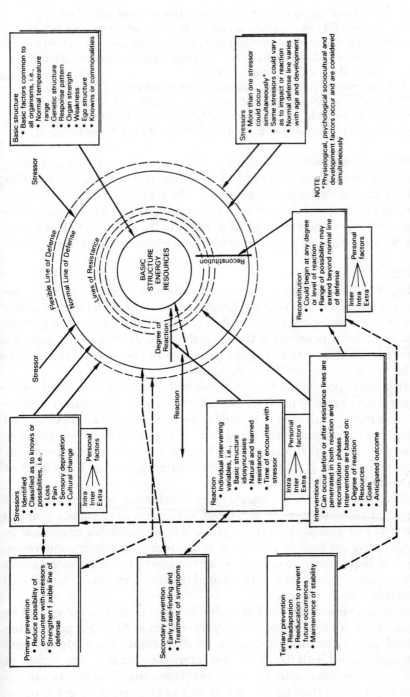

Basic structure
- Basic factors common to all organisms, i.e.,
  - Normal temperature range
  - Genetic structure
  - Response pattern
  - Organ strength
  - Weakness
  - Ego structure
  - Knowns or commonalities

Stressors
- More than one stressor could occur simultaneously*
- Same stressors could vary as to impact or reaction
- Normal defense line varies with age and development

NOTE:
*Physiological, psychological sociocultural and development factors occur and are considered simultaneously

Stressor

Flexible Line of Defense

Normal Line of Defense

Lines of Resistance

BASIC STRUCTURE ENERGY RESOURCES

Reconstitution

Degree of Reaction

Reaction

Stressor

Reconstitution
- Could begin at any degree or level of reaction
- Range of possibility may extend beyond normal line of defense

Inter
Intra → Personal factors
Extra

Stressors
- Identified
- Classified as to knows or possibilities, i.e.,
  - Loss
  - Pain
  - Sensory deprivation
  - Cultural change

Intra
Inter → Personal factors
Extra

Reaction
- Individual intervening variables, i.e.,
  - Basic structure idiosyncrasies
  - Natural and learned resistance
  - Time of encounter with stressor

Intra
Inter → Personal factors
Extra

Interventions
- Can occur before or after resistance lines are penetrated in both reaction and reconstitution phases
- Interventions are based on:
  - Degree of reaction
  - Resources
  - Goals
  - Anticipated outcome

Primary prevention
- Reduce possibility of encounter with stressors
- Strengthen flexible line of defense

Secondary prevention
- Early case-finding and
- Treatment of symptoms

Tertiary prevention
- Readaptation
- Reeducation to prevent future occurrences
- Maintenance of stability

Figure 16–1 The Neuman model: A total person approach to viewing patient problems *(From Newman, B. The Newman Systems Model,* (2nd ed). Appleton & Lange, 1989, p. 26.)

2. *Interpersonal*—forces occurring between one or more individuals, e.g., parent–child role expectations, forces between individuals that are influenced by local child-rearing practices (socio-cultural), age and development of both child and parents (biological and developmental), and feelings about the role (psychological).
3. *Intrapersonal*—forces that occur within the individual, e.g., anger: an internal force within the individual whose expression is influenced by age (developmental), peer group acceptability (socio-cultural), physical abilities (biological), and past experiences coping with anger (psychological).

Other factors will also influence the system's reaction to a stressor. What is noxious to one may not be to another. It is important to consider the number and strength of the stressors, the length of the encounter with them, and their specific meaning to this system. Therefore, careful assessment of the impact and meaning of stressors to the system as well as knowledge of past coping skills are important for adequate nursing intervention.

Reaction

Primary prevention can begin at any point at which a stressor is either suspected or identified. If a reaction has not occurred, the intervention would enter at the primary level. The goal of primary intervention is to prevent the stressor from penetrating the normal line of defense or to lessen the degree of reaction by reducing the possibility of encounter with stressors and by strengthening the line of defense.

If primary prevention is not possible and reaction has occurred, intervention would begin at the level of *secondary prevention*. Secondary prevention deals mainly with early case finding, early treatment of symptoms, and attempts to strengthen the internal lines of resistance to reduce reaction. Nursing intervention at this level can begin at any point where stress reaction is recognized. It may progress beyond or below the usual level of wellness or line of defense.

Tertiary prevention is the intervention that follows the active treatment plan when reconstitution or some reasonable degree of stabilization has occurred. The goal of the tertiary phase is to maintain this adaptation by strengthening the lines of resistance, thus preventing future occurrences. This goal is primarily accomplished by the use of re-educative measures and by optimum use of the system's total resources, including the internal and external environments.

Neuman views the model as multidimensional; that is, there must be consideration of all variables affecting the system and the "proper ranking of need priority at any given point."[22] At present, this model is being thoroughly tested both nationally and internationally in a wide variety of clinical and academic settings. As Torres points out, "The theory can describe and explain nursing practice as well as generate different propositions that can later be used for research . . . thus the theory serves a useful purpose for practice and future research and could be predictive."[23]

NEUMAN'S THEORY AND THE FOUR MAJOR CONCEPTS

The Neuman model will be viewed in terms of congruency and consistency with the four concepts of individual/human, society/environment, health/ wellness, and nursing.

Individual/Human

The focus of the Neuman model is based on the philosophy that each human is a "total person" as a client system and that this person is multidimensional, a composite of physiological, psychological, sociocultural, developmental and spiritual variables. Other variables include basic survival core characteristics possessed in common with other human beings, such as normal temperature range, genetic response patterns, ego structure, and various strengths and weaknesses of the physical body. The dynamic interaction of these variables and core characteristics along with the lines of normal defense and flexible resistance, combined with multiple stressors, provide the essence of the "total person approach." The model is based in part on general system theory, in which the whole is different from and more than the sum of its parts. Thus the concept of "wholeness" or totality is integral to Neuman's model. She states:

> We must now emphatically refuse to deal with single components, but instead relate to the concept of *wholeness*. We need to think and act systemically. Systems thinking enables us to effectively handle all parts of a system simultaneously in an interrelated manner, thus avoiding the fragmented and isolated nature of past functioning in nursing.[24]

The entire system is bound by the created-environment and its constraints, whether they be man, nursing, family, or community.

Society/Environment

Basic to the Neuman model is the concept that humans are in constant interaction with their environment. This is the fundamental phenomenon of her conceptual model. She defines environment as those internal and external forces surrounding humans at any given point in time. The created-environment is intra-, inter-, and extrapersonal. Neuman states:

> The created-environment is dynamic and represents the client's unconscious mobilization of all system variables, including the basic structure energy factors, toward system integration, stability, and integrity.[25]

In relation to environment, Neuman specifically notes similarities between her model and the field of Gestalt theories when she speaks of the occurrence of stressors and the reaction to stressors and to the organism itself. These stressors (intra-, inter-, and extrapersonal), a prominent subsystem of her model, comprise the environment in which the client system operates.

Health/Wellness

A total person definition of wellness can be derived from the Neuman model. Mayers states that "the assumption of this model can lead one to see wellness as a dynamic composite of physical, psychological, sociocultural, developmental and spiritual balance that is flexible yet retains an unbroken ability to resist disequilibrium."[26]

In her initial writings, Neuman does not define health but states that, through an interaction/adjustment process, a person retains varying degrees of balance and harmony between internal and external environments.[27] Terms used included *wellness, variances from wellness,* and *stability of the client system.* Wellness was equated with stability of the normal line of defense, and illness appeared to be variances of wellness.[27] In later writings, Neuman states that "Health. . .is equated with optimal system stability, that is, the best possible wellness state. At any given time. . .health. . .is envisioned as being at various, changing levels within a normal range, rising or falling throughout the life span because of basic structure factors and the satisfactory or unsatisfactory adjustment to environmental stressors. [Neuman] views health as living energy."[28]

Neuman continues to mention levels of wellness, which suggests she views health in a continuum rather than as a dichotomy of wellness and illness. Levels of wellness also suggest she holds a linear view rather than a holistic view, although her diagram and model attempt a view of holism.[29] In any event, nursing has as its goal those acts that conserve energy, whether the client system moves toward the wellness state or toward the illness state. Neuman illustrates this phenomenon in the paradigm shown in Figure 16–2.

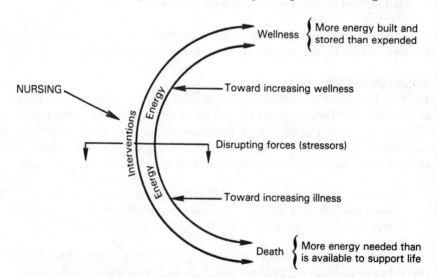

Figure 16–2. Wellness–illness based on the systems concept. *(Adapted from Neuman, B.* The Neuman Systems Model: Applications to Nursing Education and Practice, *Norwalk, Conn.: Appleton-Century-Crofts, 1982, p. 11. Used with permission.)*

Other concepts included in her writings are defined in terms of systems terminology, such as[30]:

Wellness: State of saturation; of inertness free of disruptive needs
Illness: State of insufficiency; disruptive needs are yet to be satisfied

Neuman's term *reconstitution* also needs to be addressed in relation to the concept of health. It can be inferred from her model that reconstitution can be equated with moving from "variances from wellness" to desired wellness levels and client stability. Again, reconstitution is viewed holistically as multidimensional in that the biological–psychological–sociocultural–developmental–spiritual components are affected by intra–inter–extrapersonal variables.

Nursing

In general, Neuman views nursing as a "unique profession" that concerns itself with all the variables affecting human response to stressors, with a primary concern for the total person. "The primary goal of nursing is the retention and attainment of client system stability."[31]

She defines the parameters of nursing more clearly when she states that nursing assists individuals, families, and groups to attain and maintain a maximum level of total wellness by purposeful interventions aimed at reducing stress factors and adverse conditions that affect optimal functioning in any given patient situation.[32]

As Mayers points out, nursing's purpose is to deliberately intervene where there is variance from wellness, and purposive nursing interventions are designed to produce positive changes. These changes or results should be measured according to an accepted model, theory, or wellness definition.[33] In order to facilitate movement toward the positive end of a wellness–illness continuum, the nurse needs both a philosophy and an operational model. Neuman has operationalized her model into the nursing process by providing an assessment/intervention instrument for use by practitioners. This instrument is displayed in Table 16–1.

The assessment or intervention instrument (Table 16–1) includes the various aspects of Neuman's model but is flexible enough to allow for the inclusion of any additional data deemed necessary. Factors influencing the use of the instrument would be the client, client situation, the practitioner, and the agency involved in the assessment. In Neuman's work, the instrument is accompanied by an explanatory section that includes specific rationale charts to categorize data, and plans for interventions at all levels.

THE NEUMAN MODEL AND THE NURSING PROCESS

As noted earlier, Neuman views nursing as a unique profession concerned with all the variables affecting the system's response to stressors. The cen-

TABLE 16-1. AN ASSESSMENT AND INTERVENTION TOOL

A. Intake Summary
1. Name _____
   Age _____
   Sex _____
   Marital status _____
2. Referral source and related information

B. Stressors as Perceived by Client
   (If Client is incapacitated, secure data from family or other re-sources.)
1. What do you consider your major stress area or areas of health concern? (Identify these areas.)
2. How do present circumstances differ from your usual pat-tern of living? (Identify life-style patterns.)
3. Have you ever experienced a similar problem? If so, what was that problem and how did you handle it? Were you suc-cessful? (Identify past coping patterns.)
4. What do you anticipate for yourself in the future as a conse-quence of your present situation? (Identify perceptual fac-tors, that is, reality versus distortions—expectations, present and possible future coping patterns.)
5. What are you doing and what can you do to help yourself? (Identify perceptual factors, that is, reality versus distortions—expectations, present and possible future cop-ing patterns.)
6. What do you expect care-givers, family, friends, or others to do for you? (Identify perceptual factors, that is, reality versus distortions—expectations, present and possible future cop-ing patterns.)

C. Stressors as Perceived by Caregiver
1. What do you consider to be the major stress area or areas of health concern? (Identify these areas.)
2. How do present circumstances differ from the client's usual pattern of living? (Identify life-style patterns.)
3. Has the client ever experienced a similar situation? If so, how would you evaluate what the client did? How successful do you think it was? (Identify past coping patterns.)
4. What do you anticipate for the future as a consequence of the client's present situation? (Identify perceptual factors, that is, reality versus distortions—expectations, present and possible future coping patterns.)
5. What can the client do to help himself? (Identify perceptual factors, that is, reality versus distortions—expectations, pres-ent and possible future coping patterns.)
6. What do you think the client expects from caregivers, family, friends, or other resources? (Identify perceptual factors, that is, reality versus distortions—expectations, present and possi-ble future coping patterns.)

Summary of Impressions
Note any discrepancies or distortions between the client's perception and that of the caregiver related to the situation.

D. Intrapersonal Factors
1. Physical (examples: degree of mobility, range of body func-tion.)

2. Psycho-sociocultural (examples: attitudes, values, expectations, behavior patterns, and nature of coping patterns.)
3. Developmental (examples: age, degree of normalcy, factors related to present situation)
4. Spiritual belief system (examples: hope and sustaining factors)

E. Interpersonal Factors
   Examples are resources and relationship of family, friends, or caregivers that either influence or could influence Area D.

F. Extrapersonal Factors
   Examples are resources and relationship of community facilities, finances, employment, or other areas which either influence or could influence areas D and E.

G. Forumlation of a Comprehensive Nursing Diagnosis
   Is accomplished by identify and ranking the priority of needs based on the total data obtained from the client's perception, or other resources, suchas, laboratory reports, other care givers, or agencies. The appropriate theory is related to the above data.

   With this format, reassessment is a continuous process and is related to the effectiveness of intervention based upon the prior stated goals. Effective reassessment would include the following as they relate to the total client situation:

1. Changes in nature of stressors and priority assignments
2. Changes in intrapersonal factors
3. Changes in interpersonal factors
4. Changes in extrapersonal factors

In reassessment it is important to note the change of priority of goals in relation to the primary, secondary, and tertiary prevention as intervention categories. An assessment tool of this nature should offer a current, progressive, and comprehensive analysis of the client's total circumstances and relationship of the five variables (physiological, psychological, sociocultural, developmental, and spiritual) to environmental influences.

From Neuman, B. The Neuman Systems Model. *Norwalk, Conn.: Appleton & Lange, 1989, pp. 61–63.*

tral concern of nursing is the total person or system, while the primary goal is to maintain/retain/or attain client stability.[34]

This view is reflected in the way Neuman has systematized the nursing process into the three categories of nursing diagnosis, nursing goals, and nursing outcomes (Table 16–2). She frequently refers to assessment and intervention in relation to stressors and to the three levels of prevention. An assessment instrument (Table 16–1) was included in her second revision of the model with an explanation of how to use the instrument.[35] The underlying principles are[36]:

1. Good assessment requires knowledge of all the factors influencing a client's perceptual field.
2. The meaning a stressor has to the client is validated by the client as well as the care-giver.
3. Factors in the care-giver's perceptual field that influence the assessment of the client's situation should become apparent.

Table 16–3 lists the theoretical issues involved in the three levels of prevention. Although not inclusive, it offers operational possibilities for the nursing practitioner and provides a view of the relationships between the levels of prevention and other major concepts in Neuman's model.

The Neuman model was one of the first systems that explicated an instrument (Table 16–1) that is intended to assist the practitioner in applying the model and bridging theory and practice. Neuman designed a specific format of the nursing process to facilitate the use of her systems model.

TABLE 16–2. NURSING PROCESS ACCORDING TO BETTY NEUMAN

Category	Description of Process
Nursing diagnosis	1. Based on acquisition of appropriate data base, the diagnosis identifies, assesses, classifies, and evaluates the dynamic interaction of the bio-psycho-sociocultural–developmental–spiritual variables.
	2. Variances from wellness (needs and problems) are determined by correlations and constraints through synthesis of theory and data base.
	3. Broad hypothetical interventions are determined; i.e., maintain flexible line of defense.
Nursing goals	1. Nurse–client system negotiates for prescriptive change.
	2. Nurse intervention strategies postulated to retain, attain, and maintain client system stability.
Nursing outcomes	1. Nursing intervention using one or more prevention modes.
	2. Confirmation of prescriptive change or reformulation of nursing goals.
	3. Short-term goal outcomes influence determination of intermediate and long-term goals.
	4. Client outcome validates nursing process.

TABLE 16–3. AN ASSESSMENT AND INTERVENTION TOOL DEVELOPMENT GUIDE

	Primary Prevention	Secondary Prevention	Tertiary Prevention
Stressors			
Covert or potential	Overt, actual or known	Overt, or residual-possible covert
Reaction	Hypothetical or possible, based on available knowledge	Identified symptoms or known stress factors	Hypothetical or known-residual symptoms or known stress factors
Assessment			
	Based on client assessment, experience, and theory	Determined by nature and degree of reaction	Determined by degree of stability following treatment and further potential reconstitution and possible regression factors
	Risks or possible hazards based on client and nurse perceptions	Determine internal and external available resources to resist the reaction	
	Meaning of the experience to the client	Rationale for goals–collaborative goal setting with the client	
	Life-style factors		
	Coping patterns (past, present, possible)		
	Individual differences identified		

(continued)

TABLE 16–3. (Continued)

Primary Prevention	Secondary Prevention	Tertiary Prevention
Intervention as Prevention	**Intervention as Treatment**	**Intervention as Reconstitution Following Treatment**
Strengthen client flexible line of defense	Wellness variance—overt symptoms—nursing diagnosis	Motivation
Client education and desensitization to stressors	Need priority and related goals	Education and reeducation
Stressor avoidance	Client strengths and weaknesses related to the five client variables	Behavior modification
Strengthen individual resistance factors	Shift of need priorities as client responds to treatment (primary prevention may occur simultaneously with treatment or secondary prevention.)	Reality orientation
		Progressive goal setting
	Intervention in maladaptive processes	Optimal use of internal and external available resources
	Optimal use of internal and external resources, such as energy conservation, noise reduction, and financial aid	Maintenance of client optimal functional level

From Neuman, B. The Neuman Systems Model, Norwalk, Conn.: Appleton & Lange, 1989, p. 57. Used with permission.

NEUMAN'S WORK AND THE CHARACTERISTICS OF A THEORY

In nursing literature, the terms *theoretical models, conceptual frameworks,* and *theories* are frequently used interchangeably. Although there are crucial differences between theories and frameworks and usually separate criteria to analyze them, for the purpose of this book the phenomena related to the Neuman model will be compared to the characteristics of a theory provided in Chapter 1.

1. Theories can interrelate concepts in such a way as to create a different way of looking at a particular phenomenon. The Neuman model represents a timely focus on nursing interest in the total person approach to the interaction of environment and health. The emphasis on wellness and primary prevention is unique to this framework.

The interrelationships between the concepts of person, health, nursing, and society/environment are repeatedly mentioned throughout the Neuman model and are considered to be basically adequate according to the criteria. The concepts and definition statements concerning primary, secondary, and tertiary prevention "provide the required general linkages among the concepts of the model."[37] Ziemer used such linkages as she used Neuman's System Model for her study of the effects of preoperative information on postoperative coping behaviors. Ziemer focused on primary prevention to strengthen an individual's line of defense prior to the impact of a stressor by reducing the intensity of the stressor through adequate preparation.[38]

However, some concepts need clearer definitions and further explanation. One example is the specific meaning of wellness—or "variances" thereof—and ensuing "levels of wellness." The concept of reconstitution needs to be more definitively explored.

2. Theories must be logical in nature. Neuman's model in general presents itself as logically consistent. There is a logical sequence in the process of nursing wherein emphasis on the importance of accurate data assessment is basic to the sequential steps of the nursing process. However, there are other philosophical issues that are not supported in the model. One issue involves the theoretical component of health and illness as a continuum and a dichotomy, and as negentropy and entropy. These views appear to be in conflict within and between themselves. Entropy, also, would tend to support humans as a closed system.[39]

In the logical translation of the Neuman model, there appear to be incompatible elements since the model reflects both mechanistic and organismic views of the relationship of "person" to environment. Humans as beings reacting to a stimulus in the environment is a view held by the mechanistic theorists and is essentially a stress-adaptation theory. Because the person is viewed as a reactive being, any activity is primarily the result of external forces.

On the other hand, the organismic view is one of holism where the person is an active organism in continuous interaction with the environment. This view emphasizes the whole person, not any one component or discrete part. This "world view" incorporates Neuman's use of Gestalt, field, and other philosophies that support the unity of the person.[40] However, Neuman presents her model as essentially an organismic view. Therefore some redefining of terms incorporating a more dynamic view of stress is needed to translate this model to a more logical consistency.

3. Theories should be relatively simple yet generalizable. Given the abstract nature of most conceptual models, Neuman's model is fairly simple and straightforward in approach. The terms used are easily identifiable and for the most part have definitions that are broadly accepted. The multiple use of the model in varied nursing situations (practice, curriculum, and administration) is testimony in itself to its broad applicability.[41] The potential use of this model by other health care disciplines also attests to its generalizability for use in practice.

One potential drawback in relation to simplicity is the diagrammed model (Fig. 16–1) since it presents over thirty-five variables, and tends to be awesome to the viewer as is true with many systems models. This model becomes overly complex with the specification of multiple components and multiple relationships. This complexity increases the difficulty of managing the model or evaluating effects of the model on nursing practice. In the main, the model identifies the components without specifying the *nature* of the relationships between them, which causes some difficulty in the functional use of the model.[42] Thus, at this point, the model lends itself to "reductionism" rather than "holism."

4. Theories can be the bases for hypotheses that can be tested. Neuman's model, due to its high level and breadth of abstraction, lends itself to theory development. One area for future consideration as a beginning testable theory might be the concept of prevention as intervention, subsequent to basic concept refinement in the Neuman model. Other areas for research have been developed and suggested both by Neuman and by Fawcett.[43,44]

5. Theories contribute to and assist in increasing the general body of knowledge within the discipline through the research implemented to validate them. The multidimensional nature of the model produces a framework that is attractive to many health care professionals in a variety of health care settings. The model has provided clear, comprehensive guidelines for both nursing education and practice in a variety of settings, and perhaps this is its primary contribution to nursing knowledge. Although the concepts within the guidelines are clearly explicated, and many applications of the theory have been published, little research explicitly derived from this model has been published to date. This is necessary if validity is to be established.

6. Theories can be utilized by the practitioners to guide and improve their practice. One of the most significant attributes of the Neuman model is the assessment/intervention instrument together with comprehensive guidelines for its use with the nursing process. These guidelines have provided a practical resource for many nursing practitioners and have been used extensively in a variety of settings in nursing practice, education, and administration. As Neuman points out, this multidimensional model may indeed in the future provide the "unifying" force tying together various health-related theories and behaviors, thus assisting in clarifying the relationship of variables within nursing practice.[45]

With the current emphasis on self-help, primary prevention, and increasing consumer awareness of the importance of health promotion, health care workers are moving into the arena of wellness-focused care. This is especially true of the nurse moving from illness-oriented activities to wellness-oriented settings such as clinics and ambulatory care settings. Thus, the Neuman model is very congruent with today's health care philosophies and offers some direction in wellness settings.

7. Theories must be consistent with other validated theories, laws, and principles but will leave open unanswered questions that need to be investigated. In general, there is no direct conflict with other theories. There is, however, a lack of specificity in systems concepts such as "feedback" and the exact nature of the total system "boundaries," which are indirectly addressed throughout the model. The solving of problems in these areas could be facilitated with greater exploration and clarification of definitions. Caplan's theory of the three levels of prevention as intervention leaves an interesting area to be explored.[46] Indeed, Neuman suggests exploration of how to recognize and deal with the impact of environmental forces on the nursing profession in order to develop a holistic nursing posture.[47]

SUMMARY AND CONCLUSIONS

Conceptual models are imperative to the development of nursing as a profession. Neuman's total person approach to health care is one such model. In essence, she presents an approach to viewing the person's perception of the stressors affecting the "parts" of the whole individual in constant interaction with the environment. The model is a multidimensional, total unit approach, one that can be used to describe an individual, a group, or an entire community. Inasmuch as the model emphasizes the total person, it transcends the nursing model to become a health care model, applicable to all health care disciplines.[48]

Although Neuman describes nursing as a "unique" profession, this is not clearly documented in her writings. As Venable points out, "the lack of a unique role for nursing is not necessarily seen as a detriment but rather as a call for reexamination of traditionally defined roles assigned to health care workers in general."[49]

Even though the model is interdisciplinary, it certainly has universal applicability to nursing. One of its greatest strengths is the clear direction it gives for interventions through primary, secondary, and tertiary prevention. Although society's expectation of the nursing role is tied very specifically to certain behavior in various levels of prevention (i.e., primary: community health; secondary: acute care; and tertiary: limited settings), in actuality all three levels are important aspects of care in all nursing settings. Primary and tertiary prevention will have more social congruence as society becomes increasingly aware of the emerging role of the nurse as a nucleus of the health care system.

Another strength of this model is its flexibility as a stimulus-response system model. This flexibility has lent itself to use in a variety of nursing settings as documented in Neuman's text and current use of the model.

The model has great potential for laying the groundwork for the formation of a theory, and for testing interrelationships between nursing theory, nursing research, and nursing practice.[50] Its increasing use in a variety of settings is impressive.

The primary contribution of this model has been pragmatic—in that it is a useful guide for nursing education, nursing practice, and in diverse settings. It can be useful to other service disciplines and therein lies the two-edged sword. The applicability of the model to all health disciplines could foster a common perspective and thereby fail to point out the distinctive contribution of nursing, or any other health discipline, to health care.[51]

REFERENCES

1.   Neuman, B. Family Intervention Using the Betty Neuman Health Care Systems Model, in *Family Health: A Theoretical Approach to Nursing Care*, Clements, I. & Roberts, F.B., eds., New York: Wiley, 1983, pp. 239–40.

2.   Neuman, B.M. & Young, R.J. A Model for Teaching Total Person Approach to Patient Problems, *Nursing Research*, 1972, *21*, 264–69.

3.   Neuman, B. The Betty Neuman Health-Care Systems Model: A Total Person Approach to Patient Problems, in Riehl, J.P. & Roy, Sr. C., eds., *Conceptual Models for Nursing Practice*, New York: Appleton-Century-Crofts, 1974 and 1980.

4.   Neuman, B. *The Neuman Systems Model*. Norwalk, Conn.: Appleton & Lange, 1989.

5.   Fawcett, J. Analysis and Evaluation of the Neuman Systems Model, in Neuman, B. *The Neuman Systems Model*. Norwalk, Conn.: Appleton & Lange, 1989, p. 67.

6.(a) Rogers, M.E. *An Introduction to the Theoretical Basis of Nursing*, Philadelphia: F.A. Davis Co., 1970.

6.(b) Orem, D.E. *Nursing: Concepts of Practice*, New York: McGraw-Hill, 1971.

6.(c) King, I.M. *Toward a Theory for Nursing*, New York: Wiley, 1971.

7. Peterson, C.J. Questions Frequently Asked about the Development of a Conceptual Framework, *Journal of Nursing Education*, April 1977.

8. de Chardin, P.T. *The Phenomenon of Man,* London: Collins, 1955.

9. Cornu, A. *The Origins of Marxist Thought,* Springfield, Ill.: Charles C. Thomas, Publisher, 1957.

10. Edelson, M. *Sociotherapy and Psychotherapy,* Chicago: University of Chicago Press, 1970.

11. Selye, H. *The Physiology and Pathology of Exposure to Stress,* Montreal: ACTA, Inc., 1950.

12. von Bertalanffy, L. *General System Theory,* New York: George Braziller, Inc., 1968.

13. Caplan, G. *Principles of Preventive Psychiatry,* New York: Basic Books, Inc., 1964.

14. Craddock, R.B. & Stanhope, M.K. The Neuman Health-Care Systems Model: Recommended Adaptation, in Riehl, J.P. & Roy, C., eds., *Conceptual Models for Nursing Practice* (2nd ed.), New York: Appleton-Century-Crofts, 1980, p. 159.

15. Neuman, The Betty Neuman Health Care Systems Model, p. 119.

16.(a) Neuman, *The Neuman Systems Model,* p. 35.

16.(b) Venable, J.F. The Neuman Health-Care Systems Model: An Analysis, in Riehl, J.P. & Roy, C., eds., *Conceptual Models for Nursing Practice* (2nd ed.), New York: Appleton-Century-Crofts, 1980, p. 136.

17. Neuman, *The Neuman Systems Model,* pp. 17, 21–22.

18. Lecture notes, Athens, Ohio, 1986.

19. Buchanan, B. Human Environment Interaction: A Modification of the Neuman Systems Model for Aggregates, Families, and the Community, *Public Health Nursing,* 1987, *4,* 52–64.

20. Ibid, 53.

21. Venable, The Neuman Health-Care Systems Model, p. 136.

22. Neuman, B. *The Neuman Systems Model: Application to Nursing Education and Practice,* Norwalk, Conn: Appleton-Century-Crofts, 1982, p. 16.

23. Torres, G. *Theoretical Foundation of Nursing,* Norwalk, CT: Appleton-Century-Crofts, 1986, pp. 150–151.

24. Neuman, *The Neuman Systems Model: Application,* p. 1.

25. Neuman, *The Neuman Systems Model,* p. 32.

26. Mayers, M.G. *A Systematic Approach to the Nursing Care Plan* (2nd ed.), New York: Appleton-Century-Crofts, 1978, p. 3.

27. Fawcett and others, A Framework for Analysis, and Evaluation of Conceptual Models of Nursing with Analysis and Evaluation of the Neuman Systems Model, in Neuman, B. *The Neuman Systems Model: Application to Nursing Education and Practice, Norwalk, Conn: Appleton-Century-Crofts, 1982, p. 37.*

28. Neuman, *The Neuman Systems Model,* p. 9.

29. Whall, A.L. Congruence between Existing Theories of Family Functioning and Nursing Theories, *Advances in Nursing Science,* 1980, *3,* 59–67.

30. Neuman, *The Neuman Systems Model: Application,* p. 10.

31. Fawcett and others, A Framework for Analysis, p. 37.

32. Neuman, *The Neuman Systems Model,* p. 16–17.

33. Mayers, *A Systematic Approach,* p. 2.

34. Fawcett, A Framework for Analysis, p. 72.
35. Neuman, The Betty Neuman Health-Care Systems Model, in Riehl and Roy, *Conceptual Models,* (2nd ed.), 1980, pp. 127–31.
36. Ibid, 125.
37. Fawcett, A Framework for Analysis, p. 77.
38. Fawcett, J. & Downs, F.S. *The Relationship of Theory and Research* Norwalk, Conn.: Appleton-Century-Crofts, 1986, pp. 87–88.
39. Fawcett, A Framework for Analysis, p. 76.
40. Ibid, 77–78.
41. Neuman, *The Neuman Systems Model.*
42. Stevens, B. *Nursing Theory: Analysis, Application and Evaluation* (2nd ed.), Boston: Little, Brown & Co., 1984, p. 229.
43. Fawcett and others, A Framework for Analysis, p. 41.
44. Neuman, *The Neuman Systems Model.*
45. Neuman, The Betty Neuman Health Care Systems Model, p. 125.
46. Caplan, *Principles of Preventive Psychiatry.*
47. Neuman, *The Neuman Systems Model,* p. 21.
48. Venable, The Neuman Health-Care Systems Model, p. 140.
49. Ibid, 141.
50. Koffman, M.K. From Model to Theory Construction, in Neuman, B. *The Neuman Systems Model: Application to Nursing Education and Practice,* Norwalk, Conn.: Appleton-Century-Crofts, 1982, p. 48.
51. Fawcett, A Framework for Analysis, p. 87.

CHAPTER 17

Josephine E. Paterson and Loretta T. Zderad

Susan G. Praeger
Christina R. Hogarth

Josephine E. Paterson and Loretta T. Zderad's book, Humanistic Nursing, *was published in 1976.[1] Josephine Paterson is a clinical nurse specialist at the Northport Veterans Administration Medical Center at Northport, New York. She is a graduate of Lenox Hill Hospital School of Nursing and St. John's University. She received her master's degree from Johns Hopkins School of Hygiene and Public Health, Baltimore, Maryland. Her Doctor of Nurse Science is from Boston University School of Nursing, Boston, Massachusetts, where she specialized in mental health and psychiatric nursing. Dr. Paterson has conceptualized and taught humanistic nursing to graduate students, faculty, and staff in a variety of settings. She is also currently on the faculty of the State University of New York at Stonybrook.*

Loretta T. Zderad is presently the Associate Chief for Nursing Education at the Northport Veterans Administration Medical Center, Northport, New York. She is a graduate of St. Bernard's Hospital School of Nursing and of Loyola University. She received her Master of Science degree from Catholic University, Washington, D.C. and a Doctor of Philosophy from Georgetown University, Washington, D.C. She has taught in several universities and has led groups on humanistic nursing. Dr. Zderad also serves on the faculty of the State University of New York at Stonybrook.

Josephine E. Paterson and Loretta T. Zderad have described what they call a "humanistic nursing practice" theory in several publications and presentations. It is a practice theory because they believe that the theory of a science of nursing develops from the lived experiences of the nurse and the nursed in the practice of nursing. Theory, then, becomes a response to the phenomenological experience. R.D. Laing is quoted as saying that "theory is the articulated vision of experience."[2] This means that theory becomes the philosophical perspective that is derived from the nurse's existential encounter in the health care world.

Humanistic nursing is an expression of the humanistic psychology, often called the "third force" in psychology because it was seen as an alternative response to the two dominant psychological views. Freudian psychology was seen as being limited in its orientation toward the sick personality, and behavioral psychology was seen as being too mechanistically oriented.[3] The humanistic orientation tries to take a broader view of the potential of human beings and, rather than trying to supplant other views, it is aimed toward supplementing them.[4]

There is no simple way to define the essence of humanistic nursing because it is concerned with the phenomenological experiences of individuals, the exploration of human experiences. It is rooted in existential thought.

Existentialism is a philosophical approach to understanding life. Individuals are faced with possibilities in choosing. These choices determine the direction and meaning of one's life. Like humanistic psychology, existentialism was a response to the dominant philosophies of positivism and determinism. A philosophical approach of the nineteenth century found in the writings of Kierkegaard and Nietzsche, it emerged in popularity during the twentieth century with two world wars and the threat of nuclear destruction as major social concerns.[5] Individuals needed to understand life in personally relevant terms.

The early writings provided a basis for viewing human existence in individually meaningful terms. By having the opportunity for choice, each act we choose is significant and gives meaning to our lives. One of the criticisms leveled against existentialism has been that it presents a despairing view of life.[6] Since individuals are faced with freedom of choice, there is always the possibility for making errors. Consequently, individuals experience dread as well as hope in the possible consequences of their actions.

According to Corey, there are several propositions that can be drawn from existential thought that have relevance for the helping professions. Corey says that existentialism identifies individuals as: (1) having the capacity for self-awareness; (2) having freedom and responsibility; (3) striving to find their own identity while being in relationship with others; (4) being involved in a search for meaning in life; (5) having to experience anxiety or dread if they are going to assume responsibility for their own lives; and, finally, (6) being aware of the reality of death in order to experience the significance of living.[7] Consequently, we are living in a world of many possibilities and the responsibility for making the most out of this existence rests within each of us. As a philosophy, existentialism is particularly applicable to nursing within the framework of holistic health because of the emphasis on self-determination, free choice, and self-responsibility.

Phenomenology, the study of the meaning of phenomenon to a particular individual, is often thought to have had a significant influence on the development of existentialism because existentialism requires an analysis of the human situation from the perspective of the individual's own experience.[8] When combined with humanism into an existential–phenomenological–humanistic approach, we are referring to a reverence for life that values the need for human interaction in order to determine the meaning which comes from the individual's unique way of experiencing the world. In other words, while we are ultimately alone in choosing the paths our lives will take, we can find meaning in sharing our experiences with others who are also facing the uncertain choices of daily living.

That Paterson and Zderad have been influenced by the writings of existentialists, humanistic psychologists, and phenomenologists is seen in their emphasis on the meaning of life as it is lived, the nature of dialogue, and the importance of the perceptual field. The influence of scholars, such as Buber,[9] Marcel,[10a,10b] Desan,[11] Nietzsche,[12a,12b] Hesse,[13] deChardin,[14] Jung,[15] and Bergson[16] is readily apparent in their writing. Their work, *Humanistic Nursing*, is a result of years of experience in clinical nursing, reflection, and exploration of these experiences as they have been lived with psychiatric clients, students, nurses, and other helping professionals.[17]

HUMANISTIC NURSING THEORY AND THE FOUR MAJOR CONCEPTS

Human Beings

In humanistic nursing practice theory, human beings are viewed from an existential framework of becoming through choices. "Man is an individual being necessarily related to other men in time and space. As every man is beholden to other men for his birth and development, interdependence is inherent in the human situation, . . . [and] human existence is coexistence."[18] Human beings are characterized as being capable, open to options, valuing, and the unique manifestation of their past, present, and future. It is through relationships with others that the human being becomes; this, in turn, allows for each person's unique individuality to become actualized.[18]

Health

Health is seen as a matter of personal survival, as a quality of living and dying. It is described as more than the absence of disease. Individuals have the potential for well-being, but also for more-being. Well-being implies a steady state, whereas more-being refers to being in the process of becoming all that is humanly possible.[19]

By understanding the existential premise of this theory, it becomes apparent that health is a process of finding meaning in life. Health is experienced in the process of living, of being involved in each moment. Paterson and Zderad suggest throughout their text that we become more (more-being) by being in relationships with each other. When we relate authentically to another, we are experiencing health. This conceptualization of health implies that disease, medical diagnosis, or any form of labeling does little to determine a person's capacity for health. Health can be found in a person's willingness to be open to the experiences of life regardless of his or her physical, social, spiritual, cognitive, or emotional status.

Nursing

Nursing, then, is seen within the human context. It is a nurturing response of one person to another in a time of need that aims toward the development of well-being and more-being. Nursing works toward this aim by helping to increase the possibility of making responsible choices, since this is how human beings are able to become. "The nursing situation is a particular kind of human situation in which the interhuman relating is purposely directed toward nurturing the well-being or more-being of a person with perceived needs related to the health–illness quality of living."[20] Nursing is concerned with the individual's unique being and striving toward becoming. Nursing focuses on the whole and looks beyond the categorizations of the parts. When a person is ill and the body is manifesting certain changes, these changes influence the person's world and the experience of being in the world. The client's perspective of the world is a vital consideration in nursing.

> Nursing implies a special kind of meeting of human persons. It occurs in response to a perceived need related to the health–illness quality of the human condition. Within that domain, which is shared by other health professions, nursing is directed toward the goal of nurturing well-being and more-being (human potential). Nursing, therefore does not involve a merely fortuitous encounter but rather one in which there is purposeful call and response. In this vein, humanistic nursing may be considered as a special kind of lived dialogue.[21]

Nursing is seen as a unique blend of theory and methodology. The theory may be articulated from the open framework that is derived from the human situation. This framework can be used to suggest the possible dimensions of humanistic nursing practice. Theory cannot exist without the practice of nursing, for it depends on the experience of nursing and on the reflecting of that experience. It is this practice of nursing, its methodology, that Paterson and Zderad describe as a unique blend of art and science. In an attempt to be accepted among other empirical disciplines, it is suggested that nurses have downplayed the art of nursing. However, science and art both play critical roles in humanistic nursing. If one thinks of the rules that we follow (thermoregulation, fluid and electrolyte balance, stages of grieving, growth and development) as our science, we can see that these rules guide us. They give us directions to our nursing practice, but all of those laws, principles, and theories remain meaningless unless they are applied to living situations.[22] How a nurse uses theory in response to knowing a client is the art of nursing. The art of nursing is embodied in the interaction between the nurse and the client. Like all art, that interaction is often meaningful, effective, and capable of leaving a lasting impression. Nursing, as an art, is being able to use theories within the context of life as people struggle to become all that they are capable of becoming.

The elements of the framework for humanistic nursing, as stated by Paterson and Zderad, may be described as follows:

> Incarnate men (patient and nurse) meeting (being and becoming) in a goal-directed (nurturing well-being and more-being) intersubjective transaction (being with and doing with) occurring in time and space (as measured and as lived by patient and nurse) in a world of men and things.[23]

In order to use this framework for a nursing practice theory, the authors have suggested three concepts that together provide the basis (or components) of nursing. These concepts are dialogue, community, and phenomenologic nursology. By coming together through dialogue, a community is formed through which nursing strives to nurture and comfort.

Dialogue. Nursing is a lived dialogue. It is the nurse–nursed relating creatively. Humans need nursing. Nurses need to nurse. Nursing is an intersubjective experience in which there is real sharing. Involved in this dialogue are meeting, relating, presence, and a call and response.[24]

Meeting is the coming together of human beings and is characterized by the expectation that there will be a nurse and a nursed. Factors that influence this meeting are feelings that are aroused by the anticipation of the meeting, the amount of control that the nurse or client has in coming together, the uniqueness of the nurse and the client, and the decision for disclosure and enclosure with the other.

Relating refers to the process of nurse–nursed "doing" with each other; it means being with the other. Two ways of relating are described that distinguish the human situation. We are able to relate as subject to object as well as subject to subject. "Both types of relationships are essential for genuine human existence."[25] Subject–object relating refers to how human beings use objects and know others through abstractions, conceptualizations, categorizing, labeling, etc. Subject–subject relating occurs when two persons are open to each other as fully human. The "I–Thou" relationship described by Martin Buber provides the opportunity to develop this unique potential.[26]

> Through the scientific objective approach, that is, subject–object relating, it is possible to gain certain knowledge about a person; through intersubjective, that is, subject–subject relating, it is possible to know a person in his unique individuality. Thus, both subject–subject and subject–object relationships are essential to the clinical nursing process. Both are integral elements of humanistic nursing.[27]

Presence is the quality of being open, receptive, ready, and available to another person in a reciprocal manner. Presence necessitates being open to the whole of the nursing experience; this is behavior that is difficult to achieve when the nurse at times is required to focus on specific details of the client's body or behavior. "Man is an embodied being, and the nurse, in nurturing the patient's well-being and more-being, must relate to him and his body in their mysterious interrelatedness."[28]

Call and response is an indication of the complex nature of the lived dialogue. Call and response are transactional, sequential, and simultaneous. Nurses and clients call and respond to each other, and this occurs both verbally and nonverbally. This call and response has the potential to be "all-at-once." Paterson and Zderad describe the "all-at-once" as nurses being able to relate to the subjective and objective aspects of the lived situation simultaneously. Despite the fact that we can only express this experience either verbally or in writing in succession, it is paradoxically occurring simultaneously for the nurse.[29]

It is through nursing acts that the dialogue of nursing is lived. The meaning of those acts to the nurse and to the client may differ and may act as a potential catalyst for effecting change in the dialogue.

When considering nursing as a lived dialogue, it is necessary to take into account the situation in which it occurs—the real world of other human beings and things within a framework of time and space.

Community. The phenomenon of community is the second component critical to humanistic nursing practice theory. It is two or more persons striving together, living–dying all at once. To understand community is to recognize and value uniqueness. Humanistic nursing leads to community; it occurs within a community and is affected by community. It is through the intersubjective sharing of meaning in community that human beings are comforted and nurtured. Community is the experience of persons, and it is through community, persons relating to others, that it is possible to become.[30a,30b] This component represents the strong humanistic influence of the theory. People find meaning in their existence by sharing and relating to others. Paterson and Zderad consider community as the "We" that occurs with clients, families, professional colleagues, and other health care providers.[31]

Phenomenologic nursology. Nursing, its practice and theory, would not be complete without a methodology. This methodology has been presented as phenomenologic nursology. There are five phases in this phenomenologic approach to nursing, as discussed below.

1. *Preparation of the nurse knower for coming to know.* The nurse is ever prepared and striving to be open and caring. This involves learning to take risks, being open to experiences, to one's own view of the world, and to another's perceptual framework. In order to achieve this, the nurse needs to be exposed to a wide range of experiences. Nurses can be prepared for this by immersing themselves in studies

in the humanities where different views about the nature of being are expressed. Individual experiences, as a person and a nurse, are valid and important. The wider the range of experiences that the nurse has, the wider the possibility for knowing. Relating the experiences of human beings in literature and the other arts to the nurse's experience with clients will open the way for knowing individuals in the nursing situation. Self-knowledge, the "authenticity with self," is important to knowing and can be facilitated through clinical supervision and different forms of personal growth therapy.[32]

2. *Nurse knowing the other intuitively.* This phase is the merging of the self with the rhythmic spirit of the other. Intuitive knowing of the other requires getting "inside" the other, into the rhythm of the other's experience, which results in a special, difficult to express, knowledge of the other. Intuitive knowing presumes the I–Thou relationship described by Buber.[33] It also presumes a phenomenological approach: being open to the meaning of the experience for the other. In order for the nurse to be able to intuitively grasp the phenomenon of a nursing situation, several steps can be taken to facilitate one's openness. Paterson and Zderad suggest that we go into the nursing situation without any preconceived notions, trying to avoid expectations, labeling, and judgments. It is important first to know what one's preconceptions are by being aware of one's philosophical and theoretical biases. Being aware of nursing routines and how they can dull our sensitivities can enhance one's perspective. All of these activities require a conscious effort on the part of the nurse toward self-awareness. By doing this, however, nurses can be open to all the nursing situation and will be better able to grasp intuitively the subtle nuances involved in human interaction.[34]

3. *Nurse knowing the other scientifically.* This phase implies a separateness from what is known. It requires taking the all-at-once phenomena known intuitively and looking at them, mulling them over, analyzing, sorting, comparing, contrasting, relating, interpreting, giving a name to, and categorizing them.[35] This is taking the I–Thou and reflecting on it as an "it." Paterson says, "The challenge of communicating a lived nursing reality demands authenticity with the self and rigorous effort in the selection of words, phrases, and precise grammar."[36]

4. *Nurse complementarily synthesizing known others.* This phase involves relating, comparing, and contrasting what occurs in nursing situations to enlarge one's understanding of nursing. The nurse compares and synthesizes multiple known realities and arrives at an expanded view. The nurse allows a dialogue between the realities and permits differences.[36] In this phase, the nurse uses not only personal experience but also the rich theoretical foundation of education and practice in order to put the clinical situation in perspective.

5. *Succession within the nurse from the many to the paradoxical one.* The fifth phase evolves from the descriptive process of a lived phenomenon. It is the articulated vision of experience that becomes expressed in a coherent whole. This phase is the process of refining the intuitive grasp achieved before, struggling with the known realities, and making an intuitive leap toward truth, thus forming a new hypothetical construct. Since the multiple realities and known truths are part of the nurse, the new truth is really an expression of the knower in abstract or conceptual terms beyond the individual data. It is a truth beyond the synthesis of the whole. So, the paradox rests in the fact that the nurse starts with a general notion, an intuitive grasp; then studies it, compares, contrasts, and synthesizes it in order to arrive at a truth that is uniquely personal but has meaning for all: a descriptive theoretical construct of nursing.

These last three phases (analysis, synthesis, and description) involve many of the same techniques. In each of these phases, the nurse might compare and contrast the phenomena. Commonalities in different experiences could be explored as well as the relationship between variables in the clinical situation. It would also be important to determine what distinguishes one phenomenon from another. Other techniques for analyzing, synthesizing, and describing a nursing phenomenon include stating what it is not, using analogy or metaphor. These techniques will help the nurse better understand the meaning of the experience.[37]

PHENOMENOLOGIC NURSOLOGY AND THE NURSING PROCESS

Phenomenologic nursology as developed by Paterson and Zderad is a methodology for understanding and describing nursing situations. It is a method of inquiry, as is the problem-solving approach of the nursing process. Phenomenologic nursology is a method of seeking to understand the nurse–nursed experience so that the nurse can be with the nursed in a human and therefore healing manner. The nursing process assumes the presence of a nursing problem that the nurse and client will solve together. Phenomenologic nursology assumes a perceived health need by an individual who is involved in interaction with a health care provider.

Phenomenology is a descriptive process. Theory development begins with description, and in the case of phenomenological development, the process is a "progressive intellectual intuition by which one isolates and identifies the essence."[38] Phenomenology is not concerned specifically with facts; it assumes that facts exist. Rather, it is concerned with the nature of the facts and what they mean to the individual. Phenomenology describes phenomena but does not atttempt to explain or predict their occurrence.

Nursing process and nursology are similar in many aspects. Both methodologies use a systematic approach to client interaction.

The first step of the nursing process is *assessment*. Assessment includes a collection of subjective and objective data about an individual obtained through observation, interaction with the client, and information from other sources such as laboratory studies. Phenomenologic nursology includes the collection of subjective and objective data but is broader in scope than what is traditionally meant by assessment.

Preparation of the nurse knower for coming to know as the first phase of phenomenologic nursology can be seen as a prerequisite similar to but distinct from the nursing process. Almost all nurses are educated in the humanities and sciences before beginning nursing practice in the clinical situation. The nursing process assumes that the individual undertaking the process is educated in the bio–psycho–spiritual needs of the individual. Phenomenologic nursology makes these same assumptions but also assumes that the nurse has a sensitivity to and knowledge of the human condition as well as self-knowledge. The humanistic theory and practice of nursing require that the practitioner be able to subjectively experience the other. As mentioned earlier, the nursing student can be helped to understand another's situation by studying the humanities and fine arts. Experiencing life events, through literature, drama, and the arts, enriches the student's understanding of human experiences such as love, joy, loneliness, suffering, and death. The use of guided imagery and other exercises are also helpful in developing empathy, the ability to experience the other. The development of self-awareness is important if the nurse expects to encounter others in dialogue. This can be enhanced through journaling, working in small groups, and through meditation.

Nurse knowing the other intuitively also occurs prior to the traditional assessment phase of the nursing process, even though intuition is indeed a kind of initial assessment. This phase is characterized by a "taking in" of the client in the human situation, the empathic encounter, the beginning of the I–Thou relationship wherein the nurse understands the other's experience all-at-once. It is an intuitive grasp of the other's situation.[39] The use of intuition is a significant aspect of assessment. Although intuition is not a new tool in nursing, its respectability has often been denied. In the effort to establish itself as a profession, nursing has been using an increasingly scientific, objective approach to the study of nursing and the individuals who use nursing services. The humanistic nurse, however, believes that the subjective experience of human beings is as valid as the objective experience that can be measured.

The assessment and early analysis phases of the nursing process can be compared to the *nurse knowing the other scientifically*. This phase of nursology includes the more familiar method of looking at a phenomenon from many aspects: comparing, classifying, looking for themes in relationships and among the parts. Dividing persons into biological, psychological, social, and spiritual parts is an example of classifying data. It is important to understand, in the phenomenologic method of nursology, that the call comes first, followed by intuition, then assessment, and then analysis. In the problem-solving method, a problem statement by the client is followed by scientific data collection organized by parts, and intuition is not included in the assessment or analysis.

The later stages of analysis in the nursing process are quite similar to the phase in nursology called *nurse complementarily synthesizing known others*. During the analysis portion of the nursing process, as described earlier, the nurse compares the data with other known realities such as developmental stages, Maslow's hierarchy of needs,[40] and physiologic principles. In nursology, the nurse compares "multiple known realities" with the data and the experience of the client. In other words, the nurse examines the data and experience of the client in light of scientific and subjective knowledge and then compares, contrasts, and ultimately synthesizes to an expanded view.[41] Comparisons do occur in the phenomenologic method, but the purpose of the comparisons is directed toward identifying relationships and patterns with much consideration given to opposites and polarities. The phenomenologist synthesizes opposites and patterns into a larger concept, whereas the problem solver chooses a pattern and decides whether it is a problem or not.[42]

Diagnosis refers to the step of the nursing process wherein the nurse makes a problem statement. The nurse collects data regarding the client's stated need, then analyzes the data by classifying it, comparing it to known theory and principles, and finally arriving at a conclusion that is a statement of the problem. *Succession within the nurse from the many to the paradoxical one* can be compared to the stage of identifying a diagnosis. After synthesizing the ideas, data, and experience, the nurse reaches a conclusion that is broader than the classifications and reflects the experience of the client as well as the nurse's initial intuitive grasp of the situation. This conclusion has meaning for all. The conclusion or truth is really the formation of a concept as Paterson and Zderad intended it, not the formation of a diagnosis or patient problem.[43]

The *planning* and *implementation* phases of the nursing process describe a goal or outcome to be reached by the client with steps (objectives) to be accomplished toward the goal. Specific nurse and client actions are spelled out in detail. Phenomenologic nursology does not describe the formation of a goal-directed nursing care plan. Humanistic nursing is concerned with being with another who is in need. The goal of more-being or well-being is accomplished through dialogue. In the dialogue between nurse and nursed, there is the *meeting* and the *presence* of the nurse for the other, and the *call* and *response* between the nurse and the nursed, the I–Thou relationship. This is the therapeutic relationship. Paterson and Zderad say that this relationship takes place in the nursing situation in the real world; however, they do not elaborate on incorporating the "doing" aspects of nursing into the dialogue.

The theory evolved from the authors' psychiatric nursing practice and experience where the "doing" is the relationship. However, glimpses of how they have practiced humanistic nursing are available in the rich descriptions of clinical experiences throughout the text. Examples of using touch, participating in a task such as shampooing, and spending time with clients demonstrate that any nursing interaction with a client can be a vehicle for nurturing more-being.

The *evaluation* phase of the nursing process is deciding whether the client's behavior has changed as measured by the goals and objectives. The behavior changes result from the actions of the nurse and client. By nature of being humanistic, the concern is not with the resultant behavior, but with the meaning of the experience for the client. The humanistic nurse might see a change in the client's perspective of his or her experience. A client who is able to make choices about health care activities and assume responsibility for those choices would be able to find meaning in life. By doing this with a nurse, the client would have the opportunity to affirm the humanness of the situation from his or her own perspective, resulting in personal growth, more-being, or health. For example, humanistic nursing may involve being-with another who is grieving, rather than using a series of strategies designed to assist a person toward resolution of grief work. Being-with a person who is grieving in an I–Thou relationship expands the individual's opportunities for more-being so that sadness may be shared with another. This may result in the client feeling more able to make choices and continue with life's demands. An outcome of nursing process, in contrast, may be that the client demonstrates an activity that indicates grieving is progressing, for instance, by returning to school or work.

PATERSON AND ZDERAD'S WORK AND THE CHARACTERISTICS OF A THEORY

Paterson and Zderad say that nursing is a lived dialogue between the nurse and the nursed directed toward the goal of nurturing well-being and more-being in the everyday world of men and things.[44] The authors have interrelated the four concepts of human beings, health, nursing, and society so that a different way of looking at the phenomenon of nursing (characteristic 1) has been created for using the existential philosophy and the phenomenological methodology within a humanistic framework. Nursing is described as an intersubjective transaction which has a new and different description of nursing although similar in concept to other nursing theories. Theories describe, explain, or predict phenomena. Humanistic nursing theory is descriptive; the phenomenological approach is a descriptive method.

Humanistic nursing theory is logical (characteristic 2) because Paterson and Zderad provide a framework and methodology for nursing practice. Also, the ideas and concepts fit together in a meaningful way.

Humanistic nursing theory is not simple; indeed it is somewhat difficult to grasp unless the nurse is familiar with existential philosophy and phenomenology. The theory focuses on the dialogue between the nurse and nursed as a unique encounter between two people. Knowledge gained by repeated study of this encounter will provide a generalizable concept (characteristic 3). In fact, the final step of nursology is the expression of a concept. Thus the theory is generalizable.

Paterson and Zderad's theory provides a basis for hypotheses that can be tested (characteristic 4). The authors describe several replications of the methodology and present numerous concepts that could be examined.[45] Since it is testable, phenomenologic nursology is an excellent medium for concept and theory development (characteristic 5).

Humanistic nursing theory, including phenomenologic nursology, can certainly be utilized by nurses to guide and improve practice (characteristic 6). Although nurses may find the concepts new at first, a study of humanistic psychology and existential philosophy will facilitate an understanding of the concepts and an appreciation of human potential.

Humanistic nursing theory is consistent with existentialism, humanistic psychology, and phenomenology upon which it is based (characteristic 7). Because the theory is descriptive and generalizable, it can be applied in any nursing situation and leaves the nursing situation always open for examination.

STRENGTHS AND LIMITATIONS

There are several notable strengths of this theory. The methodology is well developed and the concepts are fully described within the parameters of existential philosophy, phenomenology, and nursing. This theory broadens the possibilities for explaining and describing nursing. The study of human beings and nursing using this phenomenological method is a valid approach that enhances knowledge of nursing. An important contribution of this theory is that the methodology leads to concept formation, the basis of theory and the springboard of new inquiry. The theory provides a unique, unusual approach to the study of nursing. Another strength is the strong nursing focus. The theory developed from the lived experiences of clinical nurses and reflects that nursing perspective.

Reading the text provides an opportunity to experience the authors' own grappling with theory development. The text is written with a readable style that is often poetic in quality. While the authors tend to combine words into broader hyphenated meanings, they attempt to explain each term in a variety of ways. One of the joys of this text is sitting down to the individual essays and experiencing the possibilities that the authors suggest are available in nursing. Each chapter is inspiring and stimulates creative ideas for clinical practice. Some readers might find the text too intuitive and lacking in concrete imperatives. It is not a handy reference text that can be used to quickly solve clinical practice problems. There are no formulas for successful nursing in their theory. This is as it should be, for the theory posits that nursing is interactive and based on the moment of the interaction.

Unfortunately, some nurses might need to be well read in the humanities, particularly philosophy, in order to understand the language and the existential tone. Another difficulty may occur for new practitioners regarding the functional aspects of nursing. Nursology refers to the interaction between two people and does not address how to integrate dialogue with tasks. Since it is essentially descriptive, humanistic nursing theory provides challenges for quantitative validation that some may view as a limitation, although this would be of limited concern to a humanistic nurse or philosopher who is concerned with description.

REFERENCES

1. Paterson, J. & Zderad, L. *Humanistic Nursing*, New York: Wiley, 1976.
2. Zderad, L.T. From Hear-and-Now to Theory: Reflections on 'How', *Theory Development: What, Why, How?*, New York: National League for Nursing, 1978, p. 45.
3. Maslow, A.H. *Toward a Psychology of Being* (2nd ed.), New York: Van Nostrand Reinhold Company, 1968, pp. iii–v.
4. Bugental, J.F.T. The Third Force in Psychology, *Humanistic Psychology: A Sourcebook*, in Welch, D., Tate, G., & Richards, F., eds., Buffalo, N.Y.: Prometheus Books, 1978, p. 16.
5. Schrader, Jr., G.A. Existential Philosophy: Resurgent Humanism, *Existential Philosophers: Kierkegaard to Merleau-Ponty*, in Schrader, G. ed., New York: McGraw-Hill, 1967, p. 2.
6. Paterson & Zderad, *Humanistic Nursing*, p. 16.
7. Corey, G. *Theory and Practice of Counseling and Psychotherapy* (3rd ed.), Belmont, CA: Brooks/Cole Publishing Company, 1986, p. 78.
8. Shaffer, J.B.P. *Humanistic Psychology*, Englewood Cliffs, N.J.: Prentice-Hall, 1978, p. 21.
9. Buber, M. *The Knowledge of Man*, Friedman, M., ed., New York: Harper & Row, 1965.
10.(a) Marcel, G. *Being and Having: An Existentialist Diary*, New York: Harper Torchbooks, Harper & Row, 1965.
10.(b) Marcel, G. *The Philosophy of Existentialism*, trans. Marya Harari, New York; Citadel Press, 1956.
11. Desan, W. *The Planetary Man*, New York: Macmillan, 1972.
12.(a) Nietzsche, F. Beyond Good and Evil, trans. Helen Zimmern in *The Philosophy of Nietzsche*, New York: Random House, 1927.
12.(b) Nietsche, F. Thus Spoke Zarathustra, trans. Thomas Common in *The Philosophy of Nietzsche*, New York: Random House, 1927.
13. Hesse, H. *Steppenwolf*, New York: Holt, Rinehart & Winston, 1966.
14. de Chardin, T. *The Phenomenon of Man*, New York: Harper & Row, 1961.

15. Jung, C.G. *Modern Man in Search of a Soul,* New York: Harcourt, Brace & World, 1933.
16. Bergson, H. *The Creative Mind,* New York: The Philosophical Library, 1946.
17. Paterson & Zderad, *Humanistic Nursing,* p. 9.
18. Ibid, 16.
19. Paterson, J. & Zderad, L. Humanistic Nursing, presentation at the 2nd Annual Nurse Educator Conference, New York, N.Y., December 4–6, 1978.
20. Paterson & Zderad, *Humanistic Nursing,* p. 19.
21. Ibid, 26.
22. Ibid, 95.
23. Ibid, 23.
24. Paterson & Zderad, *Humanistic Nursing.*
25. Paterson & Zderad, *Humanistic Nursing,* p. 29.
26. Buber, M. *I and Thou,* (2nd ed.), New York: Charles Scribner's Sons, 1958, pp. 3–34.
27. Paterson & Zderad, *Humanistic Nursing,* p. 30.
28. Ibid, 32.
29. Ibid, 121.
30.(a) Paterson & Zderad, *Humanistic Nursing*
30.(b) Praeger, S.G. *Humanistic Nursing Education: Considerations and Proposals* project in lieu of dissertation, University of Northern Colorado, 1980, pp. 18–24.
31. Paterson & Zderad, *Humanistic Nursing,* p. 52.
32. Ibid, 63–66.
33. Buber, *I and Thou,* pp. 3–34.
34. Paterson & Zderad, *Humanistic Nursing,* pp. 86–87.
35. Ibid, 79.
36. Ibid, 79–80.
37. Ibid, 88–90.
38. Owens, T. *Phenomenology and Intersubjectivity,* The Hague, Netherlands: Martinus Nijhoff, 1970, p. 6.
39. Paterson & Zderad, *Humanistic Nursing,* p. 78.
40. Maslow, A. *Motivation and Personality,* New York: Harper & Row, 1954.
41. Paterson & Zderad, *Humanistic Nursing,* p. 80.
42. Oiler, C. The Phenomenological Approach to Nursing Research, *Nursing Research,* 1982, *31,* 180.
43. Paterson & Zderad, *Humanistic Nursing,* p. 23.
44. Ibid, 40.
45. Ibid, 57–70.

CHAPTER 18

Jean Watson

Barbara Talento

Jean Watson (b. 1940) received her BS in Nursing from the University of Colorado, Boulder; MS in Psychiatric-Mental Health Nursing from the University of Colorado, Denver; and her PhD in Educational Psychology from the University of Colorado, Boulder. She is currently Dean and Professor, University of Colorado School of Nursing, Denver. She has practiced nursing in private practice, as a clinical consultant, nurse researcher, faculty member, and educational administrator. She is a Fellow in the American Academy of Nursing and has received numerous other awards and honors including a Visiting Kellogg Fellowship at Western Australia Institute of Technology. She holds an honorary doctorate of Human Letters at Assumption College, Worcester, MA. Watson is the author of numerous articles, book chapters, and two books. Her research has been in the area of human caring and loss.

The foundation of Jean Watson's theory of nursing was published in 1979 in *Nursing: The Philosophy and Science of Caring.*[1] In 1985, with a re-release in 1988, her theory was published in *Nursing: Human Science and Human Care.*[2] Watson believes that the main focus in nursing is on carative factors which are derived from a humanistic perspective combined with a scientific knowledge base. For nurses to develop humanistic philosophies and value systems, a strong liberal arts background is necessary. This philosophy and value system, in turn, provide a solid foundation for the science of caring. A liberal arts base can assist nurses to expand their vision and views of the world, and to develop critical thinking skills. An expanded world view and critical thinking skills are needed in the science of caring which focuses on health promotion rather than on cure of disease.

According to Watson, curing disease is the domain of medicine. She asserts that the caring stance that nursing has always held is being threatened by the tasks and technology demands of the curative factors.[3] In Watson's works, one finds reference to existential humanists such as Maslow, Rogers, Heidegger and Erikson.[4a-4d] In addition, she uses the theories of Selye and Lazarus to delineate stress and caring, and the theories of Leininger and Henderson for nursing knowledge.[5a-5d] Overall, a humanistic value system undergirds her construction of the science of caring.

WATSON'S THEORY

Watson proposes seven assumptions about the science of caring and ten primary carative factors which form the framework for her theory. The basic assumptions are[6]:

1. Caring can be effectively demonstrated and practiced only interpersonally.
2. Caring consists of carative factors that result in the satisfaction of certain human needs.
3. Effective caring promotes health and individual or family growth.
4. Caring responses accept a person not only as he or she is now but as what he or she may become.
5. A caring environment is one that offers the development of potential while allowing the person to choose the best action for himself or herself at a given point in time.
6. Caring is more "healthogenic" than is curing. The practice of caring integrates biophysical knowledge with knowledge of human behavior to generate or promote health and to provide ministrations to those who are ill. A science of caring is therefore complementary to the science of curing.
7. The practice of caring is central to nursing.

Watson views caring as the most valuable attribute nursing has to offer to humanity, yet caring has, over time, received less emphasis than other aspects of the practice of nursing. She states:

> The human care role [in nursing] is threatened by increased medical technology, bureaucratic–managerial institutional constraints in a nuclear age society. At the same time there has been a proliferation of curing and radical treatment cure techniques often without regard to costs.[7]

In today's world, nursing seems to be responding to the various demands of the machinery with less consideration of the needs of the person attached to the machine. In Watson's view, the disease might be cured but illness would remain since, without caring, health is not attained. Caring is the essence of nursing and connotes responsiveness between the nurse and the person; the nurse coparticipates with the person. Watson contends that caring can assist the person to gain control, become knowledgeable, and promote health changes. In Watson's humanistic value system, there is a high regard for autonomy and freedom of choice. This leads to an emphasis on client self-knowledge and self-control and client as the person in charge.

The structure for the science of caring is built upon ten carative factors. These are[8]:

1. The formation of a humanistic–altruistic system of values
2. The instillation of faith–hope
3. The cultivation of sensitivity to one's self and to others
4. The development of a helping–trust relationship
5. The promotion and acceptance of the expression of positive and negative feelings
6. The systematic use of the scientific problem-solving method for decision making
7. The promotion of interpersonal teaching–learning
8. The provision for a supportive, protective and/or corrective mental, physical, sociocultural, and spiritual environment
9. Assistance with the gratification of human needs
10. The allowance for existential–phenomenological forces

Of these ten carative factors, the first three form the "philosophical foundation for the science of caring."[8] *The formation of a humanistic–altruistic value system* (carative factor 1) begins developmentally at an early age with values shared with parents. This value system is mediated through one's own life experiences, the learning one gains, and exposure to the humanities. Watson suggests that caring, based on humanistic values and altruistic behavior, can be developed through examination of one's own views, beliefs, interactions with various cultures, and personal growth experiences.[9] These are all perceived as necessary to the nurse's own maturation which then promotes altruistic behavior toward others.

Faith–hope (carative factor 2) is essential to both the carative and the curative processes. Nurses need to transcend the push toward acceptance of only Western medicine and assist the person in an understanding of alternatives such as meditation or the healing power of belief in self or in the spiritual.[10] Watson's emphasis on the spiritual, with the inclusion of the soul, is unusual in theory development.[11] When modern science has nothing further to offer the person, the nurse can continue to use faith–hope to provide a sense of well-being through those beliefs which are meaningful to the individual.

Cultivation of sensitivity to self and others (carative factor 3) explores the need of the nurse to begin to feel an emotion as it presents itself. It is only through development of one's own feelings that one can genuinely and sensitively interact with others. As nurses strive to increase their own sensitivity, they become more authentic. Becoming authentic encourages self-growth and self-actualization in both the nurse and those with whom the nurse interacts. A basic premise of Watson's is that[12]:

> A person's mind and emotions are windows to the soul. Nursing care can be and is physical, procedural, objective, and factual, but at the highest level of nursing the nurses' human care responses, the human care transactions, and the nurses' presence in the relationship transcend the physi-

cal and material world, bound in time and space, and make contact with the person's emotional and subjective world as the route to the inner self and the higher sense of self.

Further, she contends that nurses promote health and higher level functioning only when they form person-to-person relationships as opposed to manipulative relationships.[13]

In order to appreciate the remaining seven carative factors, one needs to understand that they spring from the foundation developed by these first three. Therefore, the nurse develops a humanistic–altruistic value system, believes in the instillation of faith–hope, and cultivates sensitivity to self and to others in order to develop a helping–trust relationship and the rest of the carative factors. One of the strongest tools the nurse can use in *establishing a helping-trust relationship* (carative factor 4) is a mode of communication which establishes rapport and caring. Watson uses the works of Rogers, Carkhuff, and Gazda to define the characteristics needed in the helping–trust relationship.[14a–14c] These characteristics are congruence, empathy, and warmth. Congruence implies that nurses are genuine in their interactions and do not put up facades; that nurses act in a manner which is open and honest. Empathy refers to the attempt that nurses make to tune into the feelings of their clients. Empathy may be described as "walking in another's moccasins," in that it allows the nurse to accept the client's feelings without responding defensively with anger or fear. Warmth refers to the positive acceptance of another. It is expressed most often by open body language, touch, and tone of voice.

Communication in this context includes verbal, nonverbal, and listening in a manner which connotes empathetic understanding. It is through this intense focus on communication that the nurse can center on clues and themes which can lead to an even greater depth of awareness for the person. One barrier in this process is that thoughts are often substituted for feelings which precludes the ability to reach deeper levels of awareness. *The expression of feelings, both positive and negative,* (carative factor 5) ought to be facilitated since, according to Watson, such expression improves one's level of awareness. "Feelings alter thoughts and behavior, and they need to be considered and allowed for in a caring relationship."[15] Indeed, if one can become aware of the feeling, one can often understand the behavior it engenders.

In carative factor 6, the issue of *research and systematic problem solving* is presented. Since nurses are occupied with the tasks of nursing, i.e., treatments, procedures, charts, they often fail to address the larger issues of conducting research, defining the discipline, or developing a scientific base for nursing. However, Watson believes that:

Without the systematic use of the scientific problem-solving method, effective practice is accidental at best and haphazard or harmful at worst. The scientific problem-solving method is the only method that allows for control and prediction, and that permits self-correction.[16]

While Watson makes a strong argument for the need for the absolutism of the scientific method, she also values the relative nature of nursing and makes an equally strong argument for the need to examine and develop other methods of knowing to provide an holistic perspective. The science of caring should not always be neutral and objective, two important characteristics of the scientific method.

Promotion of interpersonal teaching–learning (carative factor 7) is the factor which affords people the most control over their own health since it provides them with both information and alternatives. The caring nurse focuses on the learning process as much as the teaching process as learning offers the best way to individualize the information to be disseminated. Understanding the person's perceptions of the situation assists the nurse to prepare a cognitive plan that works within the person's framework and alleviates the stress of the event.[17]

Carative factor 8 deals with the daily, routine functions that the nurse uses to promote health, restore to health, or prevent illness. It is the factor labeled as *provision for a supportive, protective and(or) corrective mental, physical, sociocultural, and spiritual environment.* Watson divides these into external variables, such as the physical, safety, and environmental factors, and internal variables, such as mental, spiritual or cultural activities, which the nurse manipulates in order to provide support and protection for the person's mental and physical well-being.[18]

There is an interdependence between the external and the internal environments since it is the person's perceptions that render the environment as threatening or nonthreatening. While the subjective appraisal of threat can be a distortion of reality, the perception of threat is still a stressful event to the person. Events such as change of job, divorce, illness, loss of a loved one can arouse a sense of threat. Through assessment, the nurse can determine the person's appraisal of the situation and abilities to cope. Then the nurse can supply situational support, help the person develop a more accurate perception, or provide the cognitive information which can strengthen the patient's own coping mechanisms. Watson suggests that the nurse also must provide comfort, privacy, and safety as part of this carative factor. In addition, she believes that a basic element is a clean–esthetic environment. While clean, sterile surroundings might not be health promoting, esthetics can improve health through promotion of increased self-worth and dignity. A pleasant environment improves the affective state, facilitates interactions with others, and promotes a sense of satisfaction with life.[19]

Carative factor 9, *assistance with the gratification of human needs,* is grounded in a hierarchy of needs similar to that of Maslow.[20] However, Watson has created a hierarchy which she considers to be relevant to the science of caring in nursing. The following are Watson's ordering of needs[21]:

1. **Lower Order Needs (Biophysical Needs)**   Survival Needs
   The need for food and fluid
   The need for elimination
   The need for ventilation
2. **Lower Order Needs (Psychophysical Needs)**   Functional Needs
   The need for activity–inactivity
   The need for sexuality
3. **Higher Order Needs (Psychosocial Needs)**   Integrative Needs
   The need for achievement
   The need for affiliation
4. **Higher Order Need (Intrapersonal–**   Growth-seeking Need
   Interpersonal Need)
   The need for self-actualization

Establishing hierarchical needs does not preclude the necessity to view each person in the context of the whole. Meeting only lower order needs may not assist the complex human being toward self-actualization. Each need is viewed in the context of all the others and all are valued.

> Keeping in mind the holistic–dynamic framework for viewing the human needs, the carative factor assistance with the gratification of human needs leads to a more complete development of each human need. Some needs are more familiar and concrete because of the tangible ways in which they manifest themselves. Others are more abstract and elusive. They are equally important for quality nursing care and the promotion of optimal health.[22]

Overall, the theme is that, despite the hierarchical nature in which they are presented, the needs all deserve to be attended to and valued.

Research findings have established a correlation between emotional distress and illness. Therefore, an assessment that uses an holistic approach which examines the "dynamic, symbolic aspects of each need"[23] provides a more balanced portrait of the person. Watson states:

> The current thinking about holistic care emphasizes (1) that etiological components that have many factors interact and produce change through complex neurophysiological and neurochemical pathways, (2) that each psychological function has a physiological correlate, and (3) that each physiological function has a psychological correlate.[24]

As an example, disturbances found in the biophysical area of food and fluid need demonstrate the requirement for holistic care. Bulimia, anorexia, and gastrointestinal ulcers are just a few of the disorders that indicate the com-

TABLE 18-1. HOLISTIC CARE NEEDS IN BULEMIA AND ANOREXIA

Watson's Hierarchy	Application to Bulemia and Anorexia
Highest Order Need (interpersonal)	Self-actualization retarded Unrealistic sense of perfection never achieved
Higher Order Needs (psychosocial)	Diminished sense of achievement secondary to distorted body image Self-involvement leads to diminished affiliative activity, possibly impaired sexual relationships
Lower Order Needs (psychophysical)	Purge or binge or self-imposed starvation depletes cellular nutrition leading to decreased activity Body image distortion may impair sexuality
Lower Order Needs (biophysical)	Food and fluids restricted

plex interaction between the physiological and the psychological. Watson's work delineates the interrelationship in each area of her hierarchy (see Table 18-1).

Allowance for existential–phenomenological factors is carative factor 10. Phenomenology is a way of understanding people from the way things appear to them, from their frame of reference.[25] Existential psychology is the study of human existence using phenomenological analysis.[25] For the nurse, this factor helps to reconcile and mediate the incongruity of viewing the person holistically while at the same time attending to a hierarchical ordering of needs. Incorporating these factors into the science of nursing assists the nurse to understand the meaning the person finds in life or to help the person find meaning in difficult life events or both. Since there is a basic irrationality to life, illness, and death, the nurse using carative factor 10 may assist the person to find the strength or courage to confront life or death. Watson suggests that each nurse must turn inward to face his or her own existential questions before being able to assist others to cope with the human predicament.[26]

WATSON'S THEORY AND THE FOUR MAJOR CONCEPTS

Human Being

While in Watson's earlier writings she refers to her work as a philosophy and science of nursing, in her later book she clearly states that the work represents a nursing theory.[27] In that context, and using nursing's heritage, she adopts a view of the human being as:

> . . . a valued person in and of him- or herself to be cared for, respected, nurtured, understood, and assisted; in general a philosophical view of a person as a fully functional integrated self. The human is viewed as greater than, and different from, the sum of his or her parts.[28]

She believes that humans are best viewed in a developmental conflicts frame and that "systematic attention to developmental conflicts of individuals and their families is necessary for health care."[29] These conflicts, based upon Erikson's model, are primarily psychosocial and represent crises and turning points encountered throughout the human life cycle.[30] Commonly occurring, these conflicts can elicit a stress reaction that requires a coping response.[31] The nurse must understand human beings when sick, well, or under stress.

Health

While acknowledging the World Health Organization's definition of health as the positive state of physical, mental, and social well-being, Watson believes there are other factors that need to be included. She adds the following three elements[32]:

1. A high level of overall physical, mental, and social functioning
2. A general adaptive–maintenance level of daily functioning
3. The absence of illness (or the presense of efforts that lead to its absence)

Watson states that what has traditionally been called health care is a myth. That which has been called health care, the diagnosing of disease, treatment of illness, and prescription of drugs, is medical care. True health care focuses on life style, social conditions, and environment.

> Health refers to unity and harmony within the mind, body, and soul.
> Health is also associated with the degree of congruence between the self as perceived and the self as experienced.[33]

One major factor affecting health is stress or stress-related activities which are also associated with life style, social conditions, and environment. Illness, on the other hand, may not be disease but may be a disharmony between body, soul, and spirit which may lead to stress. In addition, Watson believes the individual should define his or her own state of health or illness since she prefers to view health as a subjective state within the mind of the person.

Environment/Society

One of the variables that affects society in today's world is the social environment. Society provides the values that determine how one should behave and what goals one should strive toward. These values are affected by change in the social, cultural, and spiritual arenas, which in turn affects the perception of the person and can lead to stress. People also have an intrinsic need to belong, to be part of group(s) and of society as a whole. Further, each person has a need for affection, a need to love and be loved. Stress or illness can separate the person from those who meet such affiliative or affectional needs. It is within the practice of caring that nursing can assist in meeting these needs. Watson states:

> Caring (and nursing) has existed in every society. Every society has had some people who have cared for others. A caring attitude is *not* transmitted from generation to generation by genes. It is transmitted by the culture of the profession as a unique way of coping with its environment.[34]

Nursing

According to Watson, "nursing is concerned with promoting health, preventing illness, caring for the sick, and restoring health.[35] Nursing focuses on health promotion as well as treatment of disease. She sees nursing as having to move educationally in the two areas of stress and developmental conflicts. This will provide holistic health care, which she believes is central to the practice of caring in nursing. One of Watson's assumptions is that "nursing's social, moral, and scientific contributions to humankind and society lie in its commitment to human care ideals in theory, practice, and research."[36]

In further writings Watson defines nursing as:

> ... a human science of persons and human health–illness experiences that are mediated by professional, personal, scientific, esthetic, and ethical human care transactions.[37]

Nursing in this context has its roots in the humanities as well as in the natural sciences. Nursing's goal, through the caring process, is to help people gain a high degree of harmony within the self in order to promote self-knowledge, self-healing, or to gain insight into the meaning of the happenings in life.

WATSON'S THEORY AND THE NURSING PROCESS

Watson recommends a broad approach to nursing that searches out connections rather than separations between the parts that make up the whole of the person. To accomplish this, nurses employ a scientific problem-solving method. Using this method, the nurse can draw from a data base and basic nursing principles to make nursing judgments and decisions. Watson points out that the nursing process contains the same steps as the scientific research process. The rationales for these processes are identical in that both try to solve a problem or answer a question. Both try to discover the best solution. However, she believes nurses tend to be frightened by the scientific research processes. If nurses could learn that the processes are basically the same and that they provide a framework for decision making, then nurses would derive comfort from the order established by using the scientific process. This might best be accomplished by teaching the two processes, nursing and research, at the same time, to practice them together, and to recognize that the ultimate goal in nursing is high quality patient care that can be achieved by using this systematic approach.[38]

Watson further elaborates the two processes as follows (Italics indicate the research process interwoven in the nursing process)[39]:

- *Assessment:*
  - Assessment involves *observation, identification,* and *review of the problem; use* of the applicable *knowledge in literature.*
  - It includes conceptual knowledge for the *formulation* and *conceptualization* of a *framework* in which to view and assess the problem.
  - It also includes the *formulation of hypotheses* about relationships and factors that influence the problem.
  - Assessment also includes *defining variables* that will be examined in solving the problem.
- *Plan:*
  - The plan helps to determine how variables will be *examined* or measured.
  - It includes a *conceptual approach* or design for solving problems that is referred to as the nursing care plan.
  - It also includes determining what data will be collected and on what person and how the data will be collected.
- *Intervention:*
  - Intervention is direct action and implementation of the plan.
  - It includes the collection of data.
- *Evaluation:*
  - Evaluation is the method of and the process for *analyzing data* as well as the examination of the effects of intervention based on the data.
  - It includes *interpretation* of the *results,* the degree to which a positive outcome occurred, and whether the results can be generalized beyond the situation.

Beyond that, according to Watson, evaluation may also generate additional hypotheses or possibly even lead to the generation of a nursing theory based on the problem studied and the solutions. An application of Watson's work in the nursing process is seen through the case study of Anthony M. (Table 18–2).

Situation. Anthony M. was a fourteen-year-old with a slender, almost cachectic, appearance. He weighed 85 lb and was 5'6" tall. Both his mother and father were deeply concerned about his weight loss of almost 30 pounds and upset over daily battles related to eating. Anthony was equally upset since he felt he was at just the right weight. He felt his parents had no

TABLE 18–2. WATSON'S THEORY IN THE NURSING PROCESS APPLIED TO ANTHONY M.

Nursing Process	Application of Theory
ASSESSMENT	
Lower Order Needs (biophysical)	How does Anthony M. view his body? Is he within norms for his height, weight, and age? Does he consume enough calories to maintain normal growth? Does a physical assessment indicate all systems are functioning at normal levels?
Lower Order Needs (psychophysical)	Is his body image realistic? Is he participating in the usual activities of his age? Does evaluation of laboratory tests indicate nutritional deficiencies?
Higher Order Needs (psychosocial)	Are his relationships with peers satisfactory? How does he view his nascent sexuality? Has starvation retarded puberty? Does his environment appear facilitative of personal growth? Does he feel loved or lovable? Has he established a sense of autonomy from his parents?
Highest Order Needs (intrapersonal)	How does Anthony M. feel about himself? Does he like his world? Does he feel he is accomplishing his goals?
NURSING DIAGNOSES	Disturbance in self-concept related to: Body image disturbance Powerlessness Impaired social interaction Unresolved independence or dependence
PLANNING AND IMPLEMENTATION	
Use carative factors	Establish a caring environment through empathetic understanding. Develop a helping–trust relationship by encouraging expression of feelings of fear of weight gain, anger at treatment plan, resentment of authority figures. Use warmth, empathy, and congruence to establish open communication. Promote interpersonal teaching–learning by involving patient in nutritional plan. Teach patient how to deal with conflict, issue of autonomy. Facilitate relationships within the family that foster autonomy. Encourage identification of stress factors. Assist in dealing with sexual identity. Encourage Anthony M. to assess his social interactions and develop satisfying ones. Emphasize personal satisfaction rather than perfection.
EVALUATION	Has a trusting relationship been established? Is Anthony M. developing normally in the areas assessed: biophysically, psychophysically, psychosocially, and intrapersonally? Has Anthony M. learned the skills necessary to grow and mature successfully?

right to control what or how much he ate. He was admitted to an adolescent psychiatric unit where the family's problem could be addressed.

Anthony complained that his parents were demanding and tried to control his life. He felt they did not understand him and probably did not love him. When discussing his weight, he denied being hungry, so therefore, he felt he was eating enough. He stated, "Look, I'm fat and ugly, can't they see that? Girls don't like me, I've never been invited to a boy–girl party. The guys think I'm O.K., especially since I help with their homework, but I don't hang around with anyone special."

Anthony's weight was not within the norm for his age or height. At his height, his optimal weight should range between 115 and 130 pounds. His skin appeared dry and flaky and his bones were clearly visible, there seemed to be no flesh covering them. He was listless and taciturn. His approach to food was marked by extreme disinterest.

WATSON'S WORK AND THE CHARACTERISTICS OF A THEORY

According to Watson, "a theory is an imaginative grouping of knowledge, ideas, and experience that are represented symbolically and seek to illuminate a given phenomenon."[40] She rejects traditional, quantifiable methodology when such methodology sacrifices the pursuit of new knowledge of human behavior. She sees nursing as being increasingly involved in procedures and variable manipulation while it might best be involved in a search for alternative views to study human caring, health–illness, and health promotion. She states that she views nursing as ". . . both a human science and an art, and as such it cannot be considered qualitatively continuous with traditional, reductionistic, scientific methodology."[41] Watson suggests that nursing might want to develop its own science that would not be related to the traditional sciences but rather would develop its own concepts, relationships, and methodology. Table 18–3 illustrates her ideas of nursing's context as opposed to the traditional view. Yet, her work has been developed within the traditional context and can be compared to the characteristics of a theory as delineated in Chapter 1.

1. Theories can interrelate concepts in such a way as to create a different way of looking at a particular phenomenon. The use of the term "caring" is not unique to Watson. What is unique is her basic assumptions for the science of caring in nursing and the ten carative factors that form the structure for that concept. She describes caring in both philosophical and scientific terms. Caring is placed in a hierarchical context, meeting lower order biophysical needs first and moving toward higher order psychosocial and intrapersonal needs. Watson also indicates the needs are interrelated. For example, food and fluid needs are lower order biophysical needs that must be met, yet intake of food and fluids is strongly related to love,

TABLE 18–3. DIFFERING PERSPECTIVES BETWEEN TRADITIONAL SCIENCE AND HUMAN SCIENCE

Traditional Medical Natural Science Context	Emerging Alternative Nursing Human Science and Context for Caring
Normative	Ipsative
Reductionistic	Transactional
Mechanistic	Metaphysical Humanistic—contextual
Method centered	Phenomena centered
Neutrality of values	Value laden; values acknowledged, clarified
Disease centered on pathology–physiology, the physical body	Person–experience centered Human responses to illness and personal meanings of human condition
Ethics of "science"	Human–social ethics–morality
More quantitative	More qualitative
Absolutes, givens, laws	Relativism, probabilism
Human as object	Human as subject
Objective Experiences	Subjective–intersubjective experiences
Facts	Experience, meaning
Nomothetic	Idiographic + /nomethetic
Concrete—observable	Abstract—may or may not "be seen"
Analytical	Dialectical, philosphical, metaphysical
Science as product	Science as creative process of discovery
Human = sum of parts ex. (bio–psycho–socio–cultural–spiritual–being)	Human = mind–body–spirit gestalt of whole being (not only more than sum of parts, but different)
Physical, materialistic	Existential—phenomenological–spiritual
"Real" is that which is measureable, observable, and knowable	"Real" is abstract, largely subjective as well as objective, but it may or may not ever be fully known, observable, fully measured, what is "real," holds mystery and unknowns yet to be discovered

Used with permission from Watson, J. Nursing: Human Science and Human Care. *New York: National League for Nursing, 1988, p. 10.*

security, culture, and self-concept. The science of caring suggests that the nurse recognize and assist with each of the interrelated needs in order to reach the highest order need of self-actualization.

2. Theories must be logical in nature. Watson's work is logical in that the carative factors are based on broad assumptions which provide a supportive framework. She uses these carative factors to help delineate nursing from medicine. The carative factors are logically derived from the assumptions and related to the hierarchy of needs.

3. Theories should be relatively simple yet generalizable. Watson's theory is relatively simple since it does use theories from other disciplines which are familiar to nurses. It becomes more complex when entering the area of existential-phenomenology since many nurses may not have the liberal arts background to provide the proper foundation for understanding this area. On the other hand, nurses do have the empirical knowledge of human nature, including working with persons who are dealing with pain, loss, and suffering. While the theory is relatively simple, the fact that it de-emphasizes the pathophysiological for the psychosocial diminishes its ability to be generalizable. Watson discusses this in the preface of her book when she speaks of the "trim" and "core" of nursing. She defines trim as the clinical focus, the procedures, and techniques. The core of nursing is that which is intrinsic to the nurse–client interaction that produces a therapeutic result.[42] Core mechanisms are the carative factors. Unfortunately, those are the very factors that seem to be most often sacrificed in today's technological world.

4. Theories can be the bases for hypotheses that can be tested. Watson's work is based upon phenomenological studies that generally ask questions rather than state hypotheses. Its purpose is to describe the phenomena, to analyze, and to gain an understanding.

5. Theories contribute to and assist in increasing the general body of knowledge within the discipline through research implemented to validate them. Watson has suggested that the best method for testing this theory is through field study. One example is her work in the area of loss and caring that took place in Cundeelee, Western Australia, and involved a tribe of aborigines. She first had the aborigines describe the phenomena of loss. They then defined what caring meant to them. Through analysis of the descriptive data, Watson was able to develop a theory of transpersonal caring, which states that loss creates a disharmony in three spheres, mind, body, and spirit. The nurse can enter into the process of transpersonal caring by comforting, listening, and allowing for free expression of feelings based on the culturally relevant norms of the person.[43] Since the carative factors expand on theories learned from other disciplines and mold them into uniquely nursing knowledge, continued research that involves the carative factors should increase the general body of knowledge in nursing.

6. Theories can be utilized by practitioners to guide and improve their practice. Watson's work can be used to guide and improve practice. It can provide the nurse with the most satisfying aspects of practice and can provide the client with the holistic care so necessary for human growth and development.

7. Theories must be consistent with other validated theories, laws, and principles but will leave open unanswered questions that need to be investigated. Watson's work is supported by the theoretical work of numerous humanists, philosophers, developmentalists, and psychologists. She clearly designates the theories of stress, development, communication, teaching–learning, humanistic psychology, and existential phenomenology which provide the foundation for the science of caring. She presents these in a way that provides a uniquely nursing view, which leads to further questions to be investigated.

ANALYSIS AND CONCLUSIONS

The strength of Watson's work is that it not only assists in providing the quality of care that clients ought to receive but also provides the soul satisfying care for which many nurses enter the profession. Because the science of caring ranges from the biophysical through the intrapersonal, each nurse becomes an active coparticipant in the client's struggle toward self-actualization. In addition, the client is placed in the context of the family, the community, and the culture. All of this encourages the nurse to place the client, rather than the technology, as the focus of practice. Along with that comes the nurse's responsibility and opportunity for personal growth.

The limitations may very well be the same issues. Given the acuity of illness that leads to hospitalization, the short length of stay, and the increasingly complex technology, such quality of care may be deemed impossible to give in a hospital. Bureaucratic structures are not known for their attention to much beyond the cost–benefit ratio. The rewards from within that structure are for the "trim" and not for the "core" of nursing, often placing the practitioner in an untenable position. Nurses who function in any bureaucratic structure that focuses on task accomplishment, whether that structure be in a hospital, home health or official public health agency, visiting nurse association, or any other location, are subject to the same limitations in relation to Watson's theory.

While Watson acknowledges the need for a biophysical base to nursing, this area receives little attention in her writings. The ten carative factors primarily delineate the psychosocial needs of the person. In addition, while the carative factors have a sound foundation based on other disciplines, they need further research in nursing to demonstrate their application to practice.

SUMMARY

Watson provides many useful concepts for the practice of nursing. She ties together many theories commonly used in nursing education and does so in a manner helpful to practitioners of the art and science of nursing. The detailed descriptions of the carative factors can give guidance to those who wish to employ them in practice or research. Using her theory can add a dimension to practice that is both satisfying and challenging.

REFERENCES

1. Watson, J. *Nursing: The Philosophy and Science of Caring*, Boston: Little, Brown, 1979.
2. Watson, J. *Nursing: Human Science and Human Care, A Theory of Nursing*, Norwalk, Conn.: Appleton-Century-Crofts, 1985; New York: National League for Nursing, 1988.
3. Watson, *Nursing: The Philosophy and Science of Caring*, p. 8.
4.(a) Maslow, A. *Motivation and Personality*, New York: Harper & Bros., 1954
4.(b) Rogers, C. *Person to Person: The Problem of Being Human*, California: Real People Press, 1967.
4.(c) Heidegger, M. *Being and Time*, New York: Harper & Row, 1962
4.(d) Erikson, E. *Childhood and Society* (2nd ed.), New York: Norton, 1963.
5.(a) Selye, H. *The Stress of Life*, New York: McGraw Hill, 1956.
5.(b) Lazarus, R.S. *Psychological Stress and the Coping Process*, New York: McGraw Hill, 1966.
5.(c) Leininger, M. ed., *Caring*, Thorofare, N.J.: Charles B. Slack, 1981
5.(d) Henderson, V. The Nature of Nursing, *American Journal of Nursing*, 1964,*64*, 62–68.
6. Watson, *Nursing: The Philosophy and Science of Caring*, pp. 8–9.
7. Watson, *Nursing: Human Science and Human Care*, p. 33.
8. Watson, *Nursing: The Philosophy and Science of Caring*, pp. 9–10.
9. Ibid, 11.
10. Ibid, 15.
11. Watson, *Nursing: Human Science and Human Care*, p. 49.
12. Ibid, 50.
13. Watson, *Nursing: The Philosophy and Science of Caring*, p. 18.
14.(a) Rogers, C. The Interpersonal Relationship: The Core of Guidance, *Harvard Educational Review*, 1962, *32*, 416.
14.(b) Carkhuff, R. *The Development of Human Resources in Education and Psychology and Social Change*, New York: Holt, Rhinehart & Winston, 1971.
14.(c) Gazda, G., Walters, R.P., & Childers, W.C. *Human Relations Development: A Manual for Health Sciences*, Boston: Allyn & Bacon, 1975.
15. Watson, *Nursing: The Philosophy and Science of Caring*, p. 44.
16. Ibid, 55–56.
17. Ibid, 69–79.
18. Ibid, 82.
19. Ibid, 81–100.
20. Maslow, A. *Toward a Psychology of Being* (2nd ed.), Princeton: Van Nostrand, 1968.
21. Watson, *Nursing: The Philosphy and Science of Caring*, p. 108.
22. Ibid, 109–111.
23. Ibid, 117.
24. Ibid, 117–118.
25. Ibid, 209.
26. Ibid, 208.
27. Watson, *Nursing: Human Science and Human Care*, p. 1.
28. Ibid, 14.
29. Watson, *Nursing: The Philosophy and Science of Caring*, p. 246.

30. Erikson, *Childhood and Society.*
31. Watson, *Nursing: The Philosophy and Science of Caring,* p. 246.
32. Ibid, 220.
33. Watson, *Nursing: Human Science and Human Care,* p. 48.
34. Watson, *Nursing: The Philosophy and Science of Caring,* p. 8.
35. Ibid, 7.
36. Watson, *Nursing: Human Science and Human Care,* p. 33.
37. Ibid, 54.
38. Watson, *Nursing: The Philosophy and Science of Caring,* pp. 52–56.
39. Ibid, 65–66.
40. Watson, *Nursing: Human Science and Human Care,* p. 1.
41. Ibid, 2.
42. Watson, *Nursing: The Philosophy and Science of Caring,* p. xv.
43. Watson, *Nursing: Human Science and Human Care,* pp. 87–88.

BIBLIOGRAPHY

Gaines, B., Saunders, J., & Watson, J. Philosophy of Nursing: A National Survey, *Western Journal of Nursing Research,* 1984, *6,* 401–404.

Sakalys, J. & Watson, J. Professional Educational Post-Baccalaureate Education for Professional Nursing . . . Reintegration of the Classical Liberal Arts Model, *Journal of Professional Nursing,* 1986, *2,* 91–97.

Watson, J. The Lost Art of Nursing, *Nursing Forum,* 1981, *20,* 244–249.

Watson, J. Professional Identity Crisis—Is Nursing Finally Growing Up? *American Journal of Nursing,* 1981, *81,* 1488–1490.

Watson, J. Nursing's Scientific Quest, *Nursing Outlook,* 1985, *29,* 413–416.

Watson, J. Academic and Clinical Collaboration: Advancing the Art and Science of Human Caring, *Community Nursing Research,* 1987, *20,* 1–16.

Watson, J. Nursing on the Caring Edge—Metaphorical Vignettes, *Advances in Nursing Science,* 1987, *10,* 10–18.

CHAPTER 19

Rosemarie Rizzo Parse

Janet S. Hickman

Rosemarie Rizzo Parse earned her Master's Degree in Nursing and her PhD from the University of Pittsburgh. She is currently Professor of Graduate Nursing and Coordinator, Center for Nursing Research, at Hunter College, New York City. She is the founder and President of Discovery International, Inc., Pittsburgh, Pennsylvania, a firm that provides consultation services related to nursing research, education, and practice, as well as health guidance services to individuals, families, and communities. Dr. Parse is the editor of Nursing Science Quarterly, *a Williams & Wilkins publication.*

In addition to Dr. Parse's books,[1a–1c] she has presented many papers and speeches on a wide variety of subjects related to nursing both nationally and abroad. In 1987, she was named Lynn Eminent Scholar in Nursing at Florida Atlantic University. Dr. Parse has had more than twenty years of experience in theory development, research, administration, and nursing practice and education.

Parse has created a unique theory of nursing titled "Man–Living–Health," by synthesizing principles and concepts from Rogers[2a,2b] and concepts and tenets from existential phenomenology. Parse indicates that man refers to *Homo sapiens*[3] and, thus, is a generic term for all human beings.

In 1981, Parse stated that her purpose was to posit an idea of nursing rooted in the human sciences as an alternative to ideas of nursing grounded in the natural sciences.[4] She defined natural science-based nursing as having to do with the quantification of man and illness rather than the qualification of man's total experience with health.[5]

In 1987, Parse refined this discussion by presenting two paradigms or worldviews of nursing. The first discussed is the Totality paradigm. In this paradigm, man is posited as a total summative being whose nature is a combination of bio–psycho–social–spiritual aspects. The environment is viewed as the external and internal stimuli surrounding man. Man interacts and adapts with his environment to maintain equilibrium and to achieve goals.[6] This is a refined definition of the natural or medical science approach to nursing. Parse states that the works of Peplau,[7] Henderson,[8] Hall,[9] Orlando,[10] Levine,[11] Johnson,[12] Roy,[13a,13b] Orem,[14a–14c] and King[15a,15b] are representative of the Totality Paradigm.[16]

The second worldview that Parse discusses is the Simultaneity paradigm. This paradigm views man as "a unitary being in continuous mutual interrelationship with the environment, and whose health is a negentropic unfolding . . ."[16] This is a refined definition of the human science approach to nursing. Parse states that her own work and that of Rogers[17] are representative of the Simultaneity paradigm.[18]

SUMMARY OF PARSE'S THEORY

Parse's theory relates assumptions about man and health and deduces from them the principles, concepts, and theoretical structures of Man–Living–Health. These assumptions are based on Rogers' principles and concepts and from the works of Heidegger,[19a,19b] Sartre,[20a–20c] and Merleau-Ponty[21a–21c] on existential-phenomenological thought.[22]

Parse uses Rogers' three major principles of helicy, complementarity (now called integrality), and resonancy; and her four major concepts of energy field, openness, pattern and organization, and four dimensionality as part of the theoretical basis for her own assumptions about men and health. Parse synthesizes these principles and concepts with the following tenets and concepts of existential-phenomenological thought: intentionality, human subjectivity, coconstitution, coexistence, and situation freedom.[23] It is important to remember that the process of synthesis is, by definition, the combining of elements to create something new and different. Therefore, as will be demonstrated in the discussion of Parse's assumptions, the products of her synthesis are different from the original principles, tenets, and concepts on which they were based.

ASSUMPTIONS

In her 1981 book, *Man–Living–Health: A Theory of Nursing*, Parse posited nine assumptions, each of which was based on three of the twelve previously identified principles, tenets, and concepts from Rogers' theory and existential-phenomenological thought.[23] In chart form, Parse demonstrated the three specific concepts, tenets, or principles on which each assumption was based.[24] Phillips points out that for six of the nine assumptions, two of the three concepts used as the basis for each assumption come from Rogers; this leaves three assumptions for which two of the three concepts come from existential-phenomenology.[25] Quantitatively, Phillips is implying a larger grounding of the assumptions in Rogers' theory than in existential-phenomenology. In contrast, Winkler states that their derivation is primarily from philosophical sources and secondarily from Rogers' theory.[26]

Parse's original nine assumptions are[27]:

1. Man is coexisting while coconstituting rhythmical patterns with the environment. (Based on *pattern and organization, coconstitution,* and *coexistence*).

2. Man is an open being, freely choosing meaning in situation, bearing responsibility for decisions. (Based on *energy field, openness,* and *situated freedom.*)
3. Man is a living unity continuously coconstituting patterns of relating. (Based on *energy field, pattern and organization,* and *coconstitution*).
4. Man is transcending multidimensionally with the possibles. (Based on *openness, four dimensionality,* and *situated freedom*).
5. Health is an open process of becoming, experienced by man. (Based on *openness, coconstitution,* and *situated freedom*).
6. Health is a rhythmically coconstituting process of the man–environment interrelationship. (Based on *pattern and organization, four dimensionality,* and *coconstitution*).
7. Health is man's pattern of relating value priorities. (Based on *openness, pattern and organization,* and *situated freedom*).
8. Health is an intersubjective process of transcending with the possibles. (Based on *openness, coexistence,* and *situated freedom*).
9. Health is unitary man's negentropic unfolding. (Based on *energy field, four dimensionality,* and *coexistence*).

Recently Parse has synthesized these original nine assumptions into three assumptions[28]:

1. Man–Living–Health is freely choosing personal meaning in situations in the intersubjective process of relating value priorities.
2. Man–Living–Health is cocreating rhythmical patterns of relating in open interchange with the environment.
3. Man–Living–Health is cotranscending multidimensionally with the unfolding possibles.

Parse explains that the first assumption means that Man–Living–Health is man through subject-to-subject interchange in situations where the meaning assigned to the experience reflects personal values.[29] This assumption appears to be a synthesis of numbers two, five, and seven of her original nine, which are based on the concepts of energy field, openness, situated freedom, coconstitution, and pattern and organization. It is important, however, to note that Parse is not viewing man as an energy field, but rather as an open being freely choosing personal meanings based on his values.

Parse explains that her second assumption means that Man–Living–Health and environment together create the pattern of each. Both man and environment are distinguishable, but each is a participant in the creation of the other.[30] This assumption appears to be a synthesis of original assumptions one, three, and six, which are based on the concepts of energy fields, openness, situated freedom, pattern and organization, and coconstitution.

The third assumption means that Man–Living–Health is man moving beyond self at all levels of the universe as dreams become actualities. Parse defines cotranscending as "moving beyond with others and the environment multidimensionally. Multidimensionally refers to the various levels of the universe that Man experiences all at once" and chooses possibles from in various situations.[30] This assumption appears to be a synthesis of original assumptions four, eight and nine, which are based on the concepts of openness, four dimensionality, situated freedom, coexistence, and energy field. It is important to note that Parse is viewing man as being multidimensional as opposed to four dimensional.

In this synthesized set of three assumptions, there is consistent usage of Parse's construct Man–Living–Health. In her elaborations of the assumptions, she consistently uses the phrase, "Man–Living–Health is Man . . ."[31] However, in her earlier work, she explicitly defines the hyphenated structure of Man–Living–Health to mean man's health as ongoing participation with the world.[32] It appears, by the consistent usage of the construct in the new assumptions that she intends to present the greater meaning, and her phrasing in her explanations is only to make the assumption more clearly understood.

Parse cites the following distinctives of her theory[33]:

1. The belief that man is more than and different from the sum of his parts.
2. Man evolves mutually with the environment.
3. Man participates in cocreating personal health by choosing meaning in situations.
4. Man conveys meanings that are personal values reflecting dreams and hopes.

Three main themes can be identified in Parse's assumptions: meaning, rhythmicity, and cotranscendence. Each leads to a principle of Man–Living–Health (see Fig. 19–1). These principles are[34]:

1. Structuring meaning multidimensionally is cocreating reality through the languaging of valuing and imaging.
2. Cocreating rhythmical patterns of relating is living the paradoxical unity of revealing–concealing, enabling–limiting while connecting–separating.
3. Cotranscending with the possibles is powering unique ways of originating in the process of transforming.

PRINCIPLES

I. *Structuring meaning multidimensionally is cocreating reality through the languaging of valuing and imaging.*

Parse's first principle interrelates the concepts of *imaging, valuing,* and *languaging.* This principle indicates that Man–Living–Health structures meaning to man's reality based on lived experiences. The meaning changes or is stretched to different possibilities based on

Rogers		Existential Phenomenology	
Principles	*Concepts*	*Concepts*	*Tenets*
Helicy Complemen- tarity Resonancy	Energy field Openness Pattern and orga- nization Four-dimension- ality	Coconstitution Coexistence Situated free- dom	Intentionality Human sub- jectivity

Assumptions

1. Man is coexisting while coconstituting rhythmical patterns with the environment.
2. Man is an open being, freely choosing meaning in situation, bearing responsibility of decisions.
3. Man is a living unity continuously coconstituting patterns of relating.
4. Man is transcending multidimensionally with the possibles.

5. Health is an open process of becoming, experienced by man.
6. Health is a rhythmically coconstituting process of the man–environment interrelationship.
7. Health is man's patterns of relating value priorities.
8. Health is an intersubjective process of transcending with the possibles.
9. Health is unitary man's negentropic unfolding.

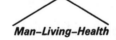

Man–Living–Health

Principles	Structuring meaning multidimensionally	Cocreating rhythmical patterns of relating	Cotranscending with the possibles
Concepts	Imaging Valuing Languaging	Revealing–concealing Enabling–limiting Connecting–separating	Powering Originating Transforming
Theoretical Structures	*Powering* is a way of *revealing and concealing imaging.* *Originating* is a manifestation of *enabling and limiting valuing.* *Transforming* unfolds in the *languaging of connecting and separating.*		

Figure 19–1. Evolution of the theory of Man–Living–Health. *(From Parse, R.R.* Man–Living–Health: A Theory of Nursing, *New York: Wiley, 1981, pp. 70–71. Used with permission.)*

lived experiences. Cocreating in this principle refers to the man/environment participation in the creation of the pattern of each. The concept of imaging is defined as "the picturing or making real of events, ideas, and people," while valuing is defined as "the living of cherished beliefs."[35] Languaging reflects images and values through speaking and moving.[35]

DIMENSIONS

Illuminating meaning is shedding light through uncovering the what was, is, and will be, as it is appearing now; it happens in *explicating* what is.

Synchronizing rhythms happens in *dwelling with* the pitch, yaw, and roll of the interhuman cadence.

Mobilizing transcendence happens in *moving beyond* the meaning moment to what is not yet.

PROCESSES

Explicating is making clear what is appearing now through languaging.

Dwelling with is giving self over to the flow of the struggle in connecting-separating.

Moving beyond is propelling toward the possibles in transforming.

Figure 19–2. Man–Living–Health Practice Methodology. *(From Parse, R.R. Nursing Science: Major Paradigms, Theories, and Critiques, Philadelphia: Saunders, 1987, p. 167. Used with permission.*

From this principle, Parse has identified a nursing practice dimension and a process (see Fig. 19–2). The practice dimension is illuminating meaning by shedding light through uncovering the what was, is, and will be, as it is appearing now. This happens by explicating or making clear what is appearing now through languaging (the process).[36] Nurses guide individuals and families to relate the meaning of a situation. In relating, individuals and families share thoughts and feelings with the nurse and each other; this sharing itself changes the meaning of a situation by making the meaning more explicit.[37]

II. *Cocreating rhythmical patterns of relating is living the paradoxical unity of revealing–concealing and enabling–limiting while connecting–separating.*

The second principle of Man–Living–Health interrelates the concepts of *revealing–concealing*, *enabling–limiting*, and *connecting–separating*. This principle speaks to Man–Living–Health again cocreating a multidimensional universe in rhythmical patterns of relating while living in a paradoxical unity. The paradoxes identified are revealing–concealing, enabling–limiting, and connecting–separating.

Connecting–separating is defined as the rhythmical process of distancing and relating. While one is relating to another or to a creative process, one is distancing oneself from another aspect of living. Within the paradox of connecting–separating are revealing–concealing and enabling–limiting. In interpersonal relationships, one reveals part of self but conceals other parts. Making choices or decisions enables an individual in some ways, but limits that person in others.[38]

The practice dimension Parse describes for this principle is the synchronizing of rhythms which happens in dwelling with the pitch, yaw, and roll of interhuman cadence. The process, an empirical activity, she identifies as the dwelling with or giving of self over to the flow of the struggle in connecting–separating.[39] In this frame of reference, the nurse would move with the flow of the individual or family, leading the family to recognize the harmony that exists within its own lived context. The nurse would not try to calm or balance rhythms or attempt to help the family adapt.[40]

III. *Contranscending with the possibles is powering unique ways of originating in the process of transforming.*

The third principle of Man–Living–Health interrelates the concepts of *powering, originating,* and *transforming.* Powering is an energizing force whose rhythm is the pushing–resisting of interhuman encounters.[41] Transforming is defined as the changing of change and is recognized by increasing diversity.[42] Powering ways of originating is man's way of distinguishing self from others.[42] Transforming is defined as the changing of change and is recognized by increasing diversity.[43a,43b]

The practice dimension identified by Parse for this principle is mobilizing transcendence which happens in moving beyond the meaning of the moment to what is not yet. The process or empirical activity she identifies is moving beyond or "propelling toward the possibles in transforming."[44] Here the nurse would guide individuals and families to plan for the changing of lived health patterns.[45]

THEORETICAL STRUCTURES

The theoretical structures of Man–Living–Health are noncausal in nature and consistent with the assumptions and principles. They are designed to guide research and practice (see Fig. 19–3). To operationalize the structures for research and practice, practice propositions must be derived. The three theoretical structures identified are[46]: (1) powering is a way of revealing–concealing imaging, (2) originating is a manifestation of enabling–limiting valuing, and (3) transforming unfolds in the languaging of connecting–separating.

In her 1987 book, Parse restates her theoretical structures at a less abstract level in order for them to be used to guide nursing practice. She explains that *"powering is a way of revealing–concealing imaging* can be stated as *struggling to live goals discloses the significance of the situation."*[47] The nursing practice focus is on illuminating the process of revealing–concealing unique

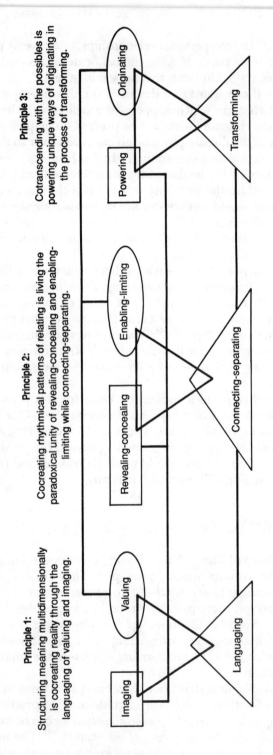

Principle 1:

Structuring meaning multidimensionally is cocreating reality through the languaging of valuing and imaging.

Principle 2:

Cocreating rhythmical patterns of relating is living the paradoxical unity of revealing-concealing and enabling-limiting while connecting-separating.

Principle 3:

Cotranscending with the possibles is powering unique ways of originating in the process of transforming.

Relationship of the concepts in the *squares*: *Powering* is a way of *revealing* and *concealing imaging*.
Relationship of the concepts in the *ovals*: *Originating* is a manifestation of *enabling* and *limiting values*.
Relationship of the concepts in the *triangles*: *Transforming* unfolds in the *languaging of connecting and separating*.

Figure 19–3. Relationship of Principles, Concepts, and Theoretical Structures of Man–Living–Health. *(From Parse, R.R. Man–Living–Health: A Theory of Nursing, New York: Wiley, 1981, p. 69. Used with permission.)*

ways a person or family can mobilize transcendence in considering new dreams, to image new possibles. Parse describes a nurse–family situation where members share their thoughts and feelings about a situation, which both reveals and conceals all they know about their struggle to meet personal goals. In disclosing the significance of the situation, the meaning of the situation changes for the family members and therefore the meaning changes for the family.[47]

According to Parse, "the second theoretical structure, *originating is a manifestation of enabling–limiting valuing* can be restated as *creating anew shows one's cherished beliefs and leads in a directional movement.*"[47] The nursing practice focus with a person or family would be on illuminating ways of being alike and different from others in changing values. By synchronizing rhythms, the members discover opportunities and limitations created by the decisions made in choosing ways to be together. Parse states that the choices of new ways of being together mobilize transcendence.[47]

As a restatement of the third theoretical structure, "*transforming unfolds in the language of connecting–separating,*" Parse suggests "*changing views emerge in speaking and moving with others.*"[47] The nursing practice focus would be on illuminating the meaning of relating ways of being together as various changing perspectives shed different light on the familiar, which gives rise to new possibles. Parse suggests that in synchronizing rhythms in a nurse–family situation, members relate their values through speech and movement. In so doing, views change and, through mobilizing transcendence, the ways of relating change.[47]

PARSE'S THEORY AND THE FOUR MAJOR CONCEPTS

The Parse theory will be discussed in terms of her beliefs about human beings, environment, health, and nursing. Parse identifies her theory, and that of Rogers, as being representative of the Simultaneity Paradigm.[48] Hence, her assumptions about the four major concepts are congruent with those of the Simultaneity Paradigm.

Human Beings/Environment/Society

Parse uses the term Man to describe human beings. Parse's theory is based on the belief that:

> Man is an open being, more than and different from the sum of parts in mutual simultaneous interchange with the environment who chooses from options and bears responsibility for choices. Man cocreates patterns of relating with the environment and is recognized by these patterns.[48]

Parse posits man as multidimensional, experiencing various levels of the universe all at once.[49]

Man is one of the three central concepts of Parse's theory. Her views about man are evident in all elements of her theory—assumptions, principles, concepts, and theoretical structures. Parse views man and environment as inseparable, each coparticipating in the creation of the experience of living. It is not possible or appropriate to define man or environment separately as together they create a lived experience greater than and different from each seen separately.

The concept of society is assumed under the larger view of man–living and is not addressed as a separate entity. In her discussion of the concept of cotranscending, Parse speaks to "moving beyond with others and the environment multidimensionally."[49] She also states what man chooses from the multiple possibles unfolds and surfaces in relationships with others and the environment.[49] While man is described as having a unique rhythmical pattern, it is difficult to interpret if there is a difference in actual pattern between individuals and the man–environment interchange. If one assumes that "others" are a part of man's environment, the interpretation becomes more clear.

Parse's view of man–living is consistent with Rogers' presentation of the person–environment as inseparable, complementary, and evolving together.[50] Her view is also consistent with the existentialist view of a person being in the world all at once and together and the phenomenological belief that the environment is made up of everything shown to the person in the lived experience.[51a,51b]

Winkler notes that while Parse states that all lived experiences are relevant, the omission of any references to biological manifestations of the person in his or her being and becoming limits Parse's theory.[52] Phillips rejects this criticism and states that the lived experience deals with the wholeness of the person.[53]

Health

Health is one of the three central concepts of Parse's theory. Health is explicitly defined in Parse's assumptions as an open process of becoming experienced by man, a rhythmically coconstituting process of the man–environment interrelationship, man's patterns of relating value priorities, an intersubjective process of transcending with the possibles, and as unitary man's negentropic unfolding.[54] Living health is an incarnation of man's choosing, experienced multidimensionally and lived uniquely.[55] Health is man's lived experiences, a nonlinear entity that cannot be qualified by terms such as good, bad, more, or less.[56] Man's health is a synthesis of values, a way of living, rather than a wellness or illness state that a man has. Disease from this perspective is a pattern that man cocreates with the world.[57]

Phillips describes Parse's theory as a way of dealing with experience, a coming to know rather than a product orientation. He states that the fundamental tenet of Parse's theory is that man participates in health.[58]

Parse's theory speaks to health as man's lived experience as it unfolds negentropically. This is a very different conceptualization of health than that of the totality paradigm theorists. From the totality world view, health is a state of balance or well-being to which man can aspire.

Parse further changes the meanings of the words man, living, and health by hyphenating them. By doing this, she demonstrates a conceptual bond among the words that creates a unity of meaning different from the individual words as they stand alone. This hyphenation "points to man's health as ongoing participation with the world."[59]

Nursing

Parse defines nursing practice as a science and art using an abstract body of knowledge in service to people. She states that nursing's responsibility to society is in the guiding of individuals and families in choosing possibilities in the changing health process. This is accomplished by intersubjective participation with people and their families. She further states that nursing practice involves innovation and creativity which are not encumbered by prescriptive rules. She posits that Man–Living–Health principles provide a broad base of abstract nursing knowledge to guide practice.[60]

This theorist contends that the goals of nursing focus on the quality of life from the person's perspective. Nursing is practiced with all individuals and families regardless of societal designations of health/illness status.[61] Parse's theory guides practice that focuses on illuminating meaning and moving beyond with the person and the family relative to changing health patterns.[62] An important aspect in regard to Parse's view of nursing is that the client, not the nurse, is the authority figure and prime decision maker. The client, guided by the nurse, determines the activities for changing health patterns. Nursing according to this theory is "a loving, true presence with the other to promote health and the quality of life."[63] The practice of nursing is not a prescriptive approach based on medical or nursing diagnoses, nor is it the offering of professional advice and opinions which stem from the personal value system of the nurse.[63]

Parse has presented a practice methodology for her theory Man–Living–Health that includes dimensions and processes (see Fig. 19–2). The dimensions are *illuminating meaning, synchronizing rhythms,* and *mobilizing transcendence.* The processes are the empirical activities of *explicating, dwelling with,* and *moving beyond.*[64] There is a clear flow of these dimensions and processes from her assumptions and principles.

Parse assigns the nurse the practice role of an interpersonal guide. While nursing practice is based on a unique body of knowledge, the nurse's role is passive. Authority, responsibility, and the consequences of decisions are accorded to the client. The traditional nursing roles of care giver, advocate, counselor, and leader do not appear to be congruent with Parse's view of nursing. The traditional nursing roles of teacher and change agent, however, are congruent. The teacher role is reflected in the dimension of illuminating meaning by explicating and the change agent role is reflected in the dimension of mobilizing transcendence by moving beyond the meaning to what is not yet.

Parse defines the contextual situations of nursing practice as being nurse–person or nurse–group participation.[64] She does not define specific practice settings as being more or less appropriate for practice application of Man–Living–Health, nor does she speak to nursing roles in disease prevention or health restoration. None of the nurse–person examples she provides deal with persons in acute care settings, but rather with mental health or health promotive situations. Winkler comments that the absence of reference to nursing roles in illness prevention and health restoration may be unacceptable to some nurses.[65] Phillips notes, in his critique of Man–Living–Health, that the empirical aspects of the theory are not as well developed as the structure. He also states that Parse has developed guidelines for the identification of emerging health patterns and activities.[66] Unfortunately, these guidelines are in an unpublished manuscript.[67]

PARSE'S THEORY AND THE NURSING PROCESS

In her book *Man–Living–Health: A Theory of Nursing* (1981), Parse presents an application of her theory to a nurse–family situation. In this example, she uses her theoretical structures to guide practice.[68] She does not at any time in her discussion refer or relate to the traditional nursing process of assessment, diagnosis, planning, implementation, and evaluation. She does state "Nursing practice is innovative and creative, unencumbered by prescriptive rules."[69] This statement implies that the use of nursing diagnoses would not be appropriate to her practice methodology.

In Parse's 1987 writing, she states that the nursing process "evolves from the discipline of philosophy and does not flow from an ontological base in the discipline of nursing."[70] She further states that the steps of the nursing process are the steps of the problem-solving process and are not unique to nursing.[70]

In addition, Parse comments that the assumptions underlying the nursing process, that the nurse is the authority on health and that the person adapts or can be "fixed," are not congruent with the theory Man–Living–Health.[71] Parse posits that as practice is the empirical life of a theory, the practice of one theory would be different from the practice of another.[72] She then explains the practice methodology she has developed for Man–Living–Health. This methodology consists of three dimensions and three processes (see Fig. 19–2). Parse's dimensions and processes flow clearly from the principles and assumptions of Man–Living–Health.

The first dimension of the practice methodology is illuminating meaning that occurs in the process of explicating. Illuminating meaning is shedding light through the uncovering of what was and what will be as it is appearing now. By explicating or making clear what is at this moment, one joins what was and what will be. The nurse guides the individual or family to relate the meaning of the situation In relating with each other, the meaning is changed and made more explicit.[73]

The second practice dimension is synchronizing rhythms which happens in the process of dwelling with the flow of interhuman cadence (the turning, spinning, and thrusting of human relationships). Rather than calming or trying to balance these rhythms, the nurse goes with the rhythms set by the individual or family. The nurse leads them, through discussion, to recognize the harmony that exists within the family's own lived context.[73]

The third practice dimension is mobilizing transcendence which happens through the process of moving beyond the meaning moment to what is not yet. This dimension focuses on the dreaming of the possibles and planning to reach the dreams. Again, the nurse guides the individual or family to plan for the changing of lived health patterns.[74]

As discussed in the summary section of this chapter, Parse has restated her theoretical structures at a less abstract level in order for them to be used to guide practice. Parse defines nursing practice as ". . . a subject-to-subject interrelationship, a loving, true presence with the other to promote health and the quality of life."[74] Parse's approach is clearly one of nurses *being with* people rather than *doing for* people.

PARSE'S WORK AND THE CHARACTERISTICS OF A THEORY

1. Theories can interrelate concepts in such a way as to create a different way of looking at a particular phenomenon. Parse's theory of Man–Living–Health creates a new way of looking at man, health, environment, and nursing. Parse has interrelated or synthesized Rogers' principles of helicy, complementarity (now called integrality), and resonancy and her four concepts of openness, energy field, pattern and organization, and four dimensionality[75] with the tenets of human subjectivity and intentionality and the concepts of coconstitution, coexistence, and situated freedom from existential phenomenological thought. This synthesis created the nine assumptions upon which Parse's theory, Man–Living–Health, is based.[76]

Parse's synthesis creates a theory in which man is an open being who, with his world, cocreates health. She views nursing as being rooted in the human sciences and focusing on man as a living unit and man's qualitative participation with health experiences.[77] Parse's goal of nursing focuses on quality of life from the person's (client's) perspective. In this worldview, the health–illness continuum is irrelevant as are care plans based on health problems. The authority, responsibility, and consequences of decision making reside with the person (client), not the nurse.[78] The nurse is presented as a guide who focuses on illuminating meaning, synchronizing rhythms, and mobilizing transcendence with the person or family relative to changing health patterns.[79]

2. Theories must be logical in nature. Parse's theory of Man–Living–Health does describe a logical sequence of events. Parse presents Rogers's principles and concepts as well as tenets and concepts from existential-phenomenological thought. She then uses the process of induction–deduction to create each of her nine assumptions. Each assumption is based on three concepts.[80] Six of the assumptions are based on two concepts from Rogers and one concept from existential phenomenology; the other three assumptions are based on two concepts from existential phenomenology and one concept from Rogers. Parse provides a clear chart to demonstrate the concept–assumption interface.[81]

Parse has recently synthesized her nine assumptions into three using the same logical precision.[82] While Parse does not take the reader through the step-by-step process of this synthesis, it is easily seen that each of the three assumptions is based on three of the earlier ones. Each of the new assumptions is based on two prior assumptions derived from two of Rogers' concepts and one existential-phenomenological concept and one prior assumption derived from two philosophical concepts and one concept from Rogers. Throughout, the development of the assumptions and their subsequent synthesis, Parse maintains a consistent, logical sequence.

The principles of Man–Living–Health are derived from the assumptions with each principle relating three concepts to each other (see Fig. 19–1). Each principle and concept is explained using support from pertinent literature.[83]

Parse then derived three theoretical structures each of which uses three concepts, one from each principle (see Fig. 19–3).[84] She defines theoretical structure as a statement that interrelates concepts in a way that can be verified.[84] Phillips points out that the stem of each theoretical structure is taken from the third principle. He speculates that greater importance might be attached to this principle, but qualifies this thought by saying that Parse makes it clear that other theoretical structures may be generated from her principles.[85]

Both Winkler and Phillips speak to the difficulty of Parse's terminology for those unfamiliar with existential-phenomenology.[86a,86b] They concur, however, that there is consistency in meaning at each level of discourse.

3. Theories should be relatively simple yet generalizable. While Parse's theory can be generalized to any lived experience, it is far from simple. Terminology which is unfamiliar to nurses is used in this theory, and the difficulty of the terminology may be confusing. The range of possibilities that exists in the lived experiences of open, interrelating beings makes this theory inherently complex.

4. Theories can be bases for hypotheses that can be tested. As Parse's theory is rooted in the human sciences rather than the natural sciences, qualitative rather than quantitative research methodologies are used to test it. Qualitative research methodologies do not pose hypotheses in the cause–effect or associative relationship tradition of quantitative research methodologies. Instead, qualitative research methods focus on entities for study that are lived experiences.[87]

Parse describes Man–Living–Health research methodology that includes the identification of major entities for study, the scientific processes of investigation, and the details of the processes appropriate for inquiry. She states that the two aspects of lived experience to consider in selecting an entity for study are nature and structure. The aspect of nature refers to common lived experiences which surface in the man–environment interrelationship and are health related; examples include "being–becoming, value priorities, negentropic unfolding, and quality of life."[88] Parse cites the example of "waiting" as being consistent with her definition of a common lived experience.

The second aspect of lived experience to consider in selecting an entity for study is structure. Parse defines structure as "the paradoxical living of the remembered, the now moment, and the not-yet all at once."[88] This is uncovered by dialogue with the participant. Thus the research question could be, what is the structure of the lived experience of waiting? The researcher would then proceed to uncover the structure of this lived experience.[89]

While quantitative research methods test hypotheses or tentative assumptions about phenomenon, the Man–Living–Health research methodology described by Parse explores research questions about the structure of lived experiences. Other examples of lived experiences to be studied include: struggling with uncovering the hidden meaning in a dialogue, struggling in cocreating possibilities for self-disclosure, being enabled and limited by a choice, being different from others, planning for the future, and shifting points of view.[90]

5. Theories contribute to and assist in increasing the general body of knowledge within the discipline through the research implemented to validate them. The book *Nursing Research: Qualitative Methods* by Parse, Coyne, and Smith[91] reports support of Man–Living–Health as a theory, through phenomenological, descriptive, and ethnographic methods. Five major qualitative studies, reported in this book, focused on the phenomenology of health, persisting in change, the lived experience of being exposed to toxic chemicals, aging, and retirement. Parse states that these five studies demonstrate similar findings that are supportive of Man–Living–Health. She reports that meaning, rhythmicity, and transcendence, the major themes in her theory, can be seen in varying ways in all of the studies.[92]

Other than this research book, the literature reveals little research using Parse's theory, and none using her recently published research methodology for Man–Living–Health. Phillips reminds the reader that qualitative research is time consuming.[93]

6. Theories can be utilized by the practitioners to guide and improve

their practice. As previously discussed, Man–Living–Health is not congruent with the traditional use of the nursing process. Man–Living–Health guides nursing practice via its own practice methodology composed of dimensions and processes. The dimensions are *illuminating meaning, synchronizing rhythms,* and *mobilizing transcendence,* while the processes are *explicating, dwelling with,* and *moving beyond.*[94] A cardinal rule of this practice methodology is that the authority and responsibility for decision making lies with the person (client), not with the nurse.[95]

Winkler states that Parse's theory would be an appropriate base for practice in situations where the focus is on the person's communicative interaction with the nurse. She also remarks that basing nursing care planning on the client's perspective of health and his or her care would encourage innovative and unique nursing activities.[96]

There is little doubt that the use of Parse's theory in practice would individualize care, but it is not impossible to imagine situations where the client is unable to interact with the nurse. In such cases, other data may guide nursing practice, but who is the decision maker? Critical care situations often require immediate action with no time for or client ability to participate in decision making. While Parse does not limit the use of Man–Living–Health to specified practice settings, the theory appears to be more applicable to those settings where clients can interrelate with the nurse.

7. Theories must be consistent with other validated theories, laws, and principles but will leave open unanswered questions that need to be investigated. Parse's theory of Man–Living–Health is consistent with Roger's principles and concepts and with the tenets and concepts of existential-phenomenological thought. However, as Phillips points out, Parse has synthesized these concepts and created a new product, which does not speak the same language as that of her sources.[97]

Consistent with other nurse theorists, Parse addresses the phenomena of human beings, health, environment, and nursing. While Parse's definition of man as an open being who cocreates health multidimensionally[98] is unique, it is similar to that of other nurse theorists. Roger, Fitzpatrick, and Newman speak to man and environment interacting to manifest health.[99a–99c] Parse's view of the importance of the lived experience and quality of life is also congruent with Rogers, Fitzpatrick, Paterson and Zderad, and Newman.[100a–100c] While Rogers' theory is based on theories across many disciplines, the theories of Parse, Fitzpatrick, and Newman synthesize Rogers' theory with specific tenets and concepts of philosophical thought. Paterson and Zderad base their theory on existentialism and phenomenology. The similarity of theoretical bases clearly contributes to the similarities and the uniqueness of these nursing theories.

As Man–Living–Health focuses on lived experiences, innumerable research questions can be posed for further investigation. Several of these were suggested in the discussion for theory criterion 4.

STRENGTHS AND WEAKNESSES

A strength of Parse's theory is the logical flow from construction of her assumptions to creation of her Man–Living–Health construct and the deductive derivation of principles and concepts. The word sequences of her theoretical structures, while logically flowing from the principles and concepts, is less clear. Phillips wonders why the stem concept for each theoretical structure comes from her third principle. He speculates that greater importance might be attached to this principle, but states that Parse makes it clear that other theoretical structures may be generated from her principles.[101] The wording of Parse's practice dimensions and processes flows directly from each of her three principles.

Another strength of Man–Living–Health is that it focuses on all individuals, not only those defined by societal norms as being ill. The individual in the nurse–person relationship discovers the meaning of his or her lived experiences as the nurse guides him or her through illuminating meaning, synchronizing rhythms, and mobilizing transcendence. In order to do this, individuals and families interrelate with the nurse on a variety of levels. One has to question the outcomes of these interrelationships when the person or client is an infant or young child, or is unconscious, in need of immediate life giving treatment, or all of these factors are present. It is not unreasonable to assume that there will be clients and families who will be unwilling to participate in such an interrelationship as well.

Phillips believes that Parse's theory of Man–Living–Health will speed the transformation from a mechanistic approach to health care to one that has a unitary perspective of the health care of humans.[102] While this is a creditable goal, there is need for a body of research to create a knowledge base about unitary man's lived experiences. The uniqueness of these lived experiences increases the complexity of this task. However, Parse does report that common elements and themes are surfacing from the current research on Man–Living–Health.[103] As these common elements and themes are validated further, they should give direction to a unitary perspective of the health care of humans.

An important strength of this theory is the assumption about man freely choosing personal meaning in the process of relating value priorities. Coupled with this assumption is the thinking that the authority and responsibility of choices resides with the person or client, not the nurse. This is an opposing stance to the tradition of paternalistic health care, where physicians make the decisions and nurses and patients accept them without question. It is a very contemporary stance. Consumers are in fact questioning health care professionals, seeking other opinions and alternative treatment modalities, and resorting to the legal system for their perceived damages. In some ways, the end results have not changed, whether one experiences a paternalistic health care system or a free choice system, the consequences of the decisions are still borne by the client or family. While Parse does not say so explicitly, one has to believe that the nurse, in being-in-true-presence with the person or client, will, via the interrelationship, establish a different and more informed knowledge base.

While Man–Living–Health provides a unique way of looking at man, and a philosophy of man and his living relationship with health, where and how nursing articulates with Man–Living–Health is less clear. Parse has defined nursing as a science and an art that uses its abstract body of knowledge in service to people,[104] with its goals focused on quality of life from the person's perspective.[105] She speaks of the need for nursing to be rooted in the human sciences, rather than the natural sciences, and therefore to be based on the themes of the man–environment interrelationship, coconstitution of health, the meaning unitary man gives to being and becoming, and man's freedom to choose alternative ways of becoming.[106] The question that arises is, Does this constitute all of nursing's knowledge base? Winkler comments that the relevance of quantitative knowledge to the understanding of the person's being and becoming is unclear.[107] This lack of clarity about nursing's knowledge base clouds expectations of what it is specifically that the nurse can and should be doing in practice.

There is also a lack of clarity as to what the natural science knowledge base of the professional nurse should be. Without a prescribed natural science knowledge base, the nurse becomes a different entity. This new entity or new nurse might not have the knowledge base to function in the roles that the profession, education, and the legal system currently ascribe to professional nursing. The roles of care giver, advocate, counselor, and leader do not appear to be congruent with Parse's view of nursing. Nor is the American Nurses' Association's definition of nursing as, "the diagnosis and treatment of human responses to actual or potential health problems,"[108] congruent with Parse's view of nursing. This new view of nursing knowledge and practice is not congruent with use of the nursing process.

Parse has clearly been successful in creating a new paradigm or worldview. Because of its incongruence with traditionally accepted definitions, roles, and nursing process, this new paradigm raises many questions and may be unacceptable as a theory of nursing to some. The strong philosophical base of Man–Living–Health and the usage of philosophical terminology makes this theory difficult for many nurses to understand, and understanding is necessary before individuals will consider a change in their worldview. However, competing paradigms do exist in the discipline of nursing. This competition is seen by scholars as a hallmark of scientific growth.[109]

REFERENCES

1.(a) Parse, R.R. *Man–Living–Health: A Theory of Nursing*, New York: Wiley, 1981.
1.(b) Parse, R.R. *Nursing Science—Major Paradigms, Theories, and Critiques*, Philadelphia: Saunders, 1987.

1.(c) Parse, R.R., Coyne, A.B., & Smith, M.J. *Nursing Research: Qualitative Methods,* Bowie, Md.: Brady Communications, 1985.

2.(a) Rogers, M.E. *The Theoretical Basis of Nursing,* Philadelphia: F.A. Davis Co., 1970, pp. 97–102.

2.(b) Rogers, M.E. Science of Unitary Human Beings: A Paradigm for Nursing, paper presented at International Nurse Theorist Conference, Edmonton, Alberta, May 2, 1984.

3. Parse, *Man–Living–Health,* p. xiii.

4. Ibid, 3.

5. Ibid, 3–4.

6. Parse, *Nursing Science,* p. 4.

7. Peplau, H.E. *Interpersonal Relations in Nursing,* New York: G.P. Putnam's Sons, 1952.

8. Henderson, V. *The Nature of Nursing,* New York: MacMillan, 1966.

9. Hall, L. Another View of Nursing Care and Quality, address given at Catholic University Workshop, Washington, D.C., 1965.

10. Orlando, I.J. *The Dynamic Nurse–Patient Relationship: Function, Process and Principles,* New York: G.P. Putnam's Sons, 1961.

11. Levine, M.E. *Introduction to Clinical Nursing* (2nd ed.), Philadelphia: F.A. Davis Co., 1973.

12. Johnson, D.E. The Behavioral System Model for Nursing, in *Conceptual Models for Nursing Practice* (2nd ed.), Riehl, J.P. & Roy, C. eds., New York: Appleton-Century-Crofts, 1980, pp. 207–216.

13.(a) Roy, C. *Introduction to Nursing: An Adaptation Model,* Englewood Cliffs, N.J.: Prentice-Hall, 1976; (b) 2nd ed., 1984.

14.(a) Orem, D.E. *Nursing: Concepts of Practice,* New York: McGraw-Hill, 1971). (b) 2nd ed., 1980; (c) 3rd ed., 1985.

15.(a) King, I.M. *Toward a Theory for Nursing: General Concepts of Human Behavior,* New York: Wiley 1971.

15.(b) King, I.M. *A Theory for Nursing: Systems, Concepts and Process,* New York: Wiley, 1981.

16. Parse, *Nursing Science,* p. 4.

17. Rogers, *The Theoretical Basis,* pp. 97–102.

18. Parse, *Nursing Science,* p. 4.

19.(a) Heidegger, M. *On Time and Being,* New York: Harper & Row, 1972.

19.(b) Heidegger, M. *Being and Time,* New York: Harper & Row, 1962.

20.(a) Sartre, J.P. *Search for a Method,* New York: Alfred A. Knopf, 1963.

20.(b) Sartre, J.P. *Nausea,* New York: New Dimensions, 1964)

20.(c) Sartre, J.P. *Being and Nothingness,* New York: Washington Square Press, 1966.

21.(a) Merleau-Ponty, M. *The Structure of Behavior,* Boston: Beacon Press, 1963.

21.(b) Merleau-Ponty, M. *The Prose of the World,* Evanston, Ill: Northwestern University Press, 1973.

21.(c) Merleau-Ponty, M. trans. by Colin Smith *Phenomenology of Perception,* New York: Humanities Press, 1974.

22. Parse, *Man–Living–Health,* p. 13.

23. Ibid, 34.

24. Ibid, 35.

25. Phillips, J.R. A Critique of Parse's Man–Living–Health Theory, in *Nursing Science: Major Paradigms, Theories, and Critiques,* Parse, R.R. ed., Philadelphia: Saunders, 1987, pp. 184–185.

26. Winkler, S. J. Parse's Theory of Nursing, in *Conceptual Models of Nursing—Analysis and Application*, Fitzpatrick, J.J. & Whall, A.L. eds., Bowie, MD: Robert J. Brady Co., 1983, p. 281.
27. Parse, *Man—Living—Health*, pp. 34–35.
28. Parse, *Nursing Science*, pp. 161–162.
29. Ibid, 161.
30. Ibid, 162.
31. Ibid, 161–162.
32. Parse, *Man—Living—Health*, p. 39.
33. Parse, *Nursing Science*, p. 162.
34. Parse, *Man—Living—Health*, p. 41.
35. Parse, *Nursing Science*, p. 164.
36. Ibid, 167.
37. Ibid, 168.
38. Ibid, 164.
39. Ibid, 167.
40. Ibid, 168.
41. Ibid, 165.
42. Parse, *Man—Living—Health*, pp. 59–60.
43.(a) Ibid, 62,
43.(b) Parse, *Nursing Science*, p. 165.
44. Parse, *Nursing Science*, p. 167.
45. Ibid, 169.
46. Parse, *Man—Living—Health*, p. 72.
47. Parse, *Nursing Science*, p. 170.
48. Ibid, 160.
49. Ibid, 162.
50. Rogers, *The Theoretical Basis*, pp. 47–54.
51.(a) Edie, J.M. Transcendental Phenomenology and Existentialism, in *Phenomenology*, Kockelmans, J.J. ed., New York: Doubleday 1967, p. 247
51.(b) Husserl, E. *Ideen*, Vol. I, p. 135.
52. Winkler, Parse's Theory, p. 289.
53. Phillips, A Critique, p. 183.
54. Parse, *Man—Living—Health*, p. 25.
55. Ibid, 30.
56. Ibid, 39.
57. Ibid, 41.
58. Phillips, A Critique, pp. 187–188.
59. Parse, *Man—Living—Health*, p. 39.
60. Ibid, 80–81.
61. Parse, *Nursing Science*, p. 136.
62. Parse, *Man—Living—Health*, p. 89.
63. Parse, *Nursing Science*, p. 169.
64. Ibid, 167.
65. Winkler, Parse's Theory, p. 277.
66. Phillips, A Critique, pp. 200–210.
67. Parse, R.R. Man—Living—Health in Practice, unpublished manuscript, Pittsburgh: Discovery International, 1984.
68. Parse, *Man—Living—Health*, pp. 83–90.

69. Ibid, 81.
70. Parse, *Nursing Science*, p. 166.
71. Ibid, 169.
72. Ibid, 166.
73. Ibid, 168.
74. Ibid, 169.
75. Rogers, *The Theoretical Basis*, pp. 97–102.
76. Parse, *Nursing Science*, p. 161.
77. Parse, *Man–Living–Health*, p. 4.
78. Parse, *Nursing Science*, p. 137.
79. Ibid, 167.
80. Parse, *Man–Living–Health*, pp. 7–25.
81. Ibid, 35.
82. Parse, *Nursing Science*, pp. 161–162.
83. Parse, *Man–Living–Health*, pp. 41–68.
84. Ibid, 68.
85. Phillips, A Critique, p. 193.
86.(a) Winkler, Parse's Theory, p. 290.
86.(b) Phillips, A Critique, p. 195.
87. Parse, *Nursing Science*, pp. 178–179.
88. Ibid, 174.
89. Ibid, 175.
90. Parse, *Man–Living–Health*, pp. 79–80.
91. Parse, R.R., Coyne, A.B., Smith, M.J. *Nursing Research: Qualitative Methods,* Bowie, MD.: Brady Communications, 1985.
92. Parse, *Nursing Science*, p. 171.
93. Ibid, 200.
94. Ibid, 167.
95. Ibid, 166–171.
96. Winkler, Parse's Theory, p. 292.
97. Phillips, A Critique, p. 196.
98. Parse, *Man–Living–Health*, p. 25.
99.(a) Rogers, *The Theoretical Base*, p. 47.
99.(b) Fitzpatrick, J.J. The Crisis Perspective: Relationship to Nursing, in *Nursing Models and Their Psychiatric Mental Health Applications,* Fitzpatrick, J.J., Whall, A.L., Johnson, R.L., & Floyd, J.A., eds., Bowie, MD.: Robert J. Brady Co., 1982, p. 33.
99.(c) Newman, M.A., *Theory Development in Nursing,* Philadelphia: F.A. Davis, 1979, p. 62.
100.(a) Rogers, M. Nursing: A Science of Unitary Man, in *Conceptual Models for Nursing Practice* (2nd ed.), Riehl, J.P. & Roy, C., eds., New York: Appleton-Century-Crofts, 1980, p. 333.
100.(b) Fitzpatrick, J.J. A Life Perspective Rhythm Model, in *Conceptual Models of Nursing: Analysis and Application,* Fitzpatrick, J.J. & Whall, A.L., eds., Bowie, MD.: Robert J. Brady Company, 1983, p. 295.
100.(c) Paterson, J.E. & Zderad, L.T., *Humanistic Nursing,* New York: Wiley, p. 16.
100.(d) Newman, *Theory Development*, p. 67.
101. Phillips, A Critique, p. 193.
102. Ibid, 201.

103.   Parse, *Nursing Science,* p. 171.
104.   Parse, *Man–Living–Health,* p. 81.
105.   Parse, *Nursing Science,* p. 136.
106.   Parse, *Man–Living–Health,* p. 13.
107.   Winkler, Parse's Theory, p. 284.
108.   American Nurses' Association, Nursing: A Social Policy Statement, Kansas City, MO.: ANA Publication, 1980, Code NP-63 35M.
109.   Meleis, A.I. *Theoretical Nursing: Development and Progress,* Philadelphia,: Lippincott, 1985.

BIBLIOGRAPHY

Bannon, J.F. *The Philosophy of Merleau-Ponty,* New York: Harcourt, Brace, and World, 1967.

Barrett, W. *What is Existentialism?,* New York: Grove Press, 1965.

Fawcett, J. On Research and the Professionalization of Nursing, *Nursing Forum,* 1980, *19,* 310–318.

Kuhn, T.S. *The Structure of Scientific Revolutions,* Chicago: University of Chicago Press, 1970.

Limandri, B.J. Review of Man–Living–Health: A Theory of Nursing, *Western Journal of Nursing Research,* 1982, *4,* 105–106.

Oiler, C.J. Qualitative Methods: Phenomenology, *New Approaches to Theory Development,* Moccia, P., ed., New York: National League for Nursing, 1986, pp. 75–103.

Parse, R.R. *Nursing Fundamentals,* Flushing, NY: Medical Examination Publishing, 1974.

Schumacher, L.P. Rosemarie Rizzo Parse: Man–Living–Health, in *Nursing Theorists and Their Work,* Marriner, A., ed., St. Louis: C.V. Mosby, 1986.

Winstead-Fry, P. The Scientific Method and its Impact on Holistic Health, *Advances in Nursing Science,* 1980, *2,* 1–7.

CHAPTER 20

Madeleine Leininger

Julia B. George

Madeleine Leininger received her basic nursing education at St. Anthony's School of Nursing, Denver, CO and graduated in 1948. In 1950 she earned a Bachelor of Science from Benedictine College, Atchison, KS; in 1953 a Master of Science in Nursing from Catholic University, Washington, DC; and in 1965 a PhD in Anthropology from the University of Washington, Seattle. She is a Fellow in the American Academy of Nursing and holds an LhD from Benedictine College.

Dr. Leininger is the founder of the transcultural subfield of nursing. She is Professor of Nursing and Anthropology, Director of the Center for Health Research, and Director of Transcultural Nursing Offerings at Wayne State University. She has held both faculty and administrative apppointments in nursing education. She has published extensively.

During the mid 1950s, Madeleine Leininger experienced what she describes as cultural shock while she was working in a child guidance home in the midwestern United States. While working as a clinical nurse specialist with disturbed children and their parents, she observed recurrent behavioral differences among the children and concluded that these differences had a cultural base. She identified a lack of knowledge of the children's cultures as the missing link in nursing to understand the variations in care of clients. This experience led her to become the first professional nurse in the world to earn a doctorate in anthropology,[1] and led to the development of the new field of transcultural nursing as a subfield of nursing.

Leininger first used the terms "transcultural nursing," "ethnonursing," and "cross-cultural nursing" in the 1960s. In 1966, at the University of Colorado, she offered the first transcultural nursing course with field experiences and has been instrumental in the development of similar courses at a number of other institutions.[2] In 1979, Leininger defined transcultural nursing as[3]:

> a learned subfield or branch of nursing which focuses upon the comparative study and analysis of cultures with respect to nursing and health–illness caring practices, beliefs, and values with the goal to provide meaningful and efficacious nursing care services to people according to their cultural values and health-illness context.

She also defined ethnonursing as[3]:

> the study of nursing care beliefs, values, and practices as cognitively perceived and known by a designated culture through their direct experience, beliefs, and value system.

The term transcultural nursing (rather than "cross-cultural") is used today to refer to the evolving knowledge and practices related to this new field of study and practice. Leininger stresses the importance of knowledge gained from direct experience or directly from those who have experienced and labels such knowledge as *emic*. She contends that *emically* derived care knowledge is essential to establish nursing's epistemological and ontological base for practice (Leininger, personal communication, 1988).

Leininger has built her theory of transcultural nursing on the premise that the peoples of each culture not only can know and define the ways in which they experience and perceive their nursing care world but also can relate these experiences and perceptions to their general health beliefs and practices. Based upon this premise, nursing care is derived and developed from the cultural context in which it is to be provided.

LEININGER'S THEORY

In 1985, Leininger published her first presentation of her work as a theory[4] and in 1988 she presented further explication of her ideas.[5] In these presentations, she provided definitions for the concepts of culture, cultural value, cultural care diversity, cultural care universality, cultural care, world view, social structure, environmental context, folk health system, health, professional health system, care/caring, cultural care preservation, cultural care accommodation, and cultural care repatterning. Some of these definitions were from earlier works and some were original to the 1985 or 1988 articles. Leininger points out that these definitions are provisional guides that may be altered as a culture is studied.[6]

In addition to the definitions she presented assumptions which support her prediction "that different cultures perceive, know, and practice care in different ways, yet there are some commonalities about care among all cultures of the world."[7] She refers to the commonalities as universality and to the differences as diversity.

Culture is the "learned, shared and transmitted values, beliefs, norms and life practices of a particular group that guides thinking, decisions and actions in patterned ways."[8] A related assumption is that human beings are cultural beings and have been able to survive over time through their ability to care for others of all ages in many environments and many ways.[9] *Cultural values* are derived from the culture and identify desirable ways of acting or knowing. These values are often held by the culture over long periods of time and serve to guide decision making for members of the culture.[10] Values may be either diverse or universal.

Cultural care diversity indicates "the variability of meanings, patterns, values or symbols of care that are culturally derived by humans for their well-being or to improve a human condition and lifeway or to face death."[11] In contrast, *cultural care universality* refers to "common, similar or uniform meanings, patterns, values or symbols of care that are culturally derived by humans for their well-being or to improve a human condition and lifeway or to face death."[11] It is assumed that, while human care is universal across cultures, caring may be demonstrated through diverse expressions, actions, patterns, lifestyles, and meanings.[12] *Cultural care* is defined as "the cognitively known values, beliefs and patterned expressions that assist, support or enable another individual or group to maintain well-being, improve a human condition or lifeway or face death and disabilities."[13] A related assumption is that cultural care is "the broadest means to know, explain, account for, and predict nursing care phenomena and to guide nursing care practices."[14]

World view is the way in which people look at the world, or at the universe, and form a "picture or value stance" about the world and their lives.[15] *Social structure* is defined as involving "the dynamic nature of interrelated structural or organizational factors of a particular culture (or society) and how these factors function to give meaning and structural order including religious, kinship, political, economic, educational, technological and cultural factors."[15] *Environmental context* is "the *totality* of an event, situation or particular experience that gives meaning to human expressions including social interactions, physical, ecological, emotional and cultural dimensions."[15] "Knowledge of meanings and practices derived from world views, social structure factors, cultural values, environmental context and language uses are essential to guide nursing and actions in providing cultural congruent care."[16]

Folk health or well being systems are "traditional or local indigenous health care or cure practices that have special meanings and uses to heal or assist people, which are generally offered in familiar home or community environmental contexts with their local practitioners."[17] *Health* is "a *state of well being* that is culturally defined, valued and practiced and which reflects the ability of individuals (or groups) to perform their daily role activities in a culturally satisfactory way."[17] *Professional health system* is defined as "professional care or cure services offered by diverse health personnel who have been prepared through formal professional programs of study in special educational institutions."[17] The related assumption is that all cultures have both professional and folk health care practices.[18]

Care as a noun is defined as those "*phenomena* related to assisting, supportive, or enabling behavior towards or for another individual (or group) with evident or anticipated needs to ameliorate or improve a human condition or lifeway."[19] Care is assumed to be a dominant, unifying and central domain of nursing and while cure cannot occur effectively without care, care may occur without cure.[20] *Care* as a verb is defined as "action directed toward assisting, supporting or enabling another individual (or group) with evident or anticipated needs to ameliorate or improve a human condition or lifeway."[21] Assumptions related to care and caring include that they are essential for the survival of humans, as well as for their development and abilities to deal with critical and recurrent life events, including illness, disability, and death. The expressions, patterns and lifestyles of care have different meanings in different cultural contexts. The phenomenon of care can be discovered or identified by examining the cultural group's view of the world, social structure, and language.[22]

Along with the universal nature of human beings as caring beings, the cultural care values, beliefs, and practices that are specific to a given culture provide a basis for the patterns, conditions, and actions associated with human care.[22] Knowledge of these provides the base for three modes of nursing care decisions and actions. *Cultural care preservation* is also known as maintenance and includes those "assistive, supportive or enabling professional actions and decisions that help clients of a particular culture to preserve or maintain a state of health, or to recover from illness, and to face death."[23] *Cultural care accommodation,* also known as negotiation, includes those "assistive, supporting or enabling professional actions and decisions that help clients of a particular culture to adapt to, or negotiate for a beneficial or satisfying health status or to face death."[23] *Cultural care repatterning,* or restructuring, includes "those assistive, supportive or enabling professional actions or decisions that help clients change their lifeways for new or different patterns that are culturally meaningful and satisfying or that support beneficial and healthy life patterns."[23]

Additional assumptions about nursing include that nursing is a transcultural care profession. Nurses provide care to people of many different cultures but often neither value nor practice from a transcultural perspective. To be effective, legitimate, and relevant to the diversity of peoples of the world, nursing needs to be based upon transcultural care knowledge and skill. Culturally based nursing care is a critical factor for effective health promotion and maintenance, as well as recovery from illness and disability.

Leininger has named her theory Cultural Care Diversity and Universality and depicts it in the Sunrise Model (see Figure 20–1). This model may be viewed as having four levels with the first level being the most abstract and the fourth level the least abstract. Levels one through three provide the knowledge base needed for the planning and delivery of culture congruent care. Level one is the world view and social system level, which directs the study of perceptions of the world outside of the culture—the suprasystem in general system terms. Leininger states this level leads to the study of the nature, meaning, and attributes of care from three perspectives. Values and social structure could be a part of each of the perspectives. The microperspective studies individuals within a culture; these studies would typi-

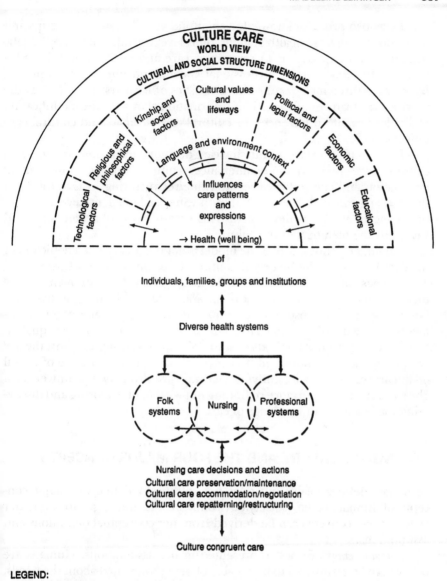

Figure 20–1. Leininger's Sunrise Model depicts dimensions of Cultural Care Diversity and Universality. *(From Leininger, M. Leininger's Theory of Nursing Cultural Care Diversity and Universality, Nursing Science Quarterly, 1988; 1, p. 157. Used with permission.)*.

cally be on a small scale. The middle perspective focuses on more complex factors in one specific culture; these studies are on a larger scale than micro-studies. The macro-studies investigate phenomena across several cultures and are large in scale.[24]

Level two provides knowledge about individuals, families, groups and institutions in diverse health systems. This level provides culturally specific meanings and expressions in relation to care and health. Level three focuses on the folk system, professional system, and nursing. Information from Level three includes the characteristics of each system as well as the specific care features of each. This information allows for the identification of similarities and differences, or cultural care diversity and cultural care universality.[24]

Level four is the level of nursing care decisions and actions and involves cultural care preservation/maintenance, cultural care accommodation/negotiation and cultural care repatterning/restructuring. It is at this level that nursing care is delivered. Within the Sunrise Model, in Level four culture congruent care is developed. This care is both congruent with and valued by the members of the culture.

Leininger points out that the model is not the theory but a depiction of the components of the theory of Cultural Care Diversity and Universality. The purpose of the model is to aid the study of how the components of the theory influence the health status of, and care provided to, individuals, families, groups and institutions within a culture. She presents cogent arguments for the use of the model to guide discovery research that uses qualitative and ethnographic methods of study. She speaks strongly against the use of operational definitions and preconceived notions, and the use of causal or linear perspectives in studying cultural care diversity and universality. She supports the importance of finding out what *is*, of exploring and discovering the essence and meanings of care.

LEININGER'S THEORY AND THE FOUR MAJOR CONCEPTS

Leininger defines health but does not specifically define the major concepts of human being, society/environment and nursing. However, her view of these concepts can be derived from her conceptual definitions and assumptions.

Human beings are best represented in her assumptions. Humans are believed to be caring and to be capable of being concerned about the needs, well-being, and survival of others. Human care is universal, that is, seen in all cultures. Humans have survived within cultures and through place and time because they have been able to care for infants, children, and the elderly in a variety of ways and in many different environments. Thus, humans are universally caring beings who survive in a diversity of cultures through their ability to provide the universality of care in a variety of ways according to differing cultures, needs, and settings.[24] Transcultural nursing also focuses beyond the individual and group to worldwide health institutions and ways to develop international nursing care policies and practices. (Leininger, personal communication, 1988).

Leininger defines *health* as "a *state of well being* that is culturally defined, valued and practiced and which reflects the ability of individuals (or groups) to perform their daily role activities in a culturally satisfactory way."[25] She speaks of health systems, health care practices, changing health patterns, health promotion and health maintenance. Health is an important concept in transcultural nursing. Because of the emphasis on the need for nurses to have knowledge that is specific to the culture in which nursing is being practiced, it is presumed that health is viewed as being universal across cultures but defined within each culture in a manner that reflects the beliefs, values, and practices of that particular culture. Thus, health is also universal and diverse.

Again, *society/environment* are not terms that are defined by Leininger; she speaks instead of world view, social structure and environmental context. However, society/environment, if viewed as being represented in culture, are a major theme of Leininger's theory. Environmental context is defined as being the totality of an event, situation or experience. Leininger's definition of culture focuses on a particular group (society) and the patterning of actions, thoughts, and decisions that occurs as the result of "learned, shared, and transmitted values, beliefs, norms, and lifeway practices."[26] This learning, sharing, transmitting, and patterning occur within a group of people who function in an identifiable setting or environment. Therefore, although Leininger does not use the specific terms of society or environment, the concept of culture is closely related to society/environment, and is a central theme of her theory.

Nursing per se is not defined by Leininger. She asserts that nursing is the phenomenon that needs to be explained.[27] She does state in her assumptions that nursing is essentially a profession that involves culture congruent care since nurses provide care to peoples of many different cultures. She expresses concern that nurses do not have adequate preparation for a transcultural perspective and that they neither value nor practice from such a perspective to the fullest extent possible. She presents three types of nursing actions that are culturally based and thus congruent with the needs and values of the clients. These are cultural care preservation/maintenance, cultural care accommodation/negotiation, and cultural care repatterning/restructuring and have been defined earlier in this chapter. These three modes of action can lead to the delivery of nursing care that best fits with the client's culture and thus decreases cultural stress and potential for conflict between client and caregiver.[28]

CULTURAL CARE DIVERSITY AND UNIVERSALITY AND THE NURSING PROCESS

After careful review of the Sunrise Model, it becomes apparent that there are parallels between the model and the nursing process. This is true, in part, because both represent a problem solving process. The focus of the nursing process is the client who is the recipient of nursing care. The client is also a focus of the Sunrise Model but the importance of knowledge and understanding of the client's culture is a major shaping force in the Model.

Gaining knowledge and understanding of another's culture may be very time consuming for the nurse who is not familiar with that culture. Leininger speaks with concern about the possibility of the nurse being involved in culture shock or cultural imposition. *Culture shock* may result when an outsider attempts to comprehend or adapt effectively to a different cultural group. The outsider is likely to experience feelings of discomfort and helplessness and some degree of disorientation because of the differences in cultural values, beliefs, and practices. Culture shock may lead to anger and can be reduced by seeking knowledge of the culture before encountering that culture. *Cultural imposition* refers to efforts of the outsider, both subtle and not so subtle, to impose his or her own cultural values, beliefs, behaviors upon an individual, family, or group from another culture. Cultural imposition has been particularly prevalent in efforts to impose.Western health care practices upon other cultures.[29]

Levels one, two, and three of the Sunrise Model involve the development of knowledge and when appropriately used could help prevent culture shock and cultural imposition. These levels are similar to the *assessment* and *diagnosis* phases of the nursing process. However, in the Sunrise Model, knowledge of the culture could be gained before identifying a specific client who would be the focus of the nursing process. In the first level, one is assessing or gathering knowledge and information about the social structure and world view of the client's culture. Other information that is needed includes the language and environmental context of the client as well as the factors of technology, religion, philosophy, kinship, social structure, cultural values and beliefs, politics, legal system, economics, and education. Much of this knowledge could be gathered before the identification of a particular client and would be useful in preventing both culture shock and cultural imposition.

Level one knowledge needs to be applied to the situation of the client, whether that client is an individual, a family, a group or a sociocultural institution (Level two). Next, it is recognized that the client exists within a health system and the values, beliefs, and behaviors of the folk, professional, and nursing portions of that health system need to be identified (Level three). Throughout this assessment process, it is important to recognize and identify those characteristics which are universal or common across cultures and those which are diverse or specific to the culture being assessed. After identifying the cultural care diversities and universalities for the culture, a nursing diagnosis can be developed based upon those areas in which the client is not meeting a cultural care diversity or universality.

Once the diagnosis has been established, *planning* and *implementation* occur within Level four, Nursing Care Decisions and Actions. Again, the nursing care decisions and actions need to be culturally based to best meet the needs of the client and provide culture congruent care. The three modes of action are cultural care preservation/maintenance, cultural care accommodation/negotiation, and cultural care repatterning/restructuring. In cultural care preservation/maintenance, the professional actions focus on supporting, assisting, or enabling clients to preserve or maintain favorable health, to recover from illness or to face death. An example would be facilitating an elderly person's access to grocery shopping so that the individual can continue to prepare healthy meals—or encouraging the sharing of those meals with another in a manner which is culturally acceptable.

Cultural care accommodation/negotiation actions focus on enabling, assisting, or supporting professional actions which represent ways to negotiate, adapt, or adjust to the client's health and care patterns for a beneficial health status or to face death. For example, in planning for prenatal classes for multigravidas in a Hispanic community, provision for child care needs to be included as Hispanic mothers place very high value on caring for their children and do not use babysitters as freely as do many mothers in American society. The Hispanic mother's care pattern is to provide care for her child and to have the child near her. She will choose to not attend the class rather than leave her child at home with a babysitter. Those who do not understand this may become involved in cultural imposition and label the mother as not caring when she does not attend meetings at which child care is not available.

Cultural care repatterning/restructuring refers to professional actions that seek to help clients change meaningful health or life patterns to patterns that will be healthier for them. For example, Charles Sanders, whose dietary pattern has been to eat a lot of fried and salted foods, is found to have hypertension and elevated blood cholesterol levels. Fried chicken with a salty batter is an important element in Mr. Sanders' diet—it is a food which appears on the menu at family celebrations and one which is frequently packed in the brown bag meal he carries to work. Fortunately, the chicken itself is one of the forms of protein which is recommended in low cholesterol diets. The repatterning which can occur relates to the way in which the chicken is prepared. The food preparer in the Sanders family could be taught to skin the chicken (helps lower the cholesterol), use a coating of herbs (rather than salt to help with the hypertension), and bake in the microwave oven with no added fat rather than fry with a salty batter (helps with both cholesterol and hypertension). Such change would repattern the preparation of a favorite food into a way that could provide for the continued inclusion of this food in the diet on a regular basis. At the same time, important changes in the way in which Mr. Sanders eats would be supported. Similar repatterning could occur with other foods, for example, instead of cooking green beans with salt pork, they could be cooked with herbs and a little polyunsaturated oil.

The Sunrise Model does not include an area identified as *evaluation*.

However, in Leininger's discussion of transcultural nursing, she places a great deal of importance upon the need for nursing care to provide ways in which care will benefit the client and on the need to systematically study nursing care behaviors to determine which care behaviors are appropriate to the lifeways and behavioral patterns of the culture for healing, health, or well-being.[30a,30b] Such study certainly is the equivalent of evaluation. Without evaluation of the outcomes of a particular plan of care that used the nursing process, or a series of such plans, the systematic study that Leininger advises cannot be completed.

CULTURAL CARE DIVERSITY AND UNIVERSALITY AND THE CHARACTERISTICS OF A THEORY

Beginning with the identification of a need to understand the culture of clients, through the introduction of the terms transcultural nursing and ethnonursing care, to the presentation of the Sunrise Model, Madeleine Leininger has developed the theory she calls Cultural Care Diversity and Universality. This theory will be discussed in relation to the characteristics of a theory presented in Chapter 1.

1. Theories can interrelate concepts in such a way as to create a different way of looking at a particular phenomenon. Leininger has developed the Sunrise Model to demonstrate the interrelationships of the concepts in her theory of Cultural Care Diversity and Universality. Level one of the model does not differ significantly from any other view of culture and its interaction with human beings, with the possible exception of the inclusion of care and health patterns. Level two focuses on individuals, families, groups and sociocultural institutions which is similar to other theories of nursing. The inclusion of the term "cultural" does provide a distinguishing feature since no other nursing theory has this emphasis on culture. Level three provides a view of health systems as including folk, professional, and nursing systems. The inclusion of the folk system is unique to the cultural care theory. Level four speaks to nursing care decisions and actions as supporting, accommodating to, or repatterning current health and care practices. The focus of nursing care decisions and actions is shared with many other theories. The division of actions into supporting, accommodating, or repatterning is specific to this theory. The Sunrise Model of Cultural Care Diversity and Universality in itself supports the concepts of diversity and universality. Levels one and two are essentially universal as they have much in common with many other theories. Levels three and four are diverse, or more specific and unique to this particular theory. Thus, Leininger has interrelated concepts in a way which provides a different way of looking at the phenomenon of nursing care.

2. Theories must be logical in nature. There is an inherent logic in the thought that as more is known about a client, the opportunity to provide care that meets that client's needs increases. Leininger has focused on a particular area of knowledge as being important—that area is the culture of the client with culture having a broad definition. The Sunrise Model has a logical order to it. This order is reflected in the movement from a world view through language and environmental context, care patterns and expressions of individuals, families, groups and institutions into diverse health systems to nursing care decisions and actions to culture congruent care (see Fig. 20–1).

3. Theories should be relatively simple yet generalizable. Leininger's theory is essentially parsimonious in that the necessary concepts are incorporated in such a manner that the theory and its model can be applied in many different settings. The theory and model are not simple in terms of being easily understood upon first contact. However, Leininger's presentations of the theory and model support the need for each of the concepts and demonstrate how the concepts are interrelated. Once the interrelationships are grasped, simplicity is more apparent. The theory and model are excellent examples of being generalizable. The concepts and relationships that are presented are at a level of abstraction which allows them to be applied in many different situations. They provide a guide for knowledge that moves from initial generation of knowledge through affirmation of substantive knowledge to application of that knowledge in a caring process. While the knowledge is to be specific to the situation in which the nursing care is to occur, the process of generating and applying the knowledge is universal.

4. Theories can be the bases for hypotheses that can be tested. During the development of the Cultural Care Diversity and Universality theory many studies have been conducted that demonstrate the theory can be the basis for research. A number of these studies were presented during four national transcultural nursing conferences held from 1975 to 1978 at the College of Nursing, University of Utah. The proceedings of these conferences are presented in *Transcultural Nursing*.[31] These proceedings reflect the importance of ethnographic research in the development of this theory. In addition, Leininger has presented a number of relational statements that provide a foundation for further study (see Table 20–1).

It is important to note that the theory of Cultural Care Diversity and Universality is based upon, and calls for, qualitative rather than quantitative research. The development of hypotheses is characteristic of positivistic, quantitative research. The development of research questions, and of relational statements is characteristic of qualitative research. Therefore, from the viewpoint of qualitative research, this criterion is met.

5. Theories contribute to and assist in increasing the general body of knowledge within the discipline through the research implemented to validate them. The research that has been conducted on transcultural nursing has contributed to the general body of knowledge within the discipline of nursing. One of the outcomes of this research is the identification of

TABLE 20–1. HYPOTHESES DERIVED FROM LEININGER'S THEORY

- There is an identifiable, positive relationship between the way people of different cultures define, interpret, and know care with their recurrent patterns of thinking and living.
- The *emic* (inside views) of cultural care values, beliefs, and practices of cultures will show a close relationship to their daily life care patterns.
- The meaning and use of cultural care concepts varies cross-culturally and influences nursing care-giver and care-receiver practices.
- There is a meaningful relationship between social structure factors and world view with folk and professional care practices.
- Nursing care subsystems are closely related to professional health care systems but differ markedly from folk health care systems.
- Nursing care decisions or actions that reflect the use of the client's cultural care values, beliefs, and practices will be positively related to client's satisfactions with nursing care.
- Nursing care actions or decisions that are based upon the use of cultural care preservation, accommodation, and/or repatterning in client care will be positively related to beneficial nursing care.
- Signs of intercultural care conflicts and stresses will be evident if caregivers fail to use cultural care values and beliefs of clients.
- Marked differences between the meanings and expressions of caregivers and care-recipients lead to dissatisfactions for both.
- High dependency of the clients upon technological nursing care activities will be closely related to cultural care that reflects decreased personalized care actions.
- Religion and kinship care factors will be more resilient to change than technological factors.
- Western views of cultural care values will be markedly different from non-Western care values.
- Self-care practices will be evident in cultures that value individualism and independence; other-care practices will be evident in cultures that support human interdependence.
- Anglo-American nurse-client teaching methods will be dysfunctional with clients of non-Western cultural value orientations.

(From Leininger, M. Transcultural Care Diversity and Universality: A Theory of Nursing, Nursing and Health Care, 1985, 6, 210, 212.)

major cultural care constructs. Leininger indicates that, as of 1988, she has identified 85 such constructs from 45 cultures. (Leininger, personal communication, 1988). These constructs have more diversity than universality of meaning. Included in these constructs are anticipation of, attentiveness to, comfort, compassion, coping, empathy, engrossment, helping, nurturance, protection, restoration, support, stimulation, stress alleviation, succorance, surveillance, tenderness, touch, and trust.[32a,32b]

Leininger has directed her research for the last three decades in the epistemological search to establish care as the essence of, and a distinct construct of, nursing. She has sought to explicate the illusive and embedded diverse culture specific and cultural universals of care. The goal of her theory is to provide *culturally congruent care* for the health or well-being of individuals, families, and institutional environments. She views transcultural nursing as the arching framework for all nursing education, theory, research, and practice as nurses are expected to *care* for all people of diverse cultures worldwide. Her ideas have moved nursing beyond unicultural reference to a multicultural perspective (Leininger, personal communication, 1988).

6. Theories can be utilized by the practitioners to guide and improve their practice. In her presentation of the theory, Leininger presents examples of research findings which can guide and improve the practice of nursing. One example presents the differences in the interpretations of care by American nurses in several general hospitals, Canadian nurses, and Polynesian nurses in Hawaii. The American nurses interpreted care as first dealing with stress alleviation and then comfort. Canadian nurses reported care as being primarily support. Polynesian nurses in Hawaii first identified care as sharing with others in personalized cultural ways and then added being generous to others to achieve signs of harmony among people and their environment. Knowing the diversity in nurses' interpretation of care supports the diversity which will be present in clients and reinforces the need to be knowledgeable about this diversity. Care is universal, the meaning of care is diverse.[33]

7. Theories must be consistent with other validated theories, laws, principles but will leave open unanswered questions that need to be investigated. Leininger's theory is certainly consistent with all theories that include the concept of the importance of knowing the client as a person rather than as a problem. Leininger's discussion of the seriousness of unintentional cultural imposition practices by nurses, and of the nurse's need to be aware of his or her own culture and its implications for the nurse–client situation,[34] is very similar to Imogene King's emphasis on the importance of perceptions and the need for the nurse to be alert to both client and personal perceptions.[35] This is but one example of areas of agreement with other theories. It is important to note that while Leininger and Watson both speak of the importance of caring, they approach caring differently.[36]

The unanswered questions that remain to be investigated are greater in number than those that have been answered. Since cultures are diverse not only among cultures but within them, and individuals, even within the same culture, respond differently to the same stimuli, each nurse–client situation provides new questions to be explored.

STRENGTHS AND LIMITATIONS

A major strength of Leininger's theory is the recognition of the importance of culture and its influence on everything that involves the recipients and providers of nursing care. The development of this theory over a number of years has allowed its concepts and constructs to be tested by a number of people in a variety of settings and cultures. The Sunrise Model provides guidance for the areas in which information needs to be collected.

Some limitations, as identified by Leininger,[37] include the limited number of graduate nurses who are academically prepared to conduct the investigations needed to provide transcultural nursing care. While there has been some increase in the number of nurses prepared in transcultural nursing, it is important to note the danger of cultural biases and cultural imposition occurring with nurses' personal cultural values. An associated concern is that too few nursing programs include courses and planned learning experiences that provide a knowledge base for transcultural nursing practice. There is also a need for research funds to support continued study of caring practices—both those that are universal and those that are particular to a culture.

In some of her writings, Leininger is not consistent in her terminology. For example, in *Transcultural Nursing,* she refers to ethnocultural care constructs[38] and then to ethnonursing care constructs.[39] In her theory presentation she refers to these same constructs as major cultural care constructs.[40] Since the constructs are listed it is relatively easy to be aware that these terms all refer to the same constructs. However, the reader's mental energy could be conserved for understanding the theory and model if the terminology were more consistent.

The complexity of the Sunrise Model can be viewed as both a strength and a limitation. The complexity is a strength in that it emphasizes the importance of the inclusion of anthropological and cultural concepts in nursing education and practice. On the other hand, the complexity can lead to misinterpretation or rejection, both of which are limitations.

SUMMARY

Madeleine Leininger has been working since the 1950s on the development of her theory of Cultural Care Diversity and Universality. In the 1960s, she first began to use the terms transcultural nursing and ethnonursing. While she has slightly different definitions of these terms, she often uses them interchangeably, an action that can be confusing to the reader.

The major concepts of her theory are culture, cultural value, cultural care diversity and universality, cultural care, world view; social structure, environmental context, folk health system, health, professional health system, care, caring, cultural care preservation, cultural care accommodation, and cultural care repatterning. She defines each of these concepts and presents assumptions that are related to them. The concepts and their interrelationships provide the basis for the Sunrise Model of this theory.

The Sunrise Model presents four levels of focus which move from the cultural and social structure through individuals, families, groups and institutions in diverse health systems to nursing care decisions and actions that are cultural care preserving, accommodating and repatterning. The Model also indicates the need to move from knowledge generation through substantive knowledge to application of the knowledge. In discussing the model, Leininger presents the idea that care patterns and processes may be universal or diverse. Universal care indicates care patterns, values, and behaviors that are common across cultures. Care diversities represent those patterns and processes that are unique or specific to an individual, family, or cultural group. Leininger believes care diversities are greater in number than are universal care patterns.[40]

The theory of Cultural Care Diversity and Universality is of significance in a society that is becoming more and more aware of the cultural diversity within its boundaries. While this theory does not provide specific directions for nursing care, it does provide guidelines for the gathering of knowledge and a framework for the making of decisions about what care is needed or would be of the greatest benefit to the client. Leininger has clearly identified what has been a major deficit in our provision of nursing care and provided a road map to begin to fill the gaps created by that deficit.

REFERENCES

1. Leininger, M. *Transcultural Nursing* New York: Masson Publishing, USA, Inc., 1979, pp. 11–12.
2. Ibid, 13–14.
3. Ibid, 15.
4. Leininger, M.M. Transcultural Care Diversity and Universality: A Theory of Nursing, *Nursing and Health Care,* 1985 *6,* 209–212.
5. Leininger, M.M. Leininger's Theory of Nursing: Cultural Care Diversity and Universality, *Nursing Science Quarterly,* 1988, *1,* 152–160.
6. Ibid, 156.
7. Leininger, Transcultural Care Diversity and Universality, p. 210.
8. Leininger, Leininger's Theory of Nursing, p. 156.
9. Leininger, Transcultural Care Diversity and Universality, p. 210.
10. Ibid, 209.
11. Leininger, Leininger's Theory of Nursing, mss. p. 13.
12. Leininger, Transcultural Care Diversity and Universality, p. 210.
13. Leininger, Leininger's Theory of Nursing, p. 156.
14. Ibid, 155.
15. Ibid, 156.
16. Ibid, 155.
17. Ibid, 156.
18. Leininger, Transcultural Care Diversity and Universality, p. 210.
19. Leininger, Leininger's Theory of Nursing, p. 156.

20.   Leininger, Transcultural Care Diversity and Universality, p. 210.
21.   Leininger, Leininger's Theory of Nursing, p. 156.
22.   Leininger, Transcultural Care Diversity and Universality, p. 210.
23.   Leininger, Leininger's Theory of Nursing, mss. p. 156.
24.   Leininger, Transcultural Care Diversity and Universality, p. 210.
25.   Leininger, Leininger's Theory of Nursing, mss. p. 156.
26.   Leininger, Transcultural Care Diversity and Universality, p. 209.
27.   Leininger, Leininger's Theory of Nursing, p. 154.
28.   Leininger, Transcultural Care Diversity and Universality, p. 210.
29.   Leininger, M. *Transcultural Nursing: Concepts, Theories, and Practices.* New York: John Wiley & Sons, 1978, p. 57.
30.(a) Leininger, *Transcultural Nursing*, p. 16.
30.(b) Transcultural Care Diversity and Universality, p. 210.
31.   Leininger, *Transcultural Nursing*.
32.(a) Leininger, *Transcultural Nursing*, p. 20.
32.(b) Leininger, Transcultural Care Diversity and Universality, p. 212.
33.   Leininger, Transcultural Care Diversity and Universality, p. 212.
34.   Leininger, *Transcultural Nursing*, p. 11.
35.   King, I. *A Theory for Nursing: Systems, Concepts, Process.* New York: John Wiley & Sons, Inc., 1981, pp. 145–146.
36.   Watson, J. *Nursing: Human Science and Human Care*, New York: National League for Nursing, 1988.
37.   Leininger, *Transcultural Nursing*, pp. 17–18.
38.   Ibid, 19.
39.   Ibid, 22.
40.   Leininger, Transcultural Care Diversity and Universality, p. 212.

BIBLIOGRAPHY

Leininger, M. ed. *Care: The Essence of Nursing and Health.* Thorofare, New Jersey: Charles B. Slack, Inc., 1984.

Leininger M. Caring: A Central Focus of Nursing and Health Care Services, *Nursing & Health Care*, 1980, 1, pp. 135–143, 176

Leininger, M. ed. *Caring: An Essential Human Need.* Thorofare, New Jersey: Charles B. Slack, Inc., 1981.

Leininger, M. ed. *Health Care Dimensions: Barriers and Facilitators to Quality Health Care.* Philadelphia: F. A. Davis Company, 1975.

Leininger, M. ed. *Health Care Dimensions: Health Care Issues.* Philadelphia: F. A. Davis Company, 1974.

Leininger, M. ed. *Health Care Dimensions: Transcultural Health Care Issues and Conditions.* Philadelphia: F. A. Davis Company, 1976.

Leininger, M. *Nursing and Anthropology: Two Worlds to Blend.* New York: John Wiley & Sons, Inc., 1970.

Leininger, M. ed. *Qualitative Research Methods in Nursing.* Orlando, Fl: Grune & Stratton, Inc., 1985.

Leininger, M. *Reference Sources for Transcultural Health and Nursing.* Thorofare, New Jersey: Charles B. Slack, 1984.

Leininger, M. Transcultural Nursing: Its Progress and Its Future, *Nursing & Health Care.* 1981, *2,* pp. 365–371.

Leininger M. Transcultural Nursing: An Overview, *Nursing Outlook,* 1984, *32,* pp. 72–73.

Leininger, M. ed. *Transcultural Nursing: Teaching, Practice and Research.* Salt Lake City: University of Utah College of Nursing, 1980.

CHAPTER 21

Nursing Theories and the Nursing Process

Marjorie Stanton
Julia B. George

The focus of this chapter is on the professional nurse's use of nursing theories or models as a framework to guide nursing practice through use in the nursing process. As professional nurses, we need to test those theories that we believe useful to practice. If nurses deliberately use the same theories or models in a variety of nursing situations, then it becomes possible to analyze the results and contribute to the body of nursing knowledge.

It is possible that a combination of these theories or models can be used so that the practicing nurse can identify new relationships and new ideas for testing. It is also possible that as we consistently use nursing theories or models in practice, we can identify those with which we as professionals feel most confident. We may also find that certain ones work better in selected situations than others. By keeping accurate records and by communicating our successes and failures to others, the practice of nursing becomes more scientific and rational.

A REVIEW OF THE EIGHTEEN THEORIES

Using various nursing theories or models, the focus of nursing practice will differ. Florence Nightingale focused on changing and manipulating the environment in order to put the patient in the best possible conditions for nature to act. She also emphasized the point that nurses should alleviate and prevent unnecessary suffering and pain. Nightingale's notions about nursing laid the groundwork for and influenced other nursing theorists (see Chapter 3).

Hildegard Peplau presents nursing as therapeutic interactions between the nurse and patient in order to clarify the patient's problems and to set mutually acceptable goals to solve those problems. Conflict may occur if the nurse and patient cannot come to agreement about the goals; however, both the patient and nurse should grow from this experience (see Chapter

4). Peplau identifies four phases in the relationship: orientation, identification, exploitation, and resolution. Her influence on the notion of nursing as interpersonal in nature in pervasive.

Virginia Henderson views nursing as doing for patients what they cannot do for themselves, and she identifies fourteen components of nursing care that need to be considered (see Chapter 5). Her view of nursing seems to foster dependence initially, although her goal is to make the patient independent. The influence of Henderson is seen in the writings of later nursing theorists.

Lydia Hall's notion of nursing centers around three components: care, core, and cure. Care represents nurturance and is exclusive to nursing. Core involves the therapeutic use of self and emphasizes the use of reflection. Cure focuses on nursing related to the physician's orders. Hall views the three components as interrelated, with one component taking precedence over the other two at varying points during the patient's course of progress. Hall's focus is primarily on the ill adult during the recovery stage (see Chapter 6).

Dorothea Orem's theory of nursing (see Chapter 7) consists of three theoretical constructs: self-care, self-care deficit, and nursing systems. The self-care construct is divided into the three self-care requisites of universal self-care, developmental self-care, and health deviation self-care. The self-care deficit construct is the core of Orem's general theory of nursing because it identifies when nursing is needed. The nursing systems construct is divided into the wholly compensatory, partly compensatory, and supportive–educative nursing systems. Orem's theoretical construct of self-care deficit has some similarity to Henderson's general concept of nursing.

Dorothy E. Johnson has developed a behavioral system model for nursing that has seven subsystems. These subsystems are: attachment or affiliative, dependency, ingestive, eliminative, sexual, aggressive, and achievement. These seven subsystems need nurturance and stimulation for growth, and they also need protection from noxious influences (see Chapter 8). Nursing problems occur when there are difficulties in the structure or function of the system or a sub-system and when behavioral functioning falls below what is considered desirable. The goal of nursing is to keep the behavioral system in balance and to maintain stability in the system. Nursing focuses on the person who is ill or is threatened with illness; and medicine, using the biological system model, focuses on the illness itself.

Faye Abdellah focuses on the nurse rather than on the patient. She provides a means for categorizing patient needs under twenty-one common nursing problems relative to caring for patients (see Chapter 9). There is some similarity to Henderson's fourteen components of basic nursing care.

Ida Jean Orlando advances to some extent Henderson's theory of nursing since she believes that the nurse helps patients meet a perceived need that the patients cannot meet for themselves. Orlando (see Chapter 10) believes that nurses provide direct assistance to meet an immediate need for help in order to avoid or to alleviate distress or helplessness. She emphasizes the need to evaluate care based on observable outcomes. Orlando indicates that nursing actions can be automatic (those chosen for reasons other than the immediate need for help) or deliberative (those resulting from validating the need for help, exploring the meaning of the need, and validating the effectiveness of actions taken to meet the need).

Ernestine Wiedenbach strongly believes that the nurse's individual philosophy lends credence to nursing care. She believes that nurses help to meet the individual's need for help. Wiedenbach also believes nursing to be a deliberative action, as does Orlando (see Chapter 11).

Myra Levine sees nursing as human interaction: the dependency of individuals on one another. She uses four conservation principles to describe nursing interventions: conservation of energy, conservation of structural integrity, conservation of personal integrity, and conservation of social integrity. She believes this provides a way to view people holistically. Levine uses the concept of organismic response to illness, which indicates to what extent adaptation is taking place (see Chapter 12).

Imogene King has developed a theory of goal attainment from an open systems framework that integrates personal systems, interpersonal systems, and social systems. The interpersonal systems provide the major emphasis in this theory of goal attainment. Nurse–client interactions are the essential component in goal setting and in identifying the means of goal achievement. King views human beings as the focus of nursing and as open systems interacting with the environment (see Chapter 13).

Martha Rogers developed the principles of homeodynamics, which focus on the wholeness of human beings and their integration with their environment. The movement of human beings toward maximum health is the purpose of nursing. Rogers believes that the science of nursing is the science of unitary human beings (see Chapter 14).

Sister Callista Roy's major emphasis is on the person as an adaptive system. To further describe the client of nursing, four adaptive modes are used: physiological needs, self-concept, role functioning, and interdependence. The person has two major internal processor subsystems, the regulator and the cognator, which are seen as mechanisms for adapting or coping. The goal of nursing is to promote adaptive responses (see Chapter 15).

Betty Neuman presents a health care systems model that focuses on the whole person and that person's reaction to stress. Her model can be used in illness or wellness. She focuses on three components in her model—man, environment, and stress—and relies on the nurse's understanding and knowledge of these components to carry out the purpose of her model (see Chapter 16).

Josephine Paterson and Loretta Zderad have developed a humanistic nursing practice theory based on their belief that nursing is an existential experience. Nursing is viewed as a lived dialogue that involves the coming together of the nurse and the person to be nursed. The essential characteristic of nursing is nurturance. Humanistic nursing cannot take place without the authentic commitment of the nurse to being with and doing with the client. Humanistic nursing also presupposes responsible choices (see Chapter 17).

Jean Watson's science of caring is built on a framework of seven assumptions and ten carative factors. She emphasizes the interpersonal nature of caring, describes the nurse as a coparticipant with the client, and includes the soul as an important consideration. She includes health promotion and treatment of illness in nursing. The goal of nursing is to help people to high degree of harmony within themselves (see Chapter 18).

Rosemarie Rizzo Parse's theory of Man–Living–Health is based on Martha Rogers' principles and concepts and on existential phenomenological thought. She emphasizes free choice of personal meaning in relating value priorities, cocreating of rhythmical patterns in exchange with the environment, and cotranscending in many dimensions as possibilities unfold. She also believes that each choice opens certain opportunities while closing others. Thus she speaks to revealing–concealing, enabling–limiting, and connecting–separating. Since each individual makes his or her own personal choices, the role of the nurse is that of guide, not decision maker (see Chapter 19).

Madeleine Leininger focuses on the importance of understanding the similarities (universalities) and differences (diversities) of peoples across cultures. She speaks to the importance of the nurse's awareness of the cultures of the client and of the nurse. She also emphasizes care and caring as the dominant and central domain of nursing (see Chapter 20).

COMPARISON OF THE THEORIES OR MODELS

A review of the theories presented indicates that there are similarities and differences among them. Most of the theorists were influenced by each other in their advancement of nursing knowledge. This fact is valuable and useful to the students of professional nursing practice. The concept of looking specifically at the environment in relation to patients or clients was initiated by Nightingale and was considered later by Johnson, King, Neuman, Orem, Roy, Rogers, and Leininger, but was not specifically considered by Henderson, Abdellah, Peplau, and Orlando. The concept of dependency and its role in nursing was identified by Henderson and was also used by Orlando, Orem, and Levine. Independence is a focus in the theories or models of Peplau, Rogers, Hall, King, and Parse. Adaptation is considered in the theories or models of Nightingale, King, Levine, Rogers, and Roy; however, where Roy views adaptation as health producing, Roger's concept of adaptation would be viewed as not being conducive to health. Peplau, Levine, Paterson and Zderad, King, Watson, Parse, and

Leininger emphasize interpersonal or interactive concepts in their writings, although these concepts are not overlooked by other theorists, e.g., Hall and Orlando. Systems theory is used specifically by Rogers, King, Roy, Johnson, Neuman, and Parse. The theories or models of Henderson, Orlando, Hall, and Levine seem primarily useful in the care of the ill, whereas those of Nightingale, Peplau, Wiedenbach, Orem, King, Rogers, Roy, Watson, and Leininger are useful for caring for the well and the ill. Abdellah's ideas seem more consistent with the technical aspects of nursing care, whereas the others' ideas do not. Caring is a particular focus of Watson and Leininger.

One way of looking at the differences among the nurse theorists is to explore the variety of ways they characterized nursing actions. A quick summary of the theorists presented identifies at least three different forms of nursing actions: (1) assuming responsibility for the person until he or she is ready to assume responsibility for self; (2) changing or manipulating the environment to facilitate health; and (3) helping the person toward some goal. The reader may be able to identify other similarities and differences.

Practitioners of nursing need to use the theories or models that are most useful in a given situation. As stated earlier, a combination of theories or models can be considered and, if used consistently, should be analyzed by the user as to their effectiveness. By using various nursing theories or models, the focus and consequences of nursing practice may differ, as discussed in the following example.

Consider the following situation: Mrs. Mary James is a sixty-eight-year-old woman recovering from a stroke that occurred three days ago. She has weakness of the left side of her body. She is left-handed and requires retraining in the following areas: balancing while standing, climbing stairs, self-feeding, bladder control, and personal hygiene activities including dressing. She is in a hospital room with four other patients and is in the bed nearest the door. There is one window in the room. Before her hospitalization for the stroke, Mrs. James maintained her own home, was quite independent, volunteered one day a week at the local hospital, and was active in the local garden club.

Table 21–1 provides a brief overview of the direction a nurse might take using the various nursing theories or models as a framework to guide nursing practice through use in the nursing process. You will note that although each theorist moves Mrs. James to some point of independence, the methods are different due to different orientations. A fully developed nursing process using any one of the theories or models as a framework would provide much more detailed and specific information about Mrs. James than is given in this table. However, the brief overview in Table 21–1 does give the reader an idea of how the process might differ if a particular theory were used. It is not intended to be an all-inclusive discussion on nursing care for Mrs. James.

The consistent use of selected nursing theories or models in nursing

TABLE 21–1. OVERVIEW OF THEORIES OR MODELS AND NURSING PROCESS

Theorist	Assessment	Nursing Diagnosis	Planning	Implementation	Evaluation
Nightingale	Focus is on environment of patient. What in environment is contributing to disability or illness of Mrs. James? What are inhibiting factors, i.e., position of bedside table; lack of flowers; too far from window; slippery, cold floor; lack of space (four-bed room); too many people in room?	Relates to environment or what is lacking in the environment as a condition to restore health, i.e., crowded, restricted environment that inhibits movement toward independence and health.	Focus is on identifying those areas of the environment needing modification or change to provide Mrs. James with the best possible conditions for nature to restore or improve health; i.e., remove restrictions, maximize use of right hand, provide sunlight and ventilation, etc.	Carries out the actions necessary to change or manipulate the environment to provide optimum conditions for restoration or improvement of health. Move Mrs. James to room with two beds for more space but with companionship; provide chair near the window; place bedside table and things needed by Mrs. James on right side of bed; provide warm, sturdy slippers or shoes; place other patient in room on Mrs. James' right; provide flowers	Relates to how well the changes in or manipulation of the environment worked to effect optimal conditions for restoration or improvement of health, i.e., able to move about room with some assistance. Sits by window and talks to patient in room. Uses right hand to feed self and care for other needs. Arranges flowers in room. Taking an interest in what is happening inside and outside the room

Peplau	Focus is on the orientation phase—Mrs. James has an expressed need for help. The nurse, family, and Mrs. James work together to clarify the problems: Mrs. James' loss of independence, her fear about what has happened to her, how will she cope, how will her family cope.	Relates to the identification of the health problem or deficit by the nurse and Mrs. James, i.e., inability to cope with dependent role caused by diminished function of left side of body.	Focus is on the nurse and Mrs. James setting mutual goals for Mrs. James to become more independent through the development of the interpersonal relationship. Mrs. James should feel comfortable in discussing how she will become more independent. This is likened to the identification phase.	Carries out plans mutually agreed upon by nurse and Mrs. James. However, Mrs. James is in control in asking for what she needs; i.e., "I don't need to be fed. Teach me to feed myself. I'm ready." The nurse helps Mrs. James to recognize and explore her feelings when she becomes frustrated in her attempts to feed herself. This can be likened to the exploitation phase.	Relates to how well Mrs. James progressed through orientation, identification, and exploitation phases. Have the needs been met? When the answer is yes, terminating the relationship (resolution phase) begins.
Henderson	Focus is on assessing Mrs. James' ability relative to the 14 components of basic nursing care; i.e., Mrs. James is left-handed with left-sided weakness (relates to component #2—"eat and drink adequately").	Relates to deficits in the ability of Mrs. James to function in each of the 14 components. Takes into consideration strength, will, and knowledge, i.e., inability to feed self due to left-handed weakness (relates to component #2).	Focus is on identifying those areas of the 14 components that Mrs. James cannot do for self and which therefore the nurse must do or assist in doing, i.e., feed Mrs. James until she is able to feed self with right hand. This should lead to independence on the part of Mrs. James.	Carries out the plan to initially feed Mrs. James while teaching her to use her right hand to feed herself.	Relates to how soon and how well Mrs. James is able to feed herself with her right hand; i.e., for the first three days she needed to be fed; by fourth day, held utensils and fed self with assistance; by seventh day, was able to feed self if food was bite-size.

(continued)

TABLE 21–1. (Continued)

Theorist	Assessment	Nursing Diagnosis	Planning	Implementation	Evaluation
Hall	Focus is on increasing Mrs. James' self-awareness through observation and reflection. Helps Mrs. James hear herself; i.e., "I'm a sick woman. I can't take care of myself. I can't even dress or feed myself. Everyone is looking at me." Biological data are also being collected; i.e., cannot grasp or hold with left hand.	Statement of Mrs. James' need or problem. Mrs. James is in control; i.e., "I need to learn to take care of myself. I need to learn to use my right hand to feed and dress myself. I need to think about myself for awhile and not worry about others."	Focus is on setting goals and priorities with Mrs. James, i.e., needs to learn to care for self: 1. Learn to use right hand to feed and dress self 2. Walk by self to bathroom 3. Improve self-concept	Carries out plans with Mrs. James. Intimate bodily care is given; i.e., help her to feed self and begin to use right hand; assist her to dress until she learns to dress self; support and listen to her.	Relates to Mrs. James' progress toward goals; i.e., able to feed self with right hand, able to dress self with assistance, able to walk to bathroom with assistance, able to state, "I think I'll be able to take care of myself."
Orem	Focus is on appraising the situation: determining why a person needs care; considering life history and life style; considering the physician's perspective and Mrs. James' perspective;—i.e., Mrs. James needs help because she has	Relating to the partly compensatory system; i.e., inability to feed self without assistance, inability to walk without assistance, ability to learn alternate methods of self-care relating to deficits identified.	Focus is on improving the self-care abilities of Mrs. James relative to eating, walking, and other deficits in activities of daily living. Identify Mrs. James' strengths, such as previous independent life style. Reach agreements with	Carries out the plan to assist Mrs. James in the performance of self-care tasks, i.e., learning to feed herself and using a walker to assist in walking.	Relates to monitoring progress of Mrs. James with regard to self-care activities and making adjustments and recommendations as necessary.

	left-sided weakness, is left-handed, and cannot feed herself or walk without assistance.	Mrs. James and family about role each will play.			
Johnson	Focus is on the behavioral subsystems to identify disturbances in structure and function of subsystems or a discrepancy in behavioral functioning. *Affiliative and dependency subsystems:* Mrs. James has no family for support and affection. Has relied on her outreach through volunteering and her relationship with garden club members for support and assistance. Limited mobility has curtailed outreach. Came to hospital alone.	Relates to a description of the behavior that is associated with an actual or potential instability in the subsystem. Diminished ability for social behavior due to immobility. Weakening of affiliative subsystem due to limited access to friends.	Focus is on identification of short- and long-term goals in the system or subsystem by modifying or changing behavior. *Long-range goal:* Diminish the effects of hospitalization and immobilization on Mrs. James. *Short-term goals:* Preserve and strengthen Mrs. James' relationships with friends to encourage and enhance her interest and caring about others.	Carries out the necessary activities to assist Mrs. James in modifying, changing, or regulating behavior so that the goal of each subsystem will be met. Behavioral objectives are used to show progress toward goal. 1. Within two days have Mrs. James contact at least two of her garden club friends. 2. Within four days have Mrs. James, with the use of the walker, visit each client in the room to begin to get to know them.	Relates to the degree of progress in achieving the goals set during planning. Mrs. James called her "dearest" friend, Ada Brown, within two days and made plans to call Mrs. Johnson by the next day. Mrs. James also visited each client in the room, using her walker, and decided that she would spend time each day with Mrs. Smith who has no visitors.

(continued)

TABLE 21-1. (Continued)

Theorist	Assessment	Nursing Diagnosis	Planning	Implementation	Evaluation
Abdellah	Focus is on each of the 21 nursing problems to collect data about Mrs. James; i.e., #7—"to facilitate maintenance of elimination." Mrs. James has not had a bowel movement in two days, has difficulty moving about, does not like fruits and vegetables.	Problems with elimination possibly due to insufficient exercise and lack of roughage in diet.	Focus is on facilitating the maintenance of elimination; i.e., assisting Mrs. James to walk at least 15 minutes twice daily and move about in bed. Also speak to dietitian regarding diet of grain cereals, sliced fruit or finger fruits, etc.	Carries out the nursing activities to assist Mrs. James to change position in bed. Encourage Mrs. James to eat diet prescribed; assist in feeding and praise her for trying fruits and vegetables.	Relates to the resolution of Mrs. James' elimination problems. Is elimination achieved and maintained?
Orlando	Focus is on collecting data relative to the immediate situation; i.e., Mrs. James has left side weakness. What are the factors identified in this situation, i.e., inability to feed self, difficulty in balancing? The nurse also clarifies own reaction to Mrs. James.	Relates to identifying Mrs. James' needs that she cannot meet by self. This is validated with her; i.e., Mrs. James needs to be taught to use her right hand to feed and bathe self.	Focus is on planning with Mrs. James and mutually setting goals; i.e., clarifying with Mrs. James that she indeed needs to learn to use her right hand in order to feed and bathe self.	Carries out the nursing activities necessary to meet Mrs. James' needs; i.e., assist Mrs. James to use her right hand to eat—do not feed her; place bedside table on her right; teach her to stand and move without assistance.	Relates to Mrs. James' behavior in terms of feeding and bathing herself using her right hand. Uses right hand to eat but needs encouragement. Able to get out of bed with assistance; can walk to bathroom; able to dress self with assistance.

Wiedenbach	Focus is on the nurse's perception and awareness of the situation; i.e., "Mrs. James must feel so helpless since she is unable to feed herself."	Relates to the situation perceived, i.e., "feeling of helplessness."	Focus is on the nurse and Mrs. James' plan to reduce Mrs. James' feeling of helplessness by teaching her how to eat with her right hand, with food prepared in bite-size pieces.	Carries out the plan of teaching after confirming it with Mrs. James. "I'll assist you in using your right hand until you can feed yourself. I'll stay with you until you learn how to feed yourself with your right hand."	Relates to validating that Mrs. James feels less helpless when she can use her right hand for feeding herself.
Levine	Focus is on using the four conservation principles as a basis for observing and interviewing Mrs. James. Using the principle relative to personal integrity, the nurse questions Mrs. James about her life style before she had the stroke: "What did you usually do each day? How did you get to the garden club?" Analysis of data reflects Mrs. James' balance of strengths and weaknesses in each of the four conservation areas.	Relates to state of illness or altered health reflecting a problem or potential problem with regard to a deficit or threatened deficit; i.e., personal integrity threatened due to increased dependency on others in caring for self.	Focus is on planning therapeutic interventions designed to promote adaptation that contributes to healing and restoration of health; i.e., plan to have Mrs. James ambulate to increase her sense of mobility and independence and conserve energy. Start out slowly—10 minutes twice a day, sitting before walking, and use of the walker.	Carries out the actions necessary based on conservation of energy, and structural, personal, and social integrity; i.e., have Mrs. James sit on the side of the bed for 2 minutes, sit in a chair for 10 minutes, walk to bathroom and back using walker, and increase time of walking as Mrs. James' strength increases.	Relates to Mrs. James' adaptation to changes in her life style that threaten personal integrity, i.e., able to walk with assistance of walker, manipulate walker very well; out of bed all day; has contacted garden club.

(continued)

TABLE 21–1. (Continued)

Theorist	Assessment	Nursing Diagnosis	Planning	Implementation	Evaluation
King	Focus is on the nurse's and Mrs. James' perception of Mrs. James' health status and her ability to adapt to stresses and to use resources to achieve potential for daily living. Mrs. James is viewed as a reacting being, a time-oriented being, and a social being; i.e., "I hate being dependent on others to feed and dress me, even to go to the bathroom." Left-handed, no strength in left hand, left-sided weakness.	Relates to the nurse's understanding and analysis of the data about Mrs. James' social system, perceptions, interpersonal relations, and health; i.e., difficulty coping with feelings of dependency.	Focus is on mutual goal setting with clear communication necessary for setting goals to move Mrs. James toward health. Working with Mrs. James, the nurse and Mrs. James identify ways to increase Mrs. James' independence in the hospital; i.e., learn to feed self with right hand; learn to walk with walker; progress to using cane; learn to use elevator.	Carries out the activities necessary for Mrs. James to achieve increased independence; i.e., teach Mrs. James to eat with right hand. Prepare food so she can do so. Stay with Mrs. James until she feels confident. Assist Mrs James to use and manipulate walker in walking and using elevator.	Relates to how well the interpersonal process of nursing assisted Mrs. James in meeting the basic activities of daily living and to cope with health and illness; i.e., feels less dependent now that she can feed self with right hand; ambulation allows Mrs. James to move out of four-bed room and relate to others; using elevator decreases feelings of dependency. "I feel so much better now that I can go to the bathroom by myself and feed myself."

Rogers				
Focus is on collecting data and opinions about the person and the environment relative to principles of integrality, helicy, resonancy; i.e., How is Mrs. James interacting with the hospital environment? Mrs. James reports difficulty in sleeping in the hospital. Until she was hospitalized, she slept 6–7 hours a night. Was very active, gardened. How has the life process of Mrs. James progressed to date? What kind of patterns characterize Mrs. James?	Relates to rhythms, patterns, and life process and reflects the principles of homeodynamics, i.e., alteration in sleep pattern.	Focuses on promoting dynamic repatterning with regard to alteration in Mrs. James' sleeping pattern. Plans are to provide an environment conducive to sleeping; increase activity during the day based on Mrs. James' previous life style; use relaxation techniques to promote readiness for sleep.	Carries out the strategies necessary to strengthen the integrity of the individual–environment relationship. Ask Mrs. James to tend plants on unit, thus increasing walking and providing a purpose. Air and smooth her bed; use appropriate pillows; flex her knees to reduce any pulling on her back muscles.	Relates to optimum state of health; i.e., What is Mrs. James' pattern of sleeping by the third day following nursing implementation? How long is she sleeping? How well is she sleeping? Does she wake at night? Does she need sleep medication? How does Mrs. James feel and look?

(continued)

TABLE 21–1. (Continued)

Theorist	Assessment	Nursing Diagnosis	Planning	Implementation	Evaluation
Roy	*First level:* Focus is on collecting data related to each adaptation mode. Physiological mode: Mrs. James' behavior related to rest and sleep. "I'm having trouble sleeping at night. I'm used to 7 hours sleep a night." Nurses during the night note Mrs. James is awake two to three times each night asking for something to sleep. *Second level:* Focal stimuli—Mrs. James is in a new environment. Contextual stimuli—other three people in room snore. Residual stimuli—Mrs. James' internal response to all the recent changes in her life.	Relates to the deficits, or excesses, of basic needs leading to ineffective behavior; i.e., inability to sleep throughout the night due to change in environment.	Focus is on promoting Mrs. James' adaptation in relation to the four modes. Physiological mode: goal is Mrs. James will sleep if an environment conducive to sleeping is created.	Carries out activities necessary to manipulate the environment by removing, increasing, decreasing, or altering stimuli. The resulting behavior should be adaptive; i.e., provide for fresh air, freshen room at bedtime, reduce light and noise, encourage Mrs. James to fall asleep before others to reduce disturbance from others' snoring. Introduce Mrs. James to relaxation techniques before sleeping.	Relates to Mrs. James' goal achievement. After two nights, check with Mrs. James about restful sleep. Has sleeping improved? Does she look and feel rested in the morning? Review the night nurses' notes relating to Mrs. James' wakefulness.

Neuman				
Focus is on Mrs. James' reaction to known or possible stressors—intra-, inter-, extrapersonal. Also looks at lines of defense and resistance. *Intrapersonal:* Mrs. James is left-handed with muscle weakness of left arm and hand and left leg. Incontinent at times. *Interpersonal:* Separated from friends. *Extrapersonal:* Unable to engage in gardening or do volunteer work. Nurse asks Mrs. James, "What are you doing and what can you do to help yourself?" "I'm being fed, but I think I can feed myself. I want to walk to the bathroom."	Relates to stressors identified in each area—intra-, inter-, extrapersonal; i.e., immobility due to left-sided weakness; intermittent lack of bladder control; diminished socialization due to immobility.	Focus is on setting priorities to facilitate Mrs. James' adaptive behaviors to stress. Teach Mrs. James to feed herself with right hand. Teach Mrs. James to use walker to become more mobile. Begin exercises for bladder control. Encourage Mrs. James to use walker to get to bathroom.	Carries out the necessary actions to achieve highest level of reconstitution. Focus is on primary, secondary, and tertiary prevention; i.e., primary prevention—reduce the possibility of Mrs. James becoming depressed by increasing independence and assisting her to feed herself immediately. Get Mrs. James out of bed and using walker to go to the bathroom. Introduce her to others in the room. Tell her how much she has accomplished. Praise her for her accomplishments.	Relates to the degree of reconstitution achieved. Mrs. James is able to feed self with right hand with little assistance. Needs help to cut meat. Able to use the walker to use the bathroom. Incontinence is occurring less frequently. Mrs. James tries hard to improve the strength of her right side. She is determined to go home as quickly as possible. She tries to cheer the other people in the room.

(continued)

TABLE 21–1. (Continued)

Theorist	Assessment	Nursing Diagnosis	Planning	Implementation	Evaluation
Paterson and Zderad	Focus is on describing what is and confirming it with Mrs. James. This begins the interdependent relationship between the nurse and the nursed. Mrs. James is a strong, independent woman who has weakness in the left side of her body. She is left handed, cannot feed or dress herself, cannot walk without help. Depends on garden club friends, has no family. "Mrs. James, I'm Sue Ryan, your nurse. Can you tell me what is happening with you?" "Well, I've had a stroke and I can't do anything without help. My friends don't know where I am—I'm a mess."	Based on assessment and relates to comfort–discomfort level. Bruised self-image due to change in body function. Limited support system due to lack of family.	Identification of ways to reduce discomfort and increase comfort to help nursed become all she can be. Assist Mrs. James to become more independent by teaching her how to feed self with right hand and how to use walker to become more mobile. This will give her more control over her life and will increase her comfort. Encourage contact with her garden club friends for needed support system.	The nurse becomes truly present to Mrs. James and behaves in ways to reduce discomfort and relieve tension. Have Mrs. James call at least two of her garden club friends. Be there for Mrs. James. Feed her when necessary. Share feelings with her. Teach her to use right hand. Encourage Mrs. James to use walker to increase her mobility and independence. Discuss her plans for the future.	The nurse examines how effective her relationship and action with Mrs. James have been in reducing discomfort and alleviating tension. *Increased independence:* Mrs. James learned to eat with her right hand within two days. Now uses walker with ease. Visits people in room with her. Uses bathroom without assistance. *Decreased discomfort and relieved tension:* Now has more control over her situation. Has decided to return home. Sharing her plans for the next few months. Mrs. James and nurse have been

Watson	Use the human needs model to guide assessment. *Lower Order Needs:* *Biophysical:* Is she able to obtain adequate food and fluids? Mrs. James needs assistance in this area due to limited use of her dominant left hand. *Elimination needs?* Mrs. James has difficulties with both bowel and bladder control.	Plan care around the ten carative factors. Include instilling faith and hope, establishing a helping–trust relationship, acceptance of feelings, interpersonal teaching–learning, a supportive–protective–corrective environment, meeting human needs.	Based on assessment and related to human needs. Areas of need include adequacy of food and fluid, bowel and bladder control, ventilation, activity and rest, self-image, and interaction with others.	Arrange meeting with therapists to explain what they can do to help Mrs. James regain function. Have a person who has recovered from a stroke visit with Mrs. James. Encourage Mrs. James to discuss her feelings about herself, her stroke, and her current abilities. Arrange environment to maximize use of her right hand—	truly present with each other. Mrs. James' self-confidence has been bolstered, and she has learned ways to become independent and in control. She has discussed care after discharge. Mrs. James and nurse have planned contact after her discharge. Are Mrs. James' human needs being met? Is her food and fluid intake adequate? Is she regaining bowel and bladder control? Is her pattern of sleep nearer to her normal pattern? Is she moving around safely with her walker? How does she describe herself? Is she interacting with other patients, with her friends?

(continued)

TABLE 21–1. (Continued)

Theorist	Assessment	Nursing Diagnosis	Planning	Implementation	Evaluation
Watson	*Ventilation?* She is in a multibed unit with only one window. *Psycho-physical: Activity or Inactivity?* Mrs. James's left-sided weakness limits her ability to walk alone. She reports difficulty sleeping. *Sexuality?* Mrs. James describes herself as "a mess." *Higher Order Needs: Psychosocial—Achievement?* Mrs. James is worried about whether or not she will be able to continue to care for her home and to serve as a hospital volunteer. *Affiliation?* Mrs James misses her regular contact with her friends in the Garden Club.			water pitcher to right of her bed, walker available, etc. With Mrs. James, plan a toileting schedule to help her regain bowel and bladder control. Move her to a smaller room so there will be fewer interruptions to her sleep.	

Intrapersonal? Mrs. James is concerned about whether others will continue to value her if she can no longer be independent.

Parse	Assessment and Diagnosis do not fit with this theory as Parse states the nurse-client interaction is not limited by pre-scriptions.	See Assessment.	Nurse is a guide, not a decision maker. Interaction is evolving.	Nurse serves as a guide to illuminate meaning—guides Mrs. James to identify the personal meaning of the situation to her; to synchronize rhythms—lead Mrs. James to recognize the harmony within her existence; and to mobilize transcendence—guide Mrs. James to move from the present to what is not yet, to dream of the possibles for her.	Because the interaction is not limited by prescription, standards of evaluation cannot be created. Essentially, the nurse can evaluate if Mrs. James has identified personal meaning, recognized harmony, and dreamed of the possibles.
Leininger	Based on Levels I, II, and III of the Sunrise Model. Level I: Social structure and culture—Mrs. James is American, active	Based on areas of cultural diversity or universality which are not being met. Includes need for independence in mobil-	Based on cultural care preservation, accommodation, repatterning, or any combination of the three.	Include preservation through helping Mrs. James continue contact with members of her Garden Club; accommo-	Are cultural diversities and universalities being met? Does Mrs. James view herself as continuing to be independent?

(continued)

TABLE 21-1. (Continued)

Theorist	Assessment	Nursing Diagnosis	Planning	Implementation	Evaluation
Leininger (continued)	in a Garden Club and as a hospital volunteer. Language—American English. Environment—until illness lived in own home; currently in multibed ward. Technology—car is stick shift model. Religion—religious preference is unknown. Philosophy—believes independence and service to others are important. Kinship—widow, two children live over 1000 miles away. Social structure—interacts primarily with her own age group. Cultural values and beliefs—values independence, believes children should not have to support parents. Politics—is not politically involved.	ity, feeding, toileting, sleep, and need for interaction with others of her own age group.		dation through helping her learn to use a walker for mobility and keeping the walker available for her; repatterning through assisting her in learning to eat with her right hand—arranging her tray to enhance use of her right hand, cutting food into bite size pieces, encouraging her to butter her own bread.	

Legal system—lives in a historic neighborhood that does not allow for external modification of dwellings. Economics—income from a trust fund; has insurance that will cover all costs associated with this illness. Education.—college graduate. Level II: Client is an individual. Level III: Health Systems: Folk—believes use of professional health services is important. Professional—physician is head of the team, various therapists are part of the team. Nursing—part of the team. Identifies needs for care due to limited use of previously dominant side—include eating, toileting, mobility, interaction.

practice provides a way to validate and test these theories or models. The transmission of such knowledge by practicing nurses and nurse researchers adds to the unique body of knowledge necessary to a profession.

The systematic use of nursing theories or models provides a structure and discipline for nursing practice. It also provides a framework for teaching professional nursing students how to base practice on knowledge.

CHAPTER 22
Other Extant Theories
Julia B. George

A number of other nurses have proposed theories of or for nursing. These theories either have not received as wide an audience or been as thoroughly developed as those presented in this text, or they focus on one of the major concepts of concern to nursing. Some of these will be explored in this chapter.

The intent of this chapter is to provide an overview of these theories. Therefore, each theory will be presented briefly without the indepth discussion found in the oher theory chapters in this text. The theories to be included are those of Adam, Fitzpatrick, Hadley, and Newman. Each of these has built upon, or been influenced by one of the theories presented in this text. Adam was influenced by Dorothy Johnson and built her work upon the work of Virginia Henderson, Hadley developed what she calls the Johnson–Hadley Connection, and Fitzpatrick and Newman were both students of Martha Rogers.

EVELYN ADAM

Evelyn Adam, (b.1929) a Canadian nurse, received her undergraduate nursing education in Canada. She earned her masters in nursing from the University of California at Los Angeles. While at UCLA, she met Dorothy Johnson, who served as a strong influence on her professional life.[1] Adam differentiates between a theory and a conceptual model in part by indicating that a theory may be useful to more than one discipline but a conceptual model is discipline specific.[2] Therefore, Adam developed concepts from the work of Virginia Henderson into a conceptual model.[3]

There are six major units in Adam's conceptual model.[4] The first is the *goal of the profession,* that which members of the profession seek to achieve. Adam defines the goal of nursing as seeking to maintain or restore the client's independence in meeting fourteen fundamental needs. Each need has dimensions that are biological, psychological, and sociocultural. The second unit is the *beneficiary,* that person or group of persons toward whom professional activity is directed. For nursing, this is the client or patient.

The third unit is *role*, the part played by the professional. Nurses have a unique role, although they share certain functions with other health professionals. It is this unique role that society expects nurses to perform. This role is complementary–supplementary to the client's strength, will, knowledge, or all three.

The fourth unit is *source of difficulty*, the probable source of problems being experienced by the beneficiary. These problems may occur in any one or more of the fourteen fundamental needs. When needs are not met, the person is not whole. The fifth unit is *intervention*, the *focus*, or area on which the professional's attention is centered, and *modes*, the means or methods of intervention that are available to the professional. These may be associated with the implementation phase of the nursing process. The sixth unit is the *consequences*, the results of the professional's efforts toward the goal. Information for this unit may be found in the evaluation phase of the nursing process.

BETTY JO HADLEY

Betty Jo Hadley earned a BA in General Studies from the University of California, Berkeley; a diploma in nursing from the California Hospital School of Nursing; a masters in counseling and guidance from the University of Southern California; and a PhD in sociology from the University of California, Los Angeles. She has entitled her theory the Johnson–Hadley Connection,[5] as she has built her conceptions upon those of Dorothy Johnson. These conceptions were first published in 1969.[6] Hadley has conducted research using her theory as a framework and has guided graduate students in similar research.

Hadley believes the focus of nursing is to prevent or reduce the tensions associated with entrance into the health care system. She defines entrance into the health care system as any contact with a health care provider from a question over the back fence to a neighbor who is a nurse to a hospital admission through the emergency room. She views man as a bio–psycho–social being who functions in a physical and a psycho–social environment. Man has patterned ways of achieving goals within these environments, as well as patterned ways of coping with the stresses of everyday life. Disruptions of these patterned behaviors lead to the primary stress of illness while the stresses of everyday life offer the threat of illness. Either illness or the threat of illness may lead to entrance into the health care system (see Fig. 22–1). Such entrance leads to changes in structure, function, the psycho–social environment and/or the physical environment which constitute the secondary stresses.

Entrance into the health care system and the secondary stresses lead to patient situations that comprise the stress syndrome of entrance. Hadley identifies patient situations as the internal and/or external environmental

A. THREAT OF ILLNESS

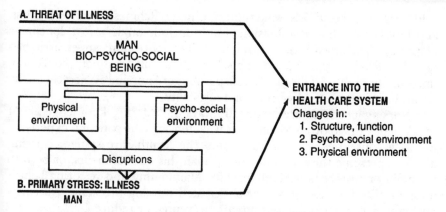

Figure 22–1. Entrance into health care system. *(From Hadley, B.J. Evolution of a Conception of Nursing.* Nursing Research, *1969,* 18, *400–405.)*

consequences of the secondary stresses (see Fig. 22–2). She also suggests these are equivalent to Johnson's Behavioral System Disturbances (personal communication). These patient situations may include such examples as body image distortions, sensory overload, affectional deprivation, immobility, inability to meet own needs, perceptual incongruence, and biochemical imbalance. The assumption which connects the patient situation with nursing problems is that stress results in tension. The nursing problems are the tensions that may include bio-physical tensions such as pain, dyspnea, tightness of skin, anorexia, nausea, bladder distension, bowel distention, hot,

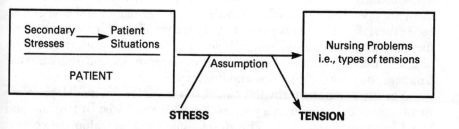

Patient Situations: Consequence of Secondary Stresses
Example: Body image distortions; sensory overload or deprivation; affectional deprivation; immobility; inability to meet needs; perceptual incongruities; biochemical imbalance; etc.

Nursing Problems: Bio–Psycho–Social Tensions
Example: Bio–physical pain; dyspnea; tightness of skin; anorexia; thirst; fatigue; etc. Psycho–social anxiety; fear; loneliness; frustration; grief; depression; anger; etc.

Figure 22–2. Consequence of Entrance. *(From Hadley, B.J. Evolution of a Conception of Nursing,* Nursing Research, *1969,* 18 *400–405.)*

cold, dizziness, sleepiness, wakefulness, hunger, itchiness, weakness, thirst, and fatigue. Psycho-social tensions would include anxiety, fear, loneliness emptiness, powerlessness, frustration, grief, depression, anger, irritableness, helplessness, self-consciousness, boredom, embarrassment, confusion, uncertainty, guilt, and disgust. These tensions are nursing's objects of analysis, and are manifested by behavioral instability.

Nursing needs to use systematic ways of ordering knowledge about man's behaviors in order to interpret what tensions the patient is experiencing as a consequence of entrance into the health care system. Nursing action represents the manipulation of man, his environments, or both to maintain or restore behavioral stability. Maintaining and restoring behavioral stability focuses on real or anticipated nursing problems. Nursing's goal is achieved when the tensions are prevented or reduced.

JOYCE FITZPATRICK

Joyce Fitzpatrick (b.1944) received her Bachelor's in Nursing from Georgetown University, Washington, D.C.; Master's in Psychiatric–Mental Health Nursing, with additional course work in Community Health Nursing from The Ohio State University, Columbus, Ohio; and PhD in nursing from New York University. She has proposed a life perspective rhythm model, based upon the work of Martha Rogers and derived from her own research on individuals' abilities to integrate crisis situations into their life perspectives. Fitzpatrick presents this model in *Conceptual Models of Nursing.*[7]

Fitzpatrick draws upon Rogers's conceptualizations of unitary man.[8a,8b] These include that man is greater than the sum of his parts; man and environment are open systems which continually exchange matter and energy with each other; the life process develops unidirectionally and irreversibly along the space-time continuum; man's wholeness is reflected in pattern and organization; and man has the ability to sense, experience emotion, think and use language, deal with abstraction and imagery.

The life perspective rhythm model, a developmental model, proposes that human development is a process that is characterized by rhythms and based in personal meaning. This development occurs within the context of continuous interaction between person and environment. Patterns of rhythm include those dealing with time, motion, consciousness, and perception. The rhythm of development has high and low points with an overall progression towards an increase in the speed of the rhythms. For example, one's perception of time moves from time progressing very slowly to time passing quickly and eventually to timelessness. Not only can the overall life process of development be described but also changes within an individual's life pattern can be identified. Within this model, health is viewed as "a continuously developing characteristic of humans with the full life potential that may characterize the process of dying—the heightened awareness of the meaningfulness of life—representing a more fully developed dimension of health."[9]

Life perspective is viewed as a dimension of health or humanness and the meaning which is attached to life is of central concern to nursing. Thus, nursing care based upon the life perspective model would focus on enhancing the developmental process in moving toward health, in encouraging individuals to develop their potential as human beings.

MARGARET NEWMAN

Margaret Newman (b.1933) earned a bachelor's degree in home economics and English from Baylor University, Waco, Texas; a bachelor's degree in nursing from the University of Tennessee, Memphis; a master's degree in medical–surgical nursing from the University of California, San Francisco; and a PhD in nursing from New York University. A student of Martha Rogers, she has developed a paradigm of health as expanding consciousness.[10]

Newman rejects the concept of health as positive and disease as negative. Rather she views disease as a manifestation of health, a meaningful aspect of the whole.[11] Health, therefore, is a process, a pattern of the whole which encompasses disease and nondisease and exists in a world of undivided wholeness. Newman's paradigm of health emphasizes pattern recognition. Pattern is characterized by the constant movement of diverse parts with a rhythm that identifies the pattern.[12] Relationships are of paramount importance as the task of nursing is not to seek to change an individual's pattern but to recognize and then relate to the pattern. Newman likens this relationship to that of the overlapping of waves that occurs when two pebbles are dropped into a pool of water and states that the task is be in touch with one's own pattern.[13]

Newman assumes that the person does not possess consciousness, but *is* consciousness which coextends in the universe and resides in all matter.[14] She defines consciousness as "the informational capacity of the system: the capacity of the system to interact with its environment."[14] This consciousness expands, or continues to evolve toward greater complexity. The pattern of consciousness is represented by the intersection of time, space, and movement. For example,

> The freedom to come and go as one pleases, when one pleases, is taken for granted until circumstances render that movement impossible or unwise. Restriction of movement forces one into a realm beyond space and time. The old ways of living and relating don't work anymore. One is confronted with one's own inner resources, the quality of one's relationships, and one's ability to live in the present. The developmental task is to allow the transformation of ourselves to occur as we move beyond space and time to higher consciousness.[15]

Newman describes assessment as consisting of exchanging, communicating, valuing, choosing, moving, perceiving, feeling, and knowing; a framework developed by the nurse theorist group of the North American Nursing Diagnosis Association. Exchanging is the interchange of matter and energy between the person and the environment and the transformation of energy from one form to another. Communicating is the interchange of information from one system to another. Relating in the connecting with other persons and the environment and valuing the assignment of worth. Choosing is the selecting of alternatives and moving the rhythmic alteration between activity and rest. Perceiving is receiving and interpreting information, feeling is sensing physical and intuitive awareness, and knowing is the personal recognition of self and world.[16] Intervention then is based on pattern recognition and identification of the rhythm characteristic of the pattern. The intent is to facilitate the pattern in the development of expanding consciousness and thus could be viewed as nonintervention since the nurse does not come into the relationship as an all-knowing problem solver.

Newman also speaks to how this new paradigm of health requires a view of nurses as "responsible providers of essential health care services."[17] She recommends that people should choose their nurse just as they choose other professionals such as their attorney and their physician. She believes that nursing should not be bound by a particular location (space) or certain circumstances (time). Such a model of practice would enable consumers to gain assistance in their efforts to recognize and facilitate their own changing patterns of expanding consciousness or health.[18]

REFERENCES

1.   Creekmur, T., DeFelice, J., Hodel, A., & Petty, C.Y. Evelyn Adam, Conceptual Model for Nursing, in Marriner, A. *Nursing Theorists and Their Work,* St. Louis: C.V. Mosby, 1986, p. 131.

2.   Adam, E. Toward More Clarity in Terminology—Frameworks, Theories and Models, *Journal of Nursing Education,* 1985, *24,* 151–155.

3.   Adam, E. *To Be a Nurse,* Philadelphia: Saunders, 1980.

4.   Ibid, 116–118.

5.   Hadley, B.J. The Author Comments, in Nicoll, L.H., ed., *Perspectives on Nursing Theory,* Boston: Little, Brown, 1986, p. 214.

6.   Hadley, B.J. Evolution of a Conception of Nursing, *Nursing Research,* 1969, *18,* 400–405.

7.   Fitzpatrick, J. A Life Perspective Rhythm Model, in Fitzpatrick, J. & Whall, A. *Conceptual Models of Nursing: Analysis and Application,* Bowie, MD: Robert J. Brady Co., 1983, pp. 295–302.

8.(a) Rogers, M.E. *An Introduction to the Theoretical Basis of Nursing,* Philadelphia: F.A. Davis Co., 1970.

8.(b) Rogers, M.E. Nursing: A Science of Unitary Man, in Riehl, J. & Roy Sr. C.,

OTHER EXTANT THEORIES** **379**

eds, *Conceptual Models for Nursing Practice* (2nd ed.), New York: Appleton-Century-Crofts, 1980.
9. Ibid, 301.
10. Newman, M.A. *Health as Expanding Consciousness*, St. Louis: C. V. Mosby, 1986.
11. Ibid, 9–10.
12. Ibid, 14.
13. Ibid, 70–71.
14. Ibid, 33.
15. Ibid, 62.
16. Ibid, 74.
17. Ibid, 87.
18. Ibid, 89.

BIBLIOGRAPHY

Chinn, P. & Jacobs, M.K. *Theory and Nursing, A Systematic Approach* (2nd ed.), St. Louis: C.V. Mosby, 1987.
Fawcett, J., *Analysis and Evaluation of Conceptual Models of Nursing*, (2nd ed.) Philadelphia: F.A. Davis Co., 1984.
Fawcett, J. & Downs, F.S. *The Relationship of Theory and Research*, Norwalk, CT: Appleton-Century-Crofts, 1986.
Fitzpatrick, J. & Whall, A., *Conceptual Models of Nursing*, (2nd ed.) Norwalk, Conn: Appleton & Lange, 1989.
Kim, H.S., *The Nature of Theoretical Thinking in Nursing*, Norwalk, CT: Appleton-Century-Crofts, 1983.
Leddy, S. & Pepper, J.M., *Conceptual Bases of Professional Nursing*, Philadelphia: Lippincott, 1985.
Marriner, A. *Nursing Theorists and Their Work*, St. Louis: C. V. Mosby, 1986.
Meleis, A.I. *Theoretical Nursing: Development & Progress*, Philadelphia: Lippincott, 1985.
Moccia, P. ed. *New Approaches to Theory Development*, New York: National League for Nursing, 1986.
National League for Nursing, *Theory Development: What, Why, How?*, New York: Author, 1978.
Nicoll, L.H., ed. *Perspectives on Nursing Theory*, Boston: Little, Brown 1986.
Riehl-Sisca, J.P. *Conceptual Models for Nursing Practice* (3rd ed.), Norwalk, Conn: Appleton & Lange, 1989.
Stevens, B.J. *Nursing Theory, Analysis, Application, Evaluation* (2nd ed.), Boston: Little, Brown, 1984.
Thibodeau, J.A. *Nursing Models: Analysis and Evaluation*, Monterey, CA: Wadsworth Health Sciences Division, 1983.
Torres, G., *Theoretical Foundations of Nursing*, Norwalk, CT: Appleton-Century-Crofts, 1986.
Walker, L. & Avant, K.C. *Strategies for Theory Construction in Nursing*, (2nd ed.) Norwalk CT: Appleton & Lange, 1988.
Winstead-Fry, P., ed. *Case Studies in Nursing Theory*, New York: National League for Nursing, 1986.

GLOSSARY*

Achievement subsystem. (Johnson) The behavioral subsystem relating to behaviors that attempt to control the environment and lead to personal accomplishment.

Adaptation. (Levine) Process of adjusting or modifying behavior or functioning to fit the situation.

Adaptation. (Rogers) Change resulting from the integration of human beings and their environment. The change occurs as an ongoing evolving process that can never return to the original state.

Adaptation. (Roy) Positive response to internal or external stimuli using bio-psycho-social mechanisms to promote personal integrity.

Adaptation level. (Roy) Condition of the person, or the individual's range of coping ability.

Adaptive responses. (Roy) Behaviors that positively affect health through promotion of the integrity of the person in terms of survival, growth, reproduction, and mastery.

Agent. (Wiedenbach) The practicing nurse, or the nurse's delegate, who serves as the propelling force in goal-directed behavior.

Aggressive subsystem. (Johnson) The behavioral subsystem that relates to behaviors concerned with protection and self-preservation.

Assumption. Statement or view that is widely accepted as true.

Assumption. (Wiedenbach) The meaning a nurse attaches to an interpretation of a sensory impression.

Attachment or affiliative subsystem. (Johnson) The behavioral subsystem that is the first formed and provides for a strong social bond.

Authority. (King) An active, reciprocal relationship that involves values, experience, and perceptions in defining, validating, and accepting the right of an individual to act within an organization.

---

* When a term relates specifically to a theorist, the name of the theorist appears in parentheses after the term.

Automatic activities. (Orlando) Nursing actions decided on for reasons other than the patient's immediate need.

Body image. (King) Individual's perceptions of their own bodies, influenced by the reactions of others.

Care. (Hall) The exclusive aspect of nursing that provides the patient bodily comfort through "laying on of hands" and provides an opportunity for closeness.

Care. (Leininger) (noun) Phenomena related to assistive, supportive, or enabling behavior toward or for another individual (or group) with evident or anticipated needs to ameliorate or improve a human condition or lifeway.

Caring. (Leininger) (verb) Action directed toward assisting, supporting, or enabling behavior another individual (or group) with evident or anticipated needs to ameliorate or improve a human condition or lifeway.

Central purpose. (Wiedenbach) The commitment of the individual nurse, based on a personal philosophy, that defines the desired quality of health and specifies the nurse's special responsibility in providing care to assist others in achieving or sustaining that quality.

Clustering of data. The grouping of data pieces that fit together and show relationships.

Cocreating. (Parse) Participation of human and environment in creating the pattern of each.

Cognator mechanism. (Roy) Coping mechanism or control subsystem that relates to the higher brain functions of perception, information processing, learning, judgment, and emotion.

Communication. (King) A direct or indirect process in which one person gives information to another.

Community. (Paterson and Zderad) Two or more persons striving together, living-dying all at once.

Concept. An abstract notion; a vehicle of thought that involves images; words that describe objects, properties, or events.

Conceptual framework. Group of interrelated concepts.

Connecting–separating. (Parse) The rhythmical process of distancing and relating.

Conservation. (Levine) Keeping together or maintaining a proper balance.

Conservation of energy. (Levine) Balancing energy output with energy input to avoid excessive fatigue.

Conservation of personal integrity. (Levine) Maintaining or restoring the patient's sense of identity and self-worth.

Conservation of social integrity. (Levine) Acknowledging the patient as a social being.

Conservation of structural integrity. (Levine) Maintaining or restoring the structure of the body.

Contextual stimuli. (Roy) Stimuli of the person's internal or external world, other than those immediately confronting the person, that influence the situation and are observable, measurable, or subjectively reported by the person.

Core. (Hall) The shared aspect with any health professional who therapeutically uses a freely offered closeness to help the patient discover who he or she is.

Covert problem. Hidden or concealed condition.

Cultural Care. (Leininger) The cognitively known values, beliefs and patterned expressions that assist, support or enable another individual or group to maintain well-being, improve a human condition or lifeway, or face death and disabilities.

Cultural care accommodation/negotiation. (Leininger) Assistive, supportive, or enabling professional actions and decisions that help clients of a particular culture to adapt to, or negotiate for a beneficial or satisfying health status, or to face death.

Cultural care diversity. (Leininger) The variability of meanings, patterns, values or symbols of care that are culturally derived by humans for their well being, or to improve a human condition or lifeway, or to face death.

Cultural care preservation/maintenance. (Leininger) Assistive, supportive or enabling professional actions and decisions that help clients of a particular culture to preserve or maintain a state of health, or to recover from illness, and to face death.

Cultural care repatterning/restructuring. (Leininger) Assistive, supportive or enabling professional actions or decisions that help clients change their lifeways for new or different patterns that are culturally meaningful and satisfying, or that support beneficial and healthy life patterns.

Cultural care universality. (Leininger) Common, similar or uniform meanings, patterns, values, or symbols of care that are culturally derived by humans for their well being or to improve a human condition and lifeway or to face death.

Cultural imposition. (Leininger) Efforts of an outsider, subtle and not so subtle, to impose his or her own cultural values, beliefs, or behaviors upon an individual, family, or group from another culture.

Cultural values. (Leininger) Values that are derived from the culture, identify desirable ways of acting or knowing, guide decision making, and are often held over long periods of time.

Culture. (Leininger) Learned, shared, and transmitted values, beliefs, norms, and lifeway practices of a particular group that guide thinking, decisions, and actions in patterned ways.

Culture. (Rogers) The integrated pattern of human behavior that includes thought, speech, action, and artifacts, and depends on man's capacity for learning and transmitting knowledge to succeeding generations.

Culture shock. (Leininger) Experiencing feelings of discomfort, helplessness, disorientation while attempting to comprehend or adapt effectively to a different cultural group.

Cure. (Hall) An aspect with medical personnel in which the nurse helps the patient and family through medical, surgical, and rehabilitative care.

Decision making in organizations. (King) An active process in which choice, directed by goals, is made and acted upon.

Deliberative actions. (Orlando) Nursing actions that ascertain or meet the patient's immediate need.

Dependency subsystem. (Johnson) The behavioral subsystem whose behaviors evoke nurturing behaviors in others.

Developmental self-care requisites. (Orem) Maintaining conditions to support life and development or to provide preventive care for adverse conditions that affect development.

Dialogue. (Paterson and Zderad) An intersubjective experience in which individuals relate creatively and have a real sharing.

Discrepancy. (Johnson) Action that does not achieve that goal intended.

Dominance. (Johnson) Primary use of one behavioral subsystem to the detriment of the other subsystems and regardless of the situation.

Eliminative subsystem. (Johnson) The behavioral subsystem that relates to socially acceptable behaviors surrounding the excretion of waste products from the body.

Emic. (Leininger) Personal knowledge or explanation of behavior; indigenous, not universal.

Empirical testing. Measurement or observation of real world events.

Enabling–limiting. (Parse) Making choices results in enabling an individual in some ways while limiting in others.

Environment. (Neuman) Those internal and external forces that surround humans at any given point in time.

Environment. (Nightingale) External conditions and influences that affect life and development.

Environment. (Rogers) Four-dimensional, negentropic energy field identified by pattern and encompassing all that is outside any given human field.

Environment. (Roy) All conditions, circumstances, and influences surrounding and affecting the development and behavior of persons or groups.

Environmental context. (Leininger) The totality of an event, situation, or particular experience that gives meaning to human expressions including physical, ecological, social interactions, emotional and cultural dimensions.

Equifinality. An open system that may attain a time-independent state independent of initial conditions and determined only by the system parameters.

Epistemology. The study of the history of knowledge, including origin, nature, methods, and limitations of knowledge development.

Ethnonursing. (Leininger) The study of nursing care beliefs, values, and practices as cognitively perceived and known by a designated culture through their direct experience, beliefs, and value system.

Existential psychology. The study of human existence using phenomenological analysis.

Exploitation phase. (Peplau) The third phase of Peplau's nurse–patient relationship. The patient takes full advantage of all available services while feeling an integral part of the helping environment. Goals are met through a collaborative effort as the patient becomes independent during convalescence.

Extrapersonal stressors. (Neuman) Forces occurring outside the system that generate a reaction or response from the system.

First level assessment. (Roy) Behavioral assessment; the gathering of output behaviors of the person in relation to the four adaptive modes.

Flexible line of defense. (Neuman) Variable and constantly changing ability to respond to stressors.

Focal stimuli. (Roy) Stimuli of the person's internal or external world that immediately confront the person.

Folk health system. (Leininger) Traditional or local indigenous health care or cure practices that have special meanings and uses to heal or assist people and are generally offered in familiar home or community environmental contexts with their local practitioners.

Framework. (Wiedenbach) The human, environmental, professional, and organizational facilities that make up the context in which nursing is practiced and constitute its currently existing limits.

General system theory. A general science of wholeness.

Goal. The end stated in broad terms to identify effective criteria for evaluating nursing action.

Goal. (Wiedenbach) Desired outcome the nurse seeks to achieve.

Growth and development. (King) The process in the lives of individuals that involves changes at the cellular, molecular, and behavioral levels and helps them move from potential to achievement.

Health deviation self-care. (Orem) Care needed by individuals who are ill or injured; may result from medical measures required to correct illness or injury.

Health problem.
Actual. Client need that currently exists.
Potential. Client need that may occur in the future and which may be averted with appropriate action.

Health. (Leininger) A state of well being that is culturally defined, valued and practiced and which reflects the ability of individuals (or groups) to perform their daily role activities in a culturally satisfactory way.

Helicy. (Rogers) The nature and direction of human and environmental change; change that is continuously innovative, probabilistic, and characterized by increasing diversity of the human field and environmental field pattern emerging out of the continuous, mutual, simultaneous interaction between the human and environmental fields and manifesting nonrepeating rhythmicities.

Holism. A theory that the universe and especially living nature are correctly seen in terms of interacting wholes that are more than the mere sum of the individual parts.

Homeodynamics. (Rogers) A way of viewing man in his wholeness. Changes in the life process of human beings are irreversible, nonrepeatable, rhythmical in nature, and evidence growing complexity of pattern. Change proceeds by continuous repatterning of both human beings and environment by resonating waves, and reflects the mutual simultaneous interaction between the two at any given point in space-time.

Humanism. (Rogers) A doctrine, attitude, or way of life centered on human interests or values. A philosophy that asserts the dignity and worth of human beings and their capacity of becoming through choices.

Identification phase. (Peplau) The second phase of Peplau's nurse–patient relationship. The perceptions and expectations of the patient and nurse become more involved while building a working relationship of further identifying the problem and deciding on appropriate plans for improved health maintenance.

Illness. (Levine) State of altered health.

Illness. (Neuman) State of insufficiency in which needs are yet to be satisfied.

Imaging. (Parse) The picturing or making real of events, ideas, and people.

Incompatibility. (Johnson) Two behavioral subsystems in the same situation being in conflict with each other.

Ineffective response. (Roy) Behaviors that do not promote the integrity of the person in terms of survival, growth, reproduction, and mastery.

Ingestive subsystem. (Johnson) The behavioral subsystem that relates to the meanings and structures of social events surrounding the occasions when food is eaten.

Insufficiency. (Johnson) A behavioral subsystem that is not functioning adequately.

Integrality. (Rogers) The continuous, mutual, simultaneous integration process between human and environmental fields.

Interactions. (King) The observable, goal-directed, behaviors of two or more persons in mutual presence.

Interpersonal stressors. (Neuman) Forces that occur between two or more individuals and evoke a reaction or response.

Intrapersonal stressors. (Neuman) Forces occurring within a person that result in a reaction or response.

Languaging. (Parse) Reflection of images and values through speaking and moving.

Lines of resistance. (Neuman) The internal set of factors that seek to stabilize the person when stressors break through the normal line of defense.

Means. (Wiedenbach) The activities and devices that enable the nurse to attain the desired goal.

Meeting. (Paterson and Zderad) The coming together of human beings characterized by the expectation that there will be a nurse and a nursed.

Model. Representation of the interactions among and between concepts which shows the patterns of these interactions.

More-being. (Paterson and Zderad) The process of becoming all that is humanly possible.

Need for help. (Orlando) A requirement for assistance in decreasing or eliminating immediate distress or in improving the sense of adequacy.

Negentropy. The open system growth process of becoming more complex and efficient.

Normal line of defense. (Neuman) The biological–psychological–sociocultural–developmental-spiritual skills developed over a lifetime to achieve stability and deal with stressors.

Nursing agency. (Orem) The specialized abilities that enable nurses to provide nursing care.

Nursing problem. (Abdellah) A condition faced by the client or client's family with which the nurse can assist through the performance of professional functions.

Nursing process. A deliberate, intellectual activity whereby the practice of nursing is approached in an orderly, systematic manner. It includes the following components:
Assessment. The process of data collection that results in a conclusion or nursing diagnosis.
Diagnosis. A behavioral statement that identifies the client's actual or potential health problem, deficit, or concern that can be affected by nursing actions.
Planning. The determination of what can be done to assist the client, including setting goals, judging priorities, and designing methods to resolve problems.
Implementation. Action initiated to accomplish defined goals.
Evaluation. The appraisal of the client's behavioral changes due to the action of the nurse.
Outcome evaluation. Evaluation based on behavioral changes.
Structure evaluation. Evaluation relating to the availability of appropriate equipment.
Process evaluation. Evaluation that focuses on the activities of the nurse.
Reassessment. The process of collecting additional data during the planning, implementing, and evaluation phases of the nursing process that may lead to immediate changes in those phases, or a change in the nursing diagnosis.

Nurturer. (Hall) A fosterer of learning, growing, and healing.

Objective. A specific means by which one proposes to accomplish or attain the goal.

Ontology. A branch of metaphysics that studies the nature of being and of reality.

Organismic response. (Levine) Changes in behavior or in the level of bodily functioning exhibited by a person adapting or attempting to adapt to the environment.

Organization. (King) An entity made up of individuals who have prescribed roles and positions and who use resources to achieve goals.

Orientation phase. (Peplau) The first phase of Peplau's nurse–patient relationship. Through assessment, the patient's health needs, expectations, and goals are explored and a care plan is devised. Concurrently, the roles of nurse and patient are being identified and clarified.

Originating. (Parse) A continuing process of growing more complex while in mutual energy exchange with the environment.

Overt problem. Apparent or obvious condition.

Paradigm. A new way of viewing a phenomenon, or group of phenomena, that attracts a group of adherents and raises many questions to be answered.

Parsimonious theory. Theory that is both simple and generalizable.

Partly compensatory system. (Orem) A situation where both nurse and patient perform care measures or other actions involving manipulative tasks or ambulation.

Perception. (King) An individual's view of reality that gives meaning to personal experience and involves the organization, interpretation, and transformation of information from sensory data and memory.

Phenomenology. The study of the meaning of phenomenon to a particular individual; a way of understanding people from the way things appear to them.

Potential comforter. (Hall) The role of the nurse seen by the patient during the care aspect of nursing.

Potential painer. (Hall) The role of the nurse seen by the patient during the cure aspect of nursing.

Power. (King) A social force and ability to use resources to influence people to achieve goals.

Powering. (Parse) An energizing force whose rhythm is the pushing–resisting of interhuman encounters.

Prescription. (Wiedenbach) A directive for activity that specifies both the nature of the action and the necessary thought process.

Prescriptive theory. (Wiedenbach) A theory that conceptualizes both the desired situation and the activities to be used to bring about the desired situation.

Presence. (Paterson and Zderad) The quality of being open, receptive, ready, and available to another in a reciprocal manner.

Primary prevention. (Neuman) The application of general knowledge in a client situation to try to identify stressors before they occur.

Problem-solving process. Identifying the problem, selecting pertinent data, formulating hypotheses, testing hypotheses through the collection of data, and revising hypotheses.

Professional health system. (Leininger) Professional care or cure services offered by diverse health personnel who have been prepared through formal professional programs of study in special educational institutions.

Professional nursing action. (Orlando) What the nurse says or does for the benefit of the patient.

Proposition. A statement explaining relationships among concepts.

Realities in the immediate situation. (Wiedenbach) At any given moment, all factors at play in the situation in which nursing actions occur; realities include the agent, the recipient, the goal, the means, and the framework.

Recipient. (Wiedenbach) The vulnerable and dependent patient who is characterized by personal attributes, problems, and capabilities, including the ability to cope.

Reflective technique. (Hall) The process of helping the patient see who he or she is by mirroring what the person's behavior says, both verbally and nonverbally.

Regulator mechanism. (Roy) Coping mechanism subsystem that includes chemical, neural, and endocrine transmitters and autonomic and psychomotor responses.

Relating. (Paterson and Zderad) The process of nurse–nursed "doing" with each other, being with each other.

Research. Formal, systematic process of gathering data to gain solutions, descriptions, answers and to interpret new ideas, facts or assumptions, and relationships.

Residual stimuli. (Roy) Characteristics of the individual that are relevant to the situation but are difficult to measure objectively.

Resolution phase. (Peplau) The fourth and final phase of Peplau's nurse–patient relationship. This phase evolves from the successful completion of the previous phases. The patient and nurse terminate their therapeutic relationship as the patient's needs are met and movement is made toward new goals.

Resonancy. (Rogers) The identification of the human field and the environmental field by wave pattern manifesting continuous change from lower frequency longer waves to higher frequency shorter waves.

Revealing–concealing. (Parse) Actions in interpersonal relationships that reveal one part of oneself and, as a result, conceal other parts.

Role. (King) The set of behaviors and rules that relate to an individual in a position in a social system.

Secondary prevention. (Neuman) Treatment of symptoms of stress reaction to lead to reconstitution.

Second level assessment. (Roy) The collection of data about focal, contextual, and residual stimuli impinging on the person.

Self-care. (Orem) Practice of activities that individuals personally initiate and perform on their own behalf to maintain life, health, and well-being.

Self-care agency. (Orem) The human ability to engage in self-care.

Self-care deficit. (Orem) The inability of an individual to carry out all necessary self-care activities.

Set. (Johnson) An individual's predisposition to behave in a certain way.

Sexual subsystem. (Johnson) The behavioral subsystem that reflects socially acceptable behaviors related to procreation.

Simultaneity paradigm. (Parse) A view of humans as unitary beings who are in continuous interrelationship with the environment and whose health is a negentropic unfolding.

Social structure. (Leininger) The dynamic nature of interrelated structural and organizational factors of a particular culture (or society) and how those factors function to give meaning and structural order including educational, technological and cultural factors.

Space. (King) A universal area, known also as *territory,* that is defined in part by the behavior of those who occupy it.

Status. (King) The relationship of an individual to a group, or a group to other groups, including identified duties, obligations, and privileges.

Stress. (King) A positive or negative energy response to interactions with the environment in an effort to maintain balance in living.

Supportive–educative system. (Orem) A situation where the patient is able to, or can and should learn to, perform required therapeutic self-care measures but needs assistance to do so.

Supportive intervention. (Levine) Action that maintains the patient's present state of altered health and prevents further health deterioration.

Synergistic wholeness. (Rogers) Cooperative action of discrete agencies such that the total effect is greater than the sum of the effects taken independently.

Tertiary prevention. (Neuman) Activities that seek to strengthen the lines of resistance after reconstitution has occurred.

Theory. A set of interrelated concepts that are testable and provide direction or prediction; systematic way of looking at the world to describe, explain, predict, or control it.

Theory. (Watson) An imaginative grouping of knowledge, ideas, and experience that are represented symbolically and seek to illuminate a given phenomenon.

Therapeutic interpersonal relationship. (Peplau) A relationship between patient and nurse in which their collaborative effort is directed toward identifying, exploring, and resolving the patient's need productively. The relationship progresses along a continuum as each experiences growth through an increasing understanding of one another's roles, attitudes, and perceptions.

Therapeutic intervention. (Levine) Action that promotes healing and restoration of health.

Therapeutic self-care demand. (Orem) The sum or total of self-actions needed, during some period of time, to meet self-care requisites.

Time. (King) The relation of one event to another, uniquely experienced by each individual.

Totality paradigm. (Parse) View of man as a summative being, a combination of bio–psycho–social–spiritual aspects, surrounded by an environment of external and internal stimuli. Man interacts with the environment to maintain equilibrium and achieve goals.

Transactions. (King) Observable behaviors between individuals and their environment that lead to the attainment of valued goals.

Transcultural nursing. (Leininger) A learned subfield or branch of nursing which focuses on the comparative study and analysis of cultures with respect to nursing and health–illness caring practices, beliefs, and values. The goal is to provide meaningful and efficacious nursing care services to people according to their cultural values and health–illness context.

Unitary humans. (Rogers) Four-dimensional, negentropic energy fields identified by pattern and manifesting characteristics and behaviors different from those of the parts, and which cannot be predicted from knowledge of the parts.

Universal self-care requisites. (Orem) Those requisites, common to all human beings throughout life, associated with life processes and the integrity of human structure and function.

Well-being. (Paterson and Zderad) A steady state.

Wholly compensatory nursing system. (Orem) A situation in which the patient has no active role in the performance of self-care.

World view. (Leininger) The way in which people look at the world, or universe, and form a value stance about the world and their lives.

INDEX